SECOND EDITION

MED-MATH

Dosage Calculation, Preparation and Administration

SECOND EDITION

MED-MATH

Dosage Calculation, Preparation and Administration

Grace Henke, S.C., R.N., M.S.N., Ed.D.
Instructor
St. Vincent's Hospital School of Nursing
New York, New York
Adjunct Professor
College of Mount St. Vincent
Riverdale, New York

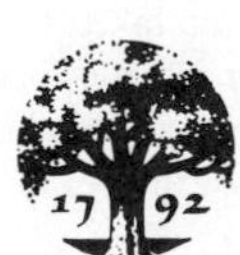

J. B. LIPPINCOTT COMPANY
Philadelphia

Sponsoring Editor: Margaret Belcher
Project Editor: Tom Gibbons
Indexer: Lynne E. Mahan
Design Coordinator: Melissa Olson
Interior Designer: Susan Hess Blaker
Cover Designer: Richard Spencer
Production Manager: Helen Ewan
Production Coordinator: Nannette Winski
Compositor: Tapsco, Incorporated
Printer/Binder: Courier Book Company/Kendallville
Cover Printer: Lehigh

2nd Edition

6 5 4 3 2 1

Library of Congress Cataloging-in-Publication Data

Henke, Grace.
Med-Math: dosage calculation, preparation and administration/
Grace Henke.—2nd ed.
p. cm.
Includes index.
ISBN 0-397-55143-6
1. Pharmaceutical arithmetic. I. Title.
[DNLM: 1. Drugs—administration & dosage—programmed instruction.
2. Drugs—administration & dosage—nurses' instruction.
3. Mathematics—nurses' instruction. 4. Mathematics—programmed instruction. QV 18 H512m 1995]
RS57.H46 1995
615.5′8′01513—dc20
DNLM/DLC
for Library of Congress 94-34069
CIP

Any procedure or practice described in this book should be applied by the healthcare practitioner under appropriate supervision in accordance with professional standards of care used with regard to the unique circumstances that apply in each practice situation. Care has been taken to confirm the accuracy of information presented and to describe generally accepted practices. However, the authors, editors, and publisher cannot accept any responsibility for errors or omissions or for any consequences from application of the information in this book and make no warranty express or implied, with respect to the contents of the book.

Every effort has been made to ensure drug selections and dosages are in accordance with current recommendations and practice. Because of ongoing research, changes in government regulations and the constant flow of information on drug therapy, reactions and interactions, the reader is cautioned to check the package insert for each drug for indications, dosages, warnings and precautions, particularly if the drug is new or infrequently used.

Dedicated to the students and faculty of St. Vincent's Hospital School of Nursing, who strive with compassion and charity to meet the challenge of caring, and who act with competence and collaboration in showing respect for the dignity of all persons.

Preface

Although **Med-Math: Dosage Calculation, Preparation and Administration, Second Edition,** is designed to meet the needs of students in every type of nursing program, this highly successful dosage calculations text has also been widely used by every health care professional who administers drugs, including practicing nurses in need of review and nurses returning to practice. Students in introductory courses should complete the chapters in order. Practicing nurses may wish to do the proficiency tests at the end of each dosage chapter to target areas of weakness for content review.

▼ KEY FEATURES OF THE TEXT

- All dosage problems are presented as physicians' orders to simulate actual clinical experience.
- All dosage problems range from simple to complex to assist the student in building a knowledge base and lasting understanding of important concepts and principles.
- Easy-to-learn formulas and a step-by-step approach aid the reader in solving problems.
- Abundant examples, practice problems, and a proficiency test at the end of each dosage chapter allow the reader to test new knowledge and skills before proceeding to the next chapter.
- Answers to all problems are provided to encourage the student to check the accuracy of answers and promote immediate reinforcement of accurate problem solution.

▼ NEW TO THIS EDITION

- Each chapter begins with Content to Master to provide an overview of key concepts in each chapter.
- **More actual manufacturers' drug labels** have been added to simulate actual drug administration settings and to assist the student to accurately calculate the correct dosage.

- **A completely revised chapter on dosage for infants and children** reflects the most current practice guidelines for administering medications to infants and children.
- **Addition of content on infusion pumps** for IVs and IVPBs provides the student with an introduction on how to ensure accurate medication delivery using these pumps.
- **Addition of computer printouts and military time** completes a comprehensive overview of the form that drug orders may take in various care settings.
- **SI units** of measurement present the international standard of measurement.
- **Expanded content on insulin and solving insulin problems** provides an introduction to a range of insulins and insulin orders.
- **Explanation of the relationship between the rule $\frac{D}{H} \times S = A$ and ratio and proportion** integrates the two methods of dosage calculation and explains why the rule is so easy to use.

Chapter 1 reviews arithmetic operations used in dosage. Multiplication and division tables are provided, along with exercises designed to test the student's knowledge of basic math. These are important and necessary drills for students who experience difficulty in calculation and even for those who find arithmetic easy. Regardless of how proficient one is in mathematics, careless medication errors can occur. No one should skip this review. Those who believe their skills are satisfactory should at least complete the practice exercises. Ratio and proportion are introduced to show the derivation of the dosage formula that is used to solve most dosage problems.

Chapter 2 explains abbreviations used in prescriptions and introduces military time and metric, household, and SI units of measurement. Some apothecary measures are covered to aid nurses who encounter orders written in grains. The chapter ends with exercises in reading and interpreting orders.

Chapter 3 explains how to interpret drug labels and discusses unit and multidose packaging for different routes of administration. Chapter 4 presents the differences among dosage measurement systems and how to convert from one system to another. Chapter 5 describes types of drug preparations and equipment, including syringes, that are used to measure doses.

Chapters 6 through 9 present dosage problems by route of administration: oral solids and liquids in Chapter 6, injections from liquids in Chapter 7, injections from powders in Chapter 8, and intravenous and "piggyback" drips in Chapter 9. The reader is encouraged to solve the problems in Chapters 6 to 8 mentally or to use paper and pencil rather than rely on a calculator. Practice of mental problem-solving promotes logical thinking and increases speed and efficiency. In Chapters 9 and 10, which consider IVs and pediatric dosage, a calculator may save time.

Chapter 11 provides information a nurse needs to administer drugs safely—drug knowledge; pregnancy categories; and pharmacokinetic, legal, and ethical considerations—and ends with tips for pouring, administering, and charting medications. Chapter 12 is a quick procedural guide to preparing and administering drugs orally, parenterally, and topically. Universal precautions, equipment, and methods of administration are given.

▼ TEACHING AID FOR INSTRUCTORS

An Instructor's Manual with Test Bank is now available for teachers who adopt this text for their course. The Instructor's Manual contains time-tested teaching aids for optimizing the teaching of dosage calculations and medication administration. The Test Bank provides test items in addition to those found in the text.

It is my hope that this second edition of *Med-Math* will be even more successful in easing the anxiety that students experience when they begin to learn dosage and calculation of medications, and prepare to administer drugs.

Sister Grace Henke

Acknowledgments

My thanks to Lippincott editor Margaret Belcher, whose enthusiasm and support guided me into undertaking this second edition, and to Kimberly Oaks and Tom Gibbons, whose patience and skill steered this project to completion. I have always thought Lippincott nursing textbooks superior; their talent confirms my belief.

A number of professional colleagues reviewed sections of the manuscript, validated content, and made pertinent suggestions: Mary Ann Dono, R.N., M.A., C.P.N.; Mary Ann Going, R.N.C., M.A.; John Jacoby III, M.D.; Curtis Kellner, M.S., R.Ph.; Maureen Meehan, R.N., M.S.N.; and Anne Marie O'Brien, R.N., B.S.N., C.I.C. I appreciate their assistance and support.

Gary Margolis and John Christopher Ramos, nursing student, sketched some of the line drawings, and Narriman Betancout typed. Thanks for listening to my concerns and doing such fine work. I am indebted to Chris Thomas of Continental Healthcare Systems for permission to use the computer printout and to the Departments of Central Distributing, Nursing and Pharmacy of St. Vincent's Hospital and Medical Center for printed forms.

Finally, my thanks to the following pharmaceutical companies for permission to use their labels and package inserts: Apothecon, a Bristol Meyers Squibb Company; Astra Pharmaceutical Products; Boots Pharmaceuticals, Inc.; Bristol Laboratories; Fujisawa Pharmaceutical Company; Glaxo Pharmaceuticals; Hoechst-Roussel Pharmaceuticals; Lederle Laboratories; Eli Lilly and Company; Merck and Company; Park Davis Division of Warner Lambert Company; Roerig-Pfizer Laboratories; SmithKline Beecham Pharmaceuticals; E. R. Squibb and Sons, Inc.; The Upjohn Company; and Wyeth Ayerst Laboratories.

Contents

SECOND EDITION

MED-MATH

Dosage Calculation, Preparation and Administration

Arithmetic Needed for Dosage

CONTENT TO MASTER

Clearing decimal points

Rounding off decimals

Using ratio and proportion

Deriving the dosage formula

When a physician's order differs from the fixed amount at which a drug is supplied, the nurse must calculate the dose needed. Calculation requires knowledge of the systems of measurement (Chapter 4) and the ability to solve arithmetic. This chapter covers those common arithmetic functions that the nurse needs for the safe administration of drugs.

Regardless of how proficient one is in mathematics, careless medication errors may occur. Therefore, *do not skip this arithmetic review.* Those who believe their skills are satisfactory should at least complete the practice exercises.

Students ask why they should perform arithmetic operations when calculators are readily available. The reason is that solving the arithmetic forces nurses to think logically about the dose ordered and evaluate the answer (the dose calculated) in relation to the order. Mentally solving dosage problems increases speed and efficiency in preparing medications. There may be occasions when a problem that requires a calculator arises in the clinical area; however, all arithmetic problems in this chapter can be completed without a calculator.

The arithmetic operations needed for dosage calculations are: multiplying whole numbers and fractions; dividing whole numbers, fractions, and decimals; reducing fractions; reading decimals; and using percentage.

▼ MULTIPLYING WHOLE NUMBERS

The multiplication table (Fig. 1-1) is provided for review. Study the table for the numbers 1 through 12. You should achieve 100% accuracy without referring to the table.

EXAMPLE Multiply 8 by 7 (8×7)

1. Find column number 8.
2. Find row number 7.
3. Read across row 7 until you intersect column number 8. The answer is 56.

1	2	3	4	5	6	7	8	9	10	11	12
2	4	6	8	10	12	14	16	18	20	22	24
3	6	9	12	15	18	21	24	27	30	33	36
4	8	12	16	20	24	28	32	36	40	44	48
5	10	15	20	25	30	35	40	45	50	55	60
6	12	18	24	30	36	42	48	54	60	66	72
7	14	21	28	35	42	49	56	63	70	77	84
8	16	24	32	40	48	56	64	72	80	88	96
9	18	27	36	45	54	63	72	81	90	99	108
10	20	30	40	50	60	70	80	90	100	110	120
11	22	33	44	55	66	77	88	99	110	121	132
12	24	36	48	60	72	84	96	108	120	132	144

Figure 1-1
The multiplication table. The numbers going down the left side (from 1 to 12) are the column numbers. The numbers going across the top (from 1 to 12) are the row numbers. To multiply any two numbers from 1 to 12, find the column for one number, find the row for the other number, and read across the row until you intersect the column.

Self-Test 1

After studying the multiplication table, write the answers to these problems. Answers are given at the end of the chapter; if you do not achieve 100%, you need more study time.

1. 2 × 6 = ________
2. 9 × 7 = ________
3. 4 × 8 = ________
4. 5 × 9 = ________
5. 12 × 9 = ________
6. 8 × 3 = ________
7. 11 × 10 = ________
8. 2 × 7 = ________
9. 8 × 6 = ________
10. 8 × 9 = ________
11. 3 × 5 = ________
12. 6 × 7 = ________
13. 4 × 6 = ________
14. 9 × 6 = ________
15. 8 × 8 = ________
16. 7 × 8 = ________
17. 2 × 9 = ________
18. 8 × 11 = ________
19. 4 × 9 = ________
20. 3 × 8 = ________
21. 12 × 11 = ________
22. 9 × 5 = ________
23. 9 × 9 = ________
24. 7 × 5 = ________

▼ DIVIDING WHOLE NUMBERS

The multiplication table is also helpful in dividing large numbers by smaller ones. Study the table for the division of numbers 2 through 12 (Fig. 1-2). Again, you should be able to achieve 100% accuracy without referring to the table; if not, study it again.

EXAMPLE Divide 108 by 12 (108 ÷ 12)

1. Find 12 (the smaller number) in the left column.
2. Read across that row until you find 108 (the larger number).
3. The number at the top of that column is the answer, 9.

Remember, because 9 × 12 = 108, then 108 ÷ 12 = 9 (see Fig. 1-2).

1	2	3	4	5	6	7	8	(9)	10	11	12
2	4	6	8	10	12	14	16	18	20	22	24
3	6	9	12	15	18	21	24	27	30	33	36
4	8	12	16	20	24	28	32	36	40	44	48
5	10	15	20	25	30	35	40	45	50	55	60
6	12	18	24	30	36	42	48	54	60	66	72
7	14	21	28	35	42	49	56	63	70	77	84
8	16	24	32	40	48	56	64	72	80	88	96
9	18	27	36	45	54	63	72	81	90	99	108
10	20	30	40	50	60	70	80	90	100	110	120
11	22	33	44	55	66	77	88	99	110	121	132
→ (12)	24	36	48	60	72	84	96	(108)	120	132	144

Figure 1-2
Division table. The numbers going down the left side (from 1 to 12) are the column numbers. The numbers going across the top (from 1 to 12) are the row numbers. To divide, find the divisor (the number performing the division) in the column. Read across the column to the dividend (the number to be divided). The number at the top of that column is the answer.

Self-Test 2

After studying the division of larger numbers by smaller numbers, write the answers to the following problems. Answers can be found at the end of the chapter.

1. 63 ÷ 7 – ________
2. 24 ÷ 6 = ________
3. 36 ÷ 12 = ________
4. 42 ÷ 6 = ________
5. 35 ÷ 5 = ________
6. 96 ÷ 12 = ________
7. 12 ÷ 3 = ________
8. 27 ÷ 9 = ________
9. 49 ÷ 7 = ________
10. 18 : 3 = ________
11. 72 ÷ 8 = ________
12. 48 ÷ 8 = ________
13. 28 ÷ 7 = ________
14. 21 ÷ 7 = ________
15. 24 ÷ 8 = ________
16. 84 ÷ 12 = ________
17. 81 ÷ 9 = ________
18. 32 ÷ 8 = ________
19. 36 ÷ 6 = ________
20. 18 ÷ 9 – ________
21. 21 ÷ 3 = ________
22. 48 ÷ 4 = ________
23. 144 ÷ 12 = ________
24. 56 ÷ 8 = ________

▼ FRACTIONS

A *fraction* is a portion of a whole number. The top number is called the *numerator*. The bottom number is called the *denominator*.

EXAMPLE 1 → numerator
4 → denominator

◀ ***Learning Aid***
The line between the numerator and the denominator is a division sign. Therefore, the fraction can be read as one divided by four.

Types of Fractions

In a *proper* fraction, the numerator is smaller than the denominator.

EXAMPLE $\frac{2}{5}$ (Read as two-fifths.)

In an *improper* fraction, the numerator is larger than the denominator.

EXAMPLE $\frac{5}{2}$ (Read as five halves.)

A *mixed number* has a whole number plus a fraction.

EXAMPLE $1\frac{2}{3}$ (Read as one and two-thirds.)

In a *complex* fraction, both the numerator and the denominator are already fractions.

EXAMPLE $\frac{\frac{1}{2}}{\frac{1}{4}}$ (Read as one-half divided by one-fourth.)

RULE

REDUCING FRACTIONS

Find the largest number that can be divided evenly into the numerator *and* the denominator.

EXAMPLE

Example 1:

Reduce $\frac{4}{12}$

$$\frac{\overset{1}{\cancel{4}}}{\underset{3}{\cancel{12}}} = \frac{1}{3}$$

Example 2:

Reduce $\frac{7}{49}$

$$\frac{\overset{1}{\cancel{7}}}{\underset{7}{\cancel{49}}} = \frac{1}{7}$$

◀ ***Learning Aid***
Check to see if the denominator is evenly divisible by the numerator. The number 7 can be evenly divided into 49.

Sometimes fractions are more difficult to reduce because the answer is not obvious.

EXAMPLE

Example 1:

Reduce $\frac{56}{96}$

$$\frac{56}{96} = \frac{\overset{1}{\cancel{8}} \times 7}{\underset{1}{\cancel{8}} \times 12} = \frac{7}{12}$$

◀ ***Learning Aid***
Your knowledge of the multiplication table can help you. Change the numbers to their multiples.

Example 2:

Reduce $\frac{54}{99}$

$$\frac{54}{99} = \frac{\overset{1}{\cancel{9}} \times 6}{\underset{1}{\cancel{9}} \times 11} = \frac{6}{11}$$

Patience is required to reduce a very large fraction. It may be difficult to find the largest number that will divide evenly into the numerator and the denominator, and you may have to reduce several times.

EXAMPLE

Example 1:

Reduce $\frac{189}{216}$

Try to divide both by 3 $\frac{\overset{63}{\cancel{189}}}{\underset{72}{\cancel{216}}} = \frac{63}{72}$

Then use multiples $\frac{63}{72} = \frac{\overset{1}{\cancel{9}} \times 7}{\underset{1}{\cancel{9}} \times 8} = \frac{7}{8}$

Example 2:

Reduce $\frac{27}{135}$

Try to divide both by 3 $\frac{\overset{9}{\cancel{27}}}{\underset{45}{\cancel{135}}} = \frac{\overset{1}{\cancel{9}}}{\underset{5}{\cancel{45}}} = \frac{1}{5}$

◀ ***Learning Aid***
Certain numbers are called prime numbers because they cannot be reduced further. Examples are 2, 3, 5, 7, and 11.
In reducing, if the last number is even or a zero, try 2.
If the last number is a zero or 5, try 5.
If the last number is odd, try 3, 7, or 11.

Self-Test 3

Reduce these fractions to their lowest terms. Answers may be found at the end of the chapter. Be patient!

1. $\frac{16}{24}$

2. $\frac{36}{216}$

3. $\frac{18}{96}$

4. $\frac{70}{490}$

5. $\frac{18}{81}$

6. $\frac{8}{48}$

7. $\frac{12}{30}$

8. $\frac{68}{136}$

9. $\frac{55}{121}$

10. $\frac{15}{60}$

Multiplying Fractions

There are two ways to multiply fractions.

First Way

Multiply the numerators across. Multiply denominators across. Reduce the answer to its lowest terms.

EXAMPLE

$\frac{2}{7} \times \frac{3}{4} = \frac{6}{28}$

$\frac{6}{28} = \frac{3 \times \overset{1}{\cancel{2}}}{14 \times \underset{1}{\cancel{2}}} = \frac{3}{14}$

◀ ***Learning Aid***
In multiplying fractions, sometimes one way will be easier. Use whichever method is more comfortable for you.

Second Way (When There Are Several Fractions)

Reduce by dividing numerators into denominators evenly. Multiply remaining numerators across. Multiply remaining denominators across. Check to see if further reductions can be made.

EXAMPLE

Example 1:

$\frac{3}{14} \times \frac{7}{10} \times \frac{5}{12} =$

$\frac{\overset{1}{\cancel{3}}}{\underset{2}{\cancel{14}}} \times \frac{\overset{1}{\cancel{7}}}{\underset{2}{\cancel{10}}} \times \frac{\overset{1}{\cancel{5}}}{\underset{4}{\cancel{12}}} = \frac{1}{16}$

◀ ***Learning Aid***
$12 \div 3 = 4$
$14 \div 7 = 2$
$10 \div 5 = 2$

Example 2:

$1\frac{1}{2} \times \frac{4}{6} =$

$\frac{\overset{1}{\cancel{3}}}{\underset{1}{\cancel{2}}} \times \frac{\overset{2}{\cancel{4}}}{\underset{2}{\cancel{6}}} = \frac{\cancel{2}}{\cancel{2}} = 1$

◀ ***Learning Aid***
Mixed numbers must be changed to improper fractions. Multiply the whole number by the denominator and add the numerator.

$1\frac{1}{2} = 1 \times 2 + 1 = \frac{3}{2}$

Example 3:

$\frac{4}{5} \times 6\frac{2}{3} =$

$\frac{4}{\underset{1}{\cancel{5}}} \times \frac{\overset{4}{\cancel{20}}}{3} = \frac{16}{3}$

◀ ***Learning Aid***
$6 \times 3 = 18 + 2 = \frac{20}{3}$

Self-Test 4

Multiply these fractions. Answers may be found at the end of the chapter.

1. $\frac{1}{6} \times \frac{4}{5} \times \frac{5}{2} =$

2. $\frac{4}{15} \times \frac{3}{2} =$

3. $1\frac{1}{2} \times 4\frac{2}{3} =$

4. $\frac{1}{5} \times \frac{15}{45} =$

5. $3\frac{3}{4} \times 10\frac{2}{3} =$

6. $\frac{7}{20} \times \frac{2}{14} =$

7. $\frac{9}{2} \times \frac{3}{2} =$

8. $6\frac{1}{4} \times 7\frac{1}{9} \times \frac{9}{5} =$

Dividing Fractions

Fractions can be divided by inverting the number after the division sign and then changing the division sign to a multiplication sign.

EXAMPLE

Example 1:

$\frac{1}{75} \div \frac{1}{150} = \frac{1}{\underset{1}{\cancel{75}}} \times \frac{\overset{2}{\cancel{150}}}{1} = 2$

Example 2:

$$\frac{\frac{1}{4}}{\frac{3}{8}} = \frac{1}{4} \div \frac{3}{8} = \frac{1}{\cancel{4}_1} \times \frac{\cancel{8}^2}{3} = \frac{2}{3}$$

◀ ***Learning Aid***
Complex fractions such as

$\frac{\frac{1}{4}}{\frac{3}{8}}$ *may be read as* $\frac{1}{4} \div \frac{3}{8}$

Remember, the long line represents a division sign.

Example 3:

$$\frac{1\frac{1}{5}}{\frac{2}{3}} = \frac{6}{5} \div \frac{2}{3} =$$

$$\frac{\cancel{6}^3}{5} \times \frac{3}{\cancel{2}_1} = \frac{9}{5}$$

Self-Test 5

Divide these fractions. This operation is important in calculating dosages correctly. Answers may be found at the end of the chapter.

1. $\frac{1}{75} \div \frac{1}{150} =$

2. $\frac{1}{8} \div \frac{1}{4} =$

3. $2\frac{2}{3} \div \frac{1}{2} =$

4. $75 \div 12\frac{1}{2} =$

5. $\frac{7}{25} \div \frac{7}{75} =$

6. $\frac{1}{2} \div \frac{1}{4} =$

7. $\frac{3}{4} \div \frac{8}{3} =$

8. $\frac{1}{60} \div \frac{7}{10} =$

Changing Fractions to Decimals

This can be accomplished by dividing the numerator by the denominator. Remember that the line between the numerator and the denominator is a division sign; hence, $\frac{1}{4}$ can be read as $1 \div 4$.

In division, the number being divided is called the *dividend;* the number that does the dividing is called the *divisor;* the answer is called the *quotient.*

```
            40. ← quotient
divisor → 16)640. ← dividend
            64
             0
```

1. Look at the fraction $\frac{1}{4}$

1 ← numerator = dividend
4 ← denominator = divisor

2. Write

$4\overline{)1}$

3. If you have difficulty setting this up, you can continue the line for the fraction and place the number above the line into the box.

$\frac{1}{4} = 4\overline{)1}$ (with the 1 above crossed out)

4. Once the division problem is set up, place a decimal point immediately after the dividend and also bring the decimal point up to the quotient.

```
 .  ← quotient
4 ) 1. ← dividend
```

Important! Failure to place decimal points carefully can lead to serious dosage errors.

◀ ***Learning Aid***
If the answer does not have a whole number, place a zero before the decimal. This prevents misreading the answer: .25 is incorrect; 0.25 is correct.
The number of places to report your answer will vary depending upon the way the stock drug comes and the equipment you use. For these exercises, carry answers to three places.

5. Carry out the division.

```
   .25 = 0.25
4 ) 1.00
     8
    20
    20
     0
```

EXAMPLE

Example 1:

```
 5       0.312
---- = 16) 5.000 = 0.312
 16        4 8
            20
            16
            40
            32
             8
```

◀ ***Learning Aid***
Note that there is a space between the 8 and the decimal point in the answer. When this occurs, place a zero in the space to complete the answer.

Example 2:

$$\frac{640}{8} = 8\overline{)640.} \;\; 80. = 80$$

Example 3:

```
 1       .013
---- = 75) 1.000 = 0.013
 75        75
           250
           225
            25
```

Self-Test 6

Divide these fractions to produce decimals. Answers will be found at the end of the chapter. Carry decimal places to three if necessary.

1. $\frac{1}{6}$

2. $\frac{6}{8}$

3. $\frac{4}{5}$

4. $\frac{9}{40}$

5. $\frac{1}{8}$

6. $\frac{1}{7}$

▼ DECIMALS

Most medication orders are written in the metric system, which uses decimals.

Reading Decimals

Count the number of places after the decimal point. As you read the decimal, you also create a fraction.

0.1 is read as one tenth $\left(\frac{1}{10}\right)$

0.01 is read as one hundredth $\left(\frac{1}{100}\right)$

0.001 is read as one thousandth $\left(\frac{1}{1000}\right)$

◀ ***Learning Aid***
The first number after a decimal point is the tenth place.
The second number after the decimal point is the 100th place.
The third number after the decimal point is the 1000th place.

EXAMPLE

0.56 = fifty-six hundredths $\left(\frac{56}{100}\right)$

0.2 = two tenths $\left(\frac{2}{10}\right)$

0.194 = one hundred and ninety-four thousandths $\left(\frac{194}{1000}\right)$

0.31 = thirty-one hundredths $\left(\frac{31}{100}\right)$

1.6 = one and six tenths $\left(1\frac{6}{10}\right)$

17.354 = seventeen and three hundred and fifty-four thousandths $\left(17\frac{354}{1000}\right)$

◀ ***Learning Aid***
In reading decimals, read the number first, then count off the decimal places.
Whole numbers preceding decimals are read in the usual way.

Self-Test 7

Write these decimals in longhand and as fractions. Answers may be found at the end of the chapter.

1. 0.25 ______________________

2. 0.004 ______________________

3. 1.7 ______________________

4. 0.5 ______________________

5. 0.334 ______________________

6. 136.75 ______________________

7. 0.1 ______________________

8. 0.150 ______________________

Dividing Decimals

Again, in division the number that is being divided is called the dividend; the number that does the dividing is called the divisor; and the answer is called the quotient.

```
             0.312→ quotient
divisor →16 )5.000→ dividend
```

Note that a decimal point is placed immediately after the dividend is written, and is also moved up to the quotient.

EXAMPLE

```
13              .
—      16 ) 13.
16
```

Division is then completed.

EXAMPLE

```
    0.812
16 )13.000
    12 8
     20
     16
      40
      32
       8
```

Clearing the Divisor of Decimal Points

Before dividing one decimal by another, the divisor must be cleared of decimal points. To do this, move the decimal point to the far right. Move the decimal point in the dividend *the same number of places* and bring the decimal point up to the quotient in the same place.

EXAMPLE

Example 1:

```
                        .
0.2 ) 0.004 = 0.2. ) 0.0.04

               0.02
Hence,  2 ) 00.04
```

Example 2:

```
                               1.262
4.3 ) 5.427  becomes  43. ) 54.270
                            43
                            11 2
                             8 6
                             2 67
                             2 58
                                90
                                86
                                 4
```

Self-Test 8

Do these problems in division of decimals. The answers may be found at the end of this chapter. If necessary, carry answer to three places.

1. $24\,\overline{)\,0.0048}$
2. $0.004\,\overline{)\,0.1}$
3. $0.02\,\overline{)\,0.2}$
4. $7.8\,\overline{)\,140}$
5. $6\,\overline{)\,140}$
6. $0.025\,\overline{)\,10}$

Rounding off Decimals

How do you determine how many places to carry your division? For the nurse, the answer must relate to the materials being used. Some syringes are marked to the tenth place, some to the hundredth place. Some tablets can be broken into halves or fourths; some liquids come in units of measurement in the tenths, hundredths, or thousandths. As you become familiar with dosage you will learn how far you need to round out your answer. At this point let us review the general rule for rounding off decimals.

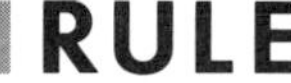 **RULE**

ROUNDING OFF DECIMALS

When the number to be dropped is 5 or more, drop the number and add 1 to the previous number. When the last number is 4 or less, drop the number.

EXAMPLE 0.864 becomes 0.86 4.562 becomes 4.56

1.55 becomes 1.6 2.38 becomes 2.4

0.33 becomes 0.3

Suppose you wanted answers to the nearest tenth. Look at the number in the hundredth place and follow the rules for rounding off.

EXAMPLE 0.12 becomes 0.1

0.667 becomes 0.7

1.46 becomes 1.5

Suppose you wanted answers to the nearest hundredth. Look at the number in the thousandth place and follow the rules for rounding off.

EXAMPLE 0.664 becomes 0.66

0.148 becomes 0.15

2.375 becomes 2.38

Suppose you wanted answers to the nearest thousandth. Look at the number in the ten-thousandth place and follow the rules for rounding off.

EXAMPLE 1.3758 becomes 1.376

0.0024 becomes 0.002

4.5555 becomes 4.556

Self-Test 9

Round off these decimals as indicated. Answers may be found at the end of the chapter.

Nearest Tenth	***Nearest Hundredth***	***Nearest Thousandth***
1. 0.25 = ______	**6.** 1.268 = ______	**11.** 1.3254 = ______
2. 1.84 = ______	**7.** 0.750 = ______	**12.** 0.0025 = ______
3. 3.27 = ______	**8.** 0.677 = ______	**13.** 0.4520 = ______
4. 0.05 = ______	**9.** 4.539 = ______	**14.** 0.7259 = ______
5. 0.63 = ______	**10.** 1.222 = ______	**15.** 0.3482 = ______

Comparing the Value of Decimals

Understanding which decimal is larger or smaller is often a help in solving dosage problems. For example, will I need more than one tablet, or less than one tablet?

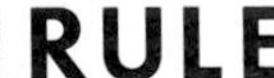 **RULE**

DETERMINING THE VALUE OF DECIMALS

The decimal with the higher number in the tenth place has the greater value.

EXAMPLE Compare 0.25 with 0.5
It is clear that 0.5 is greater because the number 5 is higher than the number 2.

Self-Test 10

In each pair, underline the decimal with the greater value. Answers may be found at the end of the chapter.

1. 0.125 and 0.25	**3.** 0.5 and 0.125	**5.** 0.825 and 0.44	**7.** 0.25 and 0.4
2. 0.04 and 0.1	**4.** 0.1 and 0.2	**6.** 0.9 and 0.5	**8.** 0.7 and 0.350

▼ PERCENT

Percent means parts per hundred. Percent is a fraction with the number becoming the numerator and 100 becoming the denominator. Whole numbers, fractions, and decimals may be written as percent. Percents may be changed to decimals or to fractions.

EXAMPLE

Whole number: 4% (four percent)

Decimal: 0.2% (two-tenths percent)

Fraction: $\frac{1}{4}$% (one-fourth percent)

Percents That Are Whole Numbers

EXAMPLE

Example 1:

Change to a fraction

$$4\% = \frac{4}{100} = \frac{1}{25}$$

Example 2:

Change to a decimal

$$4\% = \frac{4}{100} \quad 100\overline{)4.00}^{\;.04} = 0.04$$

◀ ***Learning Aid***
Note that 4% means four parts per 100. The 100th place has two decimal points. A quick rule to change a percent to a decimal is to move the decimal point two places to the left.

4% = 0.04

25% = 0.25

Percents That Are Decimals

These may be changed in three ways:

1. By using the quick rule (see Learning Aid)

   0.2% = 00.2 = 0.002

2. By keeping the decimal

   $$0.2\% = \frac{0.2}{100} \quad 100\overline{)0.200}^{\;0.002} = 0.002$$

3. By changing to a complex fraction

   $$0.2\% = \frac{\frac{2}{10}}{100} =$$

   $$\frac{2}{10} \div \frac{100}{1} =$$

   $$\frac{2}{10} \times \frac{1}{100} = \frac{2}{1000}$$

   $$\frac{\overset{1}{\cancel{2}}}{\underset{500}{\cancel{1000}}} = \frac{1}{500}$$

◀ ***Learning Aid***
Quick rule: To remove a % sign, move the decimal point two places to the left.

◀ ***Learning Aid***
Remember that the number after a division sign is inverted. The sign is changed to a multiplication sign.
Every whole number is understood to have a denominator of 1.

$$\frac{2}{10} \div 100 = \frac{2}{10} \times \frac{1}{100}$$

Percents That Are Fractions

EXAMPLE *Example 1:*

$$\frac{1}{4}\% = \frac{\frac{1}{4}}{100} = \frac{1}{4} \div \frac{100}{1}$$

$$\frac{1}{4} \div 100 = \frac{1}{4} \times \frac{1}{100} = \frac{1}{400}$$

Example 2:

$$\frac{1}{2}\% = \frac{\frac{1}{2}}{100} = \frac{1}{2} \div \frac{100}{1}$$

$$\frac{1}{2} \times \frac{1}{100} = \frac{1}{200}$$

Alternative Way. Because $\frac{1}{2} = 0.5$, $\frac{1}{2}\%$ could also be written as 0.5%. By using the quick rule of moving the decimal point two places to the left to clear a percent, you have 00.5% = 0.005.

Note that 0.005 is $\frac{5}{1000} = \frac{1}{200}$

Self-Test 11

*Change these percents to both a **fraction** and a **decimal.** Answers may be found at the end of the chapter.*

1. 10%	________	________	**4.** 20%	________	________
2. 0. 9%	________	________	**5.** 0.4%	________	________
3. $\frac{1}{5}\%$	________	________	**6.** $\frac{1}{10}\%$	________	________

▼ RATIO AND PROPORTION

A ratio indicates the relationship between two numbers. Ratios can be written as a fraction $\left(\frac{1}{10}\right)$ or as two numbers separated by a colon (1:10). (Read as *one is to ten.*)

Proportion indicates a relationship between two ratios. Proportions can be written as fractions or as two ratios separated by a double colon.

EXAMPLE $\frac{2}{8} = \frac{10}{40}$ (Read as *two is to eight as ten is to forty*)

5:30 :: 6:36 (Read as *five is to thirty as six is to thirty-six*)

Proportions written with colons can be written as fractions; therefore 5:30 :: 6:36 becomes

$$\frac{5}{30} = \frac{6}{36}$$

Solving Proportion With an Unknown

When one of the numbers in a proportion is unknown the letter x is substituted. There are three steps in determining the value of x in a proportion.

Step 1. Cross-multiply.

Step 2. Clear x.

Step 3. Reduce.

Let's see how this is done.

Proportions Expressed as Decimals

Suppose you had to solve this proportion:

$$\frac{1}{0.125} = \frac{x}{0.25}$$

Step 1. Cross-multiply numerators and denominators.

$$0.125x = 0.25$$

◀ ***Learning Aid***

$$\frac{1}{0.125} \times \frac{x}{0.25}$$

Step 2. Clear x by dividing both sides of the equation with the number preceding x.

$$x = \frac{0.25}{0.125}$$

◀ ***Learning Aid***

$$\frac{\cancel{0.125}\,x}{\cancel{0.125}} = \frac{0.25}{0.125}$$

Step 3. Reduce the number.

$$0.125\overline{)\,0.250}\quad 2.$$

$$x = 2$$

◀ ***Learning Aid***

Remember the line between the two numbers in a fraction is a division sign.

$$\frac{0.25}{0.125}$$

Can be read as 0.25 divided by 0.125.

Proportions Expressed as Two Ratios Separated by Colons

Suppose you had this proportion:

$4: 3.2 :: 7:x$

Step 1. Cross-multiply the two outside numbers (called "extremes") and the two inside numbers (called "means").

$4 : 3.2 :: 7:x$

$$4x = 22.4$$

Step 2. Clear x by dividing both sides of the equation with the number preceding x.

$$x = \frac{22.4}{4}$$

◀ ***Learning Aid***

$$\frac{\cancel{4}x}{\cancel{4}} = \frac{22.4}{4}$$

Remember that the line between two numbers in a fraction is a division sign. Read as 22.4 divided by 4.

Step 3. Reduce the number.

$x = 5.6$

◀ *Learning Aid*

$$4\overline{)22.4} = 5.6$$

EXAMPLE

$$\frac{45}{180} \times \frac{3}{x}$$

$$45x = 540$$

$$x = 12$$

◀ *Learning Aid*

$$45\overline{)540.} = 12.$$

45
90
90

EXAMPLE

11:121 :: 3:x

$$11x = 363$$

$$x = 33$$

◀ *Learning Aid*

$$11\overline{)363.} = 33.$$

33
33
33

Self-Test 12

Solve these proportions. Answers may be found at the end of the chapter.

1. $\frac{120}{4.2} = \frac{16}{x}$

2. 750:250 :: x:5

3. $\frac{14}{140} = \frac{22}{x}$

4. 2:5 :: x:10

5. $\frac{81}{3} = \frac{x}{15}$

6. 0.125 : 0.5 :: x:10

Solving Dosage Problems

When the amount of drug ordered by a physician differs from the stock, the nurse must calculate the dose to be given. Nurses use ratio and proportion to solve these problems.

EXAMPLE

Order: 0.5 mg
Stock: 0.125 mg per 4 mL

We can set this up as a fraction-ratio or as two ratios separated by colons:

$$\frac{0.5}{0.125} = \frac{x}{4} \quad \text{or}$$

0.5 : 0.125 :: x:4

To solve this problem three steps are required: cross-multiply, clear x, and reduce the number.

We can eliminate the first two steps and simplify the arithmetic by using a derivation of proportion:

$$\frac{D}{H} \times S = A$$

◀ *Learning Aid*

D = Doctor's order (0.5)
H = Strength of the drug (0.125)
S = Form of the drug (4 mL)
A = Answer; how much to give (x)

Derivation of the Dosage Formula

1. As a fraction the proportion would be

$$\frac{D}{H} = \frac{A}{S}$$

Step 1. $DS = AH \left(\frac{0.5}{0.125} = \frac{x}{4}\right)$

Step 2. $\frac{D}{H} \times S = \frac{AH}{H} \left(\frac{0.5 \times 4}{0.125} = \frac{0.125x}{0.125}\right)$

Step 3. $\frac{D}{H} \times S = A \left(\frac{0.5}{0.125} \times 4 = A\right)$

◀ ***Learning Aid***
The dosage formula is Step 3 and eliminates Steps 1 and 2.

2. As two ratios separated by colons, the proportion would be:

Step 1. D:H :: A:S

$DS = AH$

Step 2. $\frac{DS}{H} = \frac{AH}{H}$

Step 3. $\frac{DS}{H} = A$

◀ ***Learning Aid***
Note that this proportion also results in Step 3, the dosage formula.

3. Using the dosage formula $\frac{D}{H} \times S = A$

$$\frac{0.500}{0.125} \times 4 = A = 16 \text{ mL}$$

EXAMPLE

Order: 60 mg
Stock: 40 mg/tab

$$\frac{\overset{3}{\cancel{60}}}{\underset{2}{\cancel{40}}} \times 1 \text{ tab} = \frac{3}{2} = 1.5 \text{ tabs}$$

◀ ***Learning Aid***
$\frac{D}{H} \times S = A$

EXAMPLE

Order: 9 mg
Stock: 20 mg per 2 mL

$$\frac{9}{\underset{10}{\cancel{20}}} \times \overset{1}{\cancel{2}} \text{ mL} = A = 10\overline{)9.0}\ \ 0.9$$

Answer: 0.9 mL

◀ ***Learning Aid***
$\frac{D}{H} \times S = A$

Use of the dosage formula $\frac{D}{H} \times S = A$ begins in Chapter 6 to solve oral tablet and oral liquid problems.

ANSWERS

Self-Test 1

1. 12	**5.** 108	**9.** 48	**13.** 24	**17.** 18	**21.** 132
2. 63	**6.** 24	**10.** 72	**14.** 54	**18.** 88	**22.** 45
3. 32	**7.** 110	**11.** 15	**15.** 64	**19.** 36	**23.** 81
4. 45	**8.** 14	**12.** 42	**16.** 56	**20.** 24	**24.** 35

Self-Test 2

1. 9	**5.** 7	**9.** 7	**13.** 4	**17.** 9	**21.** 7
2. 4	**6.** 8	**10.** 6	**14.** 3	**18.** 4	**22.** 12
3. 3	**7.** 4	**11.** 9	**15.** 3	**19.** 6	**23.** 12
4. 7	**8.** 3	**12.** 6	**16.** 7	**20.** 2	**24.** 7

Self-Test 3

1. $\frac{16}{24}=\frac{4}{6}=\frac{2}{3}$ (divide by 4, then 2)

Alternatively: $\frac{16}{24}=\frac{2}{3}$ (divide by 8)

2. $\frac{36}{216}=\frac{6}{36}=\frac{1}{6}$ (divide by 6, then 6)

3. $\frac{18}{96}=\frac{9}{48}=\frac{3}{16}$ (divide by 2, then 3)

4. $\frac{70}{490}=\frac{7}{49}=\frac{1}{7}$ (divide by 10, then 7)

5. $\frac{18}{81}=\frac{2}{9}$ (divide by 9)

6. $\frac{8}{48}=\frac{1}{6}$ (divide by 8)

7. $\frac{12}{30}=\frac{6}{15}=\frac{2}{5}$ (divide by 2, then 3)

Alternatively: $\frac{12}{30}=\frac{2}{5}$ (divide by 6)

8. $\frac{68}{136}=\frac{34}{68}=\frac{1}{2}$ (divide by 2, then 34)

9. $\frac{55}{121}=\frac{5}{11}$ (divide by 11)

10. $\frac{15}{60}=\frac{1}{4}$ (divide by 15)

Alternatively: $\frac{15}{60}=\frac{3}{12}=\frac{1}{4}$ (divide by 5, then 3)

Self-Test 4 (Two Ways to Solve)

First Way

1. $\frac{1}{6}\times\frac{4}{5}\times\frac{5}{2}=\frac{20}{60}=\frac{1}{3}$

2. $\frac{4}{15}\times\frac{3}{2}=\frac{\cancel{12}^{2}}{\cancel{30}_{5}}=\frac{2}{5}$

(Divide by 6)

3. $1\frac{1}{2}\times4\frac{2}{3}=\frac{3}{2}\times\frac{14}{3}=\frac{42}{6}=7$

Second Way

1. $\frac{1}{\cancel{6}_{3}}\times\frac{\cancel{4}^{\cancel{2}^{1}}}{\cancel{5}_{1}}\times\frac{\cancel{5}^{1}}{\cancel{2}_{1}}=\frac{\cancel{2}^{1}}{\cancel{6}_{3}}=\frac{1}{3}$

2. $\frac{\cancel{4}^{2}}{\cancel{15}_{5}}\times\frac{\cancel{3}^{1}}{\cancel{2}_{1}}=\frac{2}{5}$

3. $1\frac{1}{2}\times4\frac{2}{3}=\frac{\cancel{3}^{1}}{\cancel{2}_{1}}\times\frac{\cancel{14}^{7}}{\cancel{3}_{1}}=7$

First Way	*Second Way*
4. $\frac{1}{5} \times \frac{15}{45} = \frac{\overset{3}{\cancel{15}}}{\underset{45}{\cancel{225}}} = \frac{3}{45} = \frac{1}{15}$ (Divide by 5)	**4.** $\frac{1}{5} \times \frac{\overset{1}{\cancel{15}}}{\underset{3}{\cancel{45}}} = \frac{1}{15}$
5. $3\frac{3}{4} \times 10\frac{2}{3} = \frac{15}{4} \times \frac{32}{3}$ (Too confusing! Use the second way.)	**5.** $\frac{\overset{5}{\cancel{15}}}{\underset{1}{\cancel{4}}} \times \frac{\overset{8}{\cancel{32}}}{\underset{1}{\cancel{3}}} = 40$
6. $\frac{7}{20} \times \frac{2}{14}$ (Too difficult. Use the second way.)	**6.** $\frac{\overset{1}{\cancel{7}}}{\underset{10}{\cancel{20}}} \times \frac{\overset{1}{\cancel{2}}}{\underset{2}{\cancel{14}}} = \frac{1}{20}$
7. $\frac{9}{2} \times \frac{3}{2} = \frac{27}{4}$ (Cannot reduce)	
8. $6\frac{1}{4} \times 7\frac{1}{9} \times \frac{9}{5} = \frac{25}{4} \times \frac{64}{9} \times \frac{9}{5}$ (Too difficult. Use the second way.)	**8.** $\frac{\overset{5}{\cancel{25}}}{\underset{1}{\cancel{4}}} \times \frac{\overset{16}{\cancel{64}}}{\underset{1}{\cancel{9}}} \times \frac{\overset{1}{\cancel{9}}}{\underset{1}{\cancel{5}}} = 80$

Self-Test 5

1. $\frac{1}{75} \div \frac{1}{150} = \frac{1}{\underset{1}{\cancel{75}}} \times \frac{\overset{2}{\cancel{150}}}{1} = 2$
2. $\frac{1}{8} \div \frac{1}{4} = \frac{1}{\underset{2}{\cancel{8}}} \times \frac{\overset{1}{\cancel{4}}}{1} = \frac{1}{2}$
3. $2\frac{2}{3} \div \frac{1}{2} = \frac{8}{3} \times \frac{2}{1} = \frac{16}{3}$
4. $75 \div 12\frac{1}{2} = 75 \div \frac{25}{2} = \overset{3}{\cancel{75}} \times \frac{2}{\underset{1}{\cancel{25}}} = 6$
5. $\frac{7}{25} \div \frac{7}{75} = \frac{\overset{1}{\cancel{7}}}{\underset{1}{\cancel{25}}} \times \frac{\overset{3}{\cancel{75}}}{\underset{1}{\cancel{7}}} = 3$
6. $\frac{1}{2} \div \frac{1}{4} = \frac{1}{\underset{1}{\cancel{2}}} \times \frac{\overset{2}{\cancel{4}}}{1} = 2$
7. $\frac{3}{4} \div \frac{8}{3} = \frac{3}{4} \times \frac{3}{8} = \frac{9}{32}$
8. $\frac{1}{60} \div \frac{7}{10} = \frac{1}{\underset{6}{\cancel{60}}} \times \frac{\overset{1}{\cancel{10}}}{7} = \frac{1}{42}$

Self-Test 6

1. $\frac{1}{6}$ $6\overline{)1.000}$ quotient .166 = 0.166
   6 / 40 / 36 / 40 / 36 / 4

2. $\frac{6}{8} = \frac{3}{4}$ $4\overline{)3.00}$ quotient .75 = 0.75
   2 8 / 20 / 20 / 0

3. $\frac{4}{5}$ $5\overline{)4.0}$ quotient .8 = 0.8
   4 0 / 0

4. $\frac{9}{40}$ $40\overline{)9.000}$ quotient .225 = 0.225
   8 0 / 1 00 / 80 / 200 / 200 / 0

5. $\frac{1}{8}$ $8\overline{)1.000}$ quotient .125 = 0.125
   8 / 20 / 16 / 40 / 40 / 0

6. $\frac{1}{7}$ $7\overline{)1.000}$ quotient .142 = 0.142
   7 / 30 / 28 / 20 / 14 / 6

Self-Test 7

1. Twenty-five hundredths $\left(\frac{25}{100}\right)$
2. Four thousandths $\left(\frac{4}{1000}\right)$
3. One and seven tenths $\left(1\frac{7}{10}\right)$
4. Five tenths $\left(\frac{5}{10}\right)$
5. Three hundred thirty-four thousandths $\left(\frac{334}{1000}\right)$
6. One hundred thirty-six and seventy-five hundredths $\left(136\frac{75}{100}\right)$
7. One tenth $\left(\frac{1}{10}\right)$
8. One hundred fifty thousandths $\left(\frac{150}{1000}\right)$. The zero at the end of 0.150 is not necessary. The number could be read as fifteen hundredths $\left(\frac{15}{100}\right)$.

Self-Test 8

1. $24\overline{)0.0048}$ quotient 0.0002 No decimals in the divisor, so no need to move the decimal in the dividend.

2. $0.004\overline{)0.100}$ (decimal moved three places) Now it is $4\overline{)100.}$ quotient 25.

3. $0.02\overline{)0.20}$ (decimal moved two places) Now it is $2\overline{)20}$ quotient 10.

4. $7.8\overline{)140.0}$ (decimal moved one place) Now it is $78\overline{)1400.000}$ quotient 17.948
   78 / 620 / 546 / 74 0 / 70 2 / 3 80 / 3 12 / 680 / 624 / 56

5. $6\overline{)140.000}$ quotient 23.333
   12 / 20 / 18 / 20 / 18 / 20 / 18 / 20 / 18 / 2

6. $0.025\overline{)10.000}$ (decimal moved three places) Now it is $25\overline{)10000.}$ quotient 400.

   Note that because there are two places between the 4 and the decimal, you had to add 2 zeros.

Self-Test 9

Nearest Tenth	*Nearest Hundredth*	*Nearest Thousandth*
1. 0.3	**6.** 1.27	**11.** 1.325
2. 1.8	**7.** 0.75	**12.** 0.003
3. 3.3	**8.** 0.68	**13.** 0.452
4. 0.1	**9.** 4.54	**14.** 0.726
5. 0.6	**10.** 1.22	**15.** 0.348

Self-Test 10

1. 0.25
2. 0.1
3. 0.5
4. 0.2
5. 0.825
6. 0.9
7. 0.4
8. 0.7

Self-Test 11

1. Fraction $10\% = \frac{\overset{1}{\cancel{10}}}{\underset{10}{\cancel{100}}} = \frac{1}{10}$

Decimal $10\% = \frac{10}{100} \quad 100\overline{)10.0}^{\,.1} = 0.1$

Quick rule decimal $10.\% = 0.1$

2. Fraction $0.9\% = \frac{\frac{9}{10}}{100} = \frac{9}{10} \div 100 = \frac{9}{10} \times \frac{1}{100} = \frac{9}{1000}$

Decimal $0.9\% = \frac{0.9}{100} \quad 100\overline{)0.900}^{\,.009} = 0.009$

Quick rule decimal $00.9 = 0.009$

3. Fraction $\frac{1}{5}\% = \frac{\frac{1}{5}}{100} = \frac{1}{5} \div 100 = \frac{1}{5} \times \frac{1}{100} = \frac{1}{500}$

Decimal $\frac{1}{5}\% = \frac{1}{5} \div 100 = \frac{1}{500} \quad 500\overline{)1.000}^{\,.002} = 0.002$

Quick rule decimal $\frac{1}{5}\% = \frac{1}{5} \quad 5\overline{)1.0}^{\,.2} = 0.2\%$

$00.2 = 0.002$

4. Fraction $\frac{\overset{1}{\cancel{20}}}{\underset{5}{\cancel{100}}} = \frac{1}{5}$

Decimal $20\% = \frac{20}{100} \quad 100\overline{)20.0}^{\,0.2}$

Quick rule decimal $20.\% = 0.2$

5. Fraction $0.4\% = \frac{\frac{4}{10}}{100} = \frac{4}{10} \div \frac{100}{1} = \frac{\overset{1}{\cancel{4}}}{10} \times \frac{1}{\underset{25}{\cancel{100}}} = \frac{1}{250}$

Decimal $0.4\% = \frac{0.4}{100} \quad 100\overline{)0.400}^{\,0.004} = 0.004$

Quick rule decimal $00.4\% = 0.004$

6. Fraction $\frac{1}{10}\% = \frac{\frac{1}{10}}{100} = \frac{1}{10} \div \frac{100}{1} = \frac{1}{10} \times \frac{1}{100} = \frac{1}{1000}$

Decimal $\frac{1}{10}\% = \frac{1}{10} \div \frac{100}{1} = \frac{1}{10} \times \frac{1}{100} = \frac{1}{1000} \quad 1000\,\overline{)\,1.000}^{\,0.001} = 0.001$

Quick rule decimal $\frac{1}{10}\% = \frac{1}{10} \quad 10\,\overline{)\,1.0}^{\,0.1} = 0.1\% = 00.1 = 0.001$

Self-Test 12

1. $\frac{120}{4.2} = \frac{16}{x}$

$120x = 67.2$

$x = 0.56$

$$120\,\overline{)\,67.20}^{\,0.56} \quad \begin{array}{r} 60\,0 \\ \hline 720 \\ 720 \\ \hline \end{array}$$

2. $750{:}250 :: x{:}\,5$

$250x = 750 \times 5$

$x = 15$

$$\frac{\overset{3}{\cancel{750}} \times 5}{\underset{1}{\cancel{250}}} = 15$$

3. $\frac{14}{140} = \frac{22}{x}$

$14x = 22 \times 140$

$x = 220$

$$\frac{22 \times \overset{10}{\cancel{140}}}{\underset{1}{\cancel{14}}} = 220$$

4. $2{:}5 :: x{:}10$

$5x = 20$

$x = 4$

5. $\frac{3}{81} = \frac{15}{x}$

$3x = 81 \times 15$

$x = 405$

$$\frac{81 \times \overset{5}{\cancel{15}}}{\underset{1}{\cancel{3}}} = 405$$

6. $0.125 : 0.5 :: x{:}10$

$0.5x = 0.125 \times 10$

$x = 2.5$

$$\frac{\overset{1}{\cancel{0.125}}}{\underset{4}{\cancel{0.500}}} \times 10 = \frac{10}{4} \quad 4\,\overline{)\,10.0}^{\,2.5}$$

Interpreting the Language of Prescriptions

CONTENT TO MASTER

Abbreviating times and routes of administration

Understanding military time—the 24-hour clock

Abbreviating metric, apothecary, and household measurements

Understanding SI units

Reading prescriptions

Terms and abbreviations for drug preparations

Every medication order contains the name and dosage of the drug and the route and time of administration. The dosage, route, and time are written in shorthand using abbreviations. Learn this shorthand to become proficient in reading and interpreting prescriptions.

In writing orders, some physicians use capital letters, whereas others use lower-case letters; some use periods after abbreviations, others do not. These variations reflect individual writing style and are not important. Concentrate on understanding the meaning of the abbreviation in the context of the order.

Here are three medication orders that will make sense to you after studying the material in this chapter:

Morphine sulfate 15 mg SC stat and 10 mg q4h prn

Neomycin ophthalmic oint OS bid

Ampicillin 1 g IVPB q6h

▼ TIME OF ADMINISTRATION OF DRUGS

The abbreviations for times of drug administration are based on Latin words. They are included here under *Learning Aid* for your information, but it is not necessary for you to study or learn the Latin words. Learn the abbreviations, their meanings, and the sample times that indicate how the abbreviations are interpreted.

Time Abbreviation	Meaning	Learning Aid
ac	Before meals	Latin, *ante cibum* **Sample time:** 7:30 AM, 11:30 AM, 4:30 PM
pc	After meals	Latin, *post cibum* **Sample time:** 10 AM, 2 PM, 6 PM
qd	Every day, daily	Latin, *quaque die* **Sample time:** 10 AM
bid	Twice a day	Latin, *bis in die* **Sample time:** 10 AM, 6 PM
tid	Three times a day	Latin, *ter in die* **Sample time:** 10 AM, 2 PM, 6 PM
qid	Four times a day	Latin, *quater in die* **Sample time:** 10 AM, 2 PM, 6 PM, 10 PM
qh	Every hour	Latin, *quaque hora* Because the drug is given every hour, it will be given 24 times in one day.
hs	At bedtime, hour of sleep	Latin, *hora somni* **Sample time:** 10 PM
qn	Every night	Latin, *quaque nocte* **Sample time:** 10 PM
stat	Immediately	Latin, *statim* **Sample time:** now!

The following time abbreviations are based on a 24-hour day. To determine the number of times a medication will be given in a day, divide 24 by the number given in the abbreviation.

Time Abbreviation	Meaning	Learning Aid
q2h or q2°	Every 2 hours	The drug will be given 12 times in a 24-hour period (24 ÷ 2). **Sample times:** even hours at 2 AM, 4 AM, 6 AM, 8 AM, 10 AM, 12 noon, 2 PM, 4 PM, 6 PM, 8 PM, 10 PM, 12 midnight
q4h or q4°	Every 4 hours	The drug will be given six times in a 24-hour period (24 ÷ 4). **Sample time:** 2 AM, 6 AM, 10 AM, 2 PM,6 PM, 10 PM
q6h or q6°	Every 6 hours	The drug will be given four times in a 24-hour period (24 ÷ 6). **Sample times:** 6 AM, 12 noon, 6 PM, 12 midnight
q8h or q8°	Every 8 hours	The drug will be given three times in a 24-hour period (24 ÷ 8). **Sample times:** 6 AM, 2 PM, 10 PM
q12 h or q12°	Every 12 hours	The drug will be given twice in a 24-hour period (24 ÷ 12). **Sample times:** 6 AM, 6 PM

There are four additional time abbreviations that require explanation. They are as follows:

Time Abbreviation	Meaning	Learning Aid
qod	Every other day	Latin, *quaque otra die* This abbreviation is interpreted by the days of the **month:** the nurse writes on the medication record: qod odd days of the month **Sample time:** 10 AM on the first, third, fifth day, and so on The nurse might write: qod even days of the month **Sample time:** 10 AM on the second, fourth, sixth day, and so on
prn	As needed	Latin, *pro re nata* **This abbreviation is usually combined with a time abbreviation.** **Example:** q4h prn (every 4 hours as needed). This permits the nurse to assess the patient and make a nursing judgment about whether or not to administer the medication. **Sample:** acetaminophen 650 mg po q4h prn (650 milligrams of acetaminophen by mouth, every 4 hours as needed) for pain) The nurse assesses the patient for pain every 4 hours; if the patient has pain, the nurse may administer the drug. This abbreviation has three administration implications: 1. The nurse **must wait** 4 hours before giving the next dose. 2. Once 4 hours has elapsed, the dose may be given at any time thereafter. 3. Sample times are not given because the nurse does not know when the patient will need the drug.
tiw	Three times per week	Latin, *ter in vicis* Time relates to days of the **week.** **Sample time:** 10 AM on Monday, Wednesday, Friday Do not confuse with tid (three times per **day**).
biw	Twice per week	Latin, *bis in vicis* Time relates to days of the **week.** **Sample time:** 10 AM on Monday, Thursday Do not confuse with bid (twice per **day**).

Self-Test 1

After studying the abbreviations for times of administration, give the meaning of the following terms. Include sample times. Answers are given at the end of the chapter.

1. tid ____________
2. qn ____________
3. pc ____________
4. qod ____________
5. bid ____________
6. hs ____________
7. stat ____________
8. qid ____________
9. q4h ____________
10. ac ____________
11. qd ____________
12. q8h ____________
13. qh ____________
14. prn ____________
15. q4h prn ____________

Military Time: The 24-Hour Clock

Confusion about times of administration can arise by misinterpreting handwriting as AM or PM. To prevent error many institutions have converted from the traditional 12-hour clock to a 24-hour clock, referred to as military time.

The 24-hour clock begins at midnight as 0000. The hours from 1 AM to 12 noon are the same as traditional time; colons and the terms AM and PM are omitted. For example:

Traditional	*Military*
12 midnight	0000
1 AM	0100
5 AM	0500
7:30 AM	0730
11:45 AM	1145
12:00 noon	1200

◀ ***Learning Aid***
In military time, minutes are written in tenths, hours in hundredths or thousandths.

The hours from 1 PM continue numerically; 1 PM becomes 1300. For example:

Traditional	*Military*
1 PM	1300
2:30 PM	1430
5 PM	1700
7:15 PM	1915
10:45 PM	2245
11:59 PM	2359

◀ ***Learning Aid***
To change traditional time to military time from 1 PM on add 12.

Self-Test 2

A. Change these traditional times to military time. Answers may be found at the end of the chapter.

1. 2 PM ________ **5.** 1:30 AM ________
2. 9 AM ________ **6.** 9:15 PM ________
3. 4 PM ________ **7.** 4:50 AM ________
4. 12 noon ________ **8.** 6:20 PM ________

B. Change these military times to traditional times. Answers may be found at the end of this chapter.

1. 0130 ________ **5.** 1910 ________
2. 1745 ________ **6.** 0600 ________
3. 1100 ________ **7.** 2450 ________
4. 2015 ________ **8.** 1000 ________

◀ ***Learning Aid***
To change military time to traditional time from 1300 on, subtract 12.

▼ ROUTES OF ADMINISTRATION

Some of these abbreviations are based on Latin words, whereas others are not. Again, the Latin words are included for your information, but it is not necessary to study them. Alternative abbreviations are given in parentheses.

Route Abbreviation	Meaning	Learning Aid
IM	Intramuscularly	The injection is given at a 90° angle into a muscle.
IV	Intravenously	The injection is given into a vein.
IVPB	Intravenous piggyback	Medication prepared in a small volume of fluid is attached to an IV (which is already infusing fluid into a patient's vein) at specified times (Fig. 2-1).
NGT (ng)	Nasogastric tube	Medication is placed in the stomach through a tube in the nose.
OD	In the right eye	Latin, *oculus dextra*
OS	In the left eye	Latin, *oculus sinister*
OU	In both eyes	Latin, *oculi utrique*
po (PO)	By mouth	Latin, *per os*
pr (PR)	In the rectum	Latin, *per rectum*
SC (SQ)	Subcutaneously	The injection is usually given at a 45° angle into subcutaneous tissue.
SL	Sublingual, under the tongue	Latin, *sub lingua*
S & S	Swish and swallow	By using tongue and cheek muscles, the patient coats his mouth with a liquid medication.

Self-Test 3

After studying the abbreviations for route of administration, give the meaning of the following terms. Answers are given at the end of the chapter.

1. SL ______
2. OU ______
3. NGT ______
4. IV ______
5. po ______
6. OD ______
7. IVPB ______
8. OS ______
9. IM ______
10. pr ______
11. S&S ______
12. SC ______

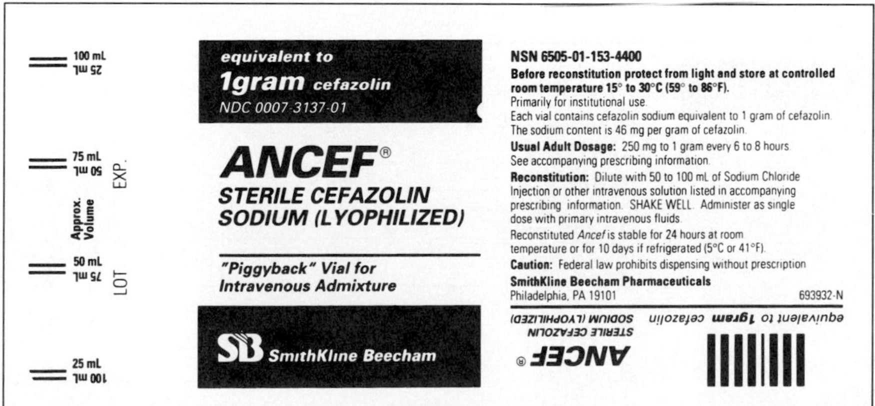

Figure 2-1
Label states the route of administration. (Courtesy of Smith Kline Beecham Pharmaceuticals)

▼ METRIC AND SI ABBREVIATIONS

Metric abbreviations in dosage relate to a drug's weight or volume and are the most common measures in dosage. The International System of Units (Systèm International d'Unités; SI) was adapted from the metric system in 1960. Most developed countries except the United States have adopted SI nomenclature to provide a standard language of measurement.

Differences between metric and SI systems do not occur in dosage. The meaning and abbreviations for weight and volume are the same. Weight measures are based on the gram; volume measures are based on the liter.

Study the meaning of the abbreviations listed in the following table. Under *Learning Aid,* one equivalent is given for each abbreviation in order to help you understand what kinds of quantities are involved; it is not yet necessary to study the equivalents (equivalents are discussed in Chapter 4). The preferred abbreviation is listed first; variations are given in parentheses.

Metric Abbreviation	Meaning	Learning Aid
cc	Cubic centimeter	This is a measure of volume. It is now usually reserved for measuring gases; however you may still find it used as a liquid measure. (One cubic centimeter is approximately equal to 16 drops from a medicine dropper.)
g (gm, Gm)	Gram	This is a solid measure of weight. (One gram is approximately equal to the weight of two paper clips.)
kg (Kg)	Kilogram	This is a weight measure. (One kilogram equals 2.2 pounds.)
L	Liter	This is a liquid measure. (One liter is a little more than a quart.)
μg (mcg)	Microgram	This is a measure of weight. (One thousand micrograms make up 1 milligram: 1000 μg = 1 mg)
mEq	Milliequivalent	No equivalent necessary. Drugs are prepared and ordered in this weight measure.
mg	Milligram	This is a measure of weight. (One thousand milligrams make up 1 gram: 1000 mg = 1 g)
mL (ml)	Milliliter	This is a liquid measure. The terms *cubic centimeter* (cc) and *milliliter* (mL) are interchangeable in dosage (1 cc = 1 mL).
unit (U)	Unit	This is a measure of biologic activity. Nurses do not calculate this measure. **Example:** penicillin potassium 300,000 units *Important:* It is considered safer to write the word *unit* rather than use the abbreviation, because the *U* could be read as a zero and a medication error might result.

Self-Test 4 *After studying metric abbreviations, write the meaning of the following terms. Answers can be found at the end of the chapter.*

1. 0.3 g ____________ **6.** 0.25 mg ____________

2. 150 mcg ____________ **7.** 14 kg ____________

3. 80 U ____________ **8.** 20 mEq ____________

4. 0.5 mL ____________ **9.** 1.5 L ____________

5. 1.7 cc ____________ **10.** 50 μg ____________

▼ APOTHECARY ABBREVIATIONS

The archaic apothecary system of measures has largely been replaced by the more precise metric system. However, because some physicians still order in apothecary terms, several of these abbreviations are listed in the following table. The meanings given are commonly accepted interpretations used in nursing practice. The system requires notation in Roman numerals and fractions.

Apothecary Abbreviation	Meaning	Learning Aid
ʒ	Dram	This is a liquid measure. It is slightly less than a household teaspoon. (One dram equals 4 milliliters: ʒi = 4 mL [see below])
℥	Ounce	This is a liquid measure, It is slightly more than a household ounce. (One ounce equals 32 milliliters: ℥i = 32 mL)
gr	Grain	Latin, *granum*. This solid measure was based on the weight of a grain of wheat in ancient times. There is no commonly used equivalent to the grain in the metric system.
gtt	Drop	Latin, *guttae*. This liquid measure was based on a drop of water. (One drop equals 1 minim)
m (M, Mx)	Minim	Latin, *minim*. (One minim equals one drop: 1 m = 1 gtt; Fig. 2-2)
ṡṡ	One-half	Latin, *semis*
i	One	**Example:** gr i = grains I; ʒi = 4 mL
i ṡṡ	One-and-a-half	**Example:** gr i ṡṡ = grains $1\frac{1}{2}$
ii	Two	**Example:** gr ii = grains 2
iii	Three	**Example:** gr iii = grains 3
iv	Four	**Example:** gr iv = grains 4 ʒ iv = drams 4
v	Five	**Example:** gr v = grains 5 m v = minims 5
vii	Seven	**Example:** gr vii = grains 7
vii ṡṡ	Seven-and-a-half	**Example:** gr vii ṡṡ = grains $7\frac{1}{2}$
x	Ten	**Example:** gr x = grains 10 m x = minims 10
xv	Fifteen	**Example:** gr xv = grains 15 m xv = minims 15

Self-Test 5

After studying the apothecary abbreviations, write the meaning of the following terms. Answers can be found at the end of the chapter.

1. m x ______________
2. ʒ ii ______________
3. gr v ______________
4. gtt x ______________
5. ℥ i ______________
6. ʒ viii ______________
7. ℥ ṡṡ ______________
8. gr x ______________
9. m v ______________
10. gr i ṡṡ ______________

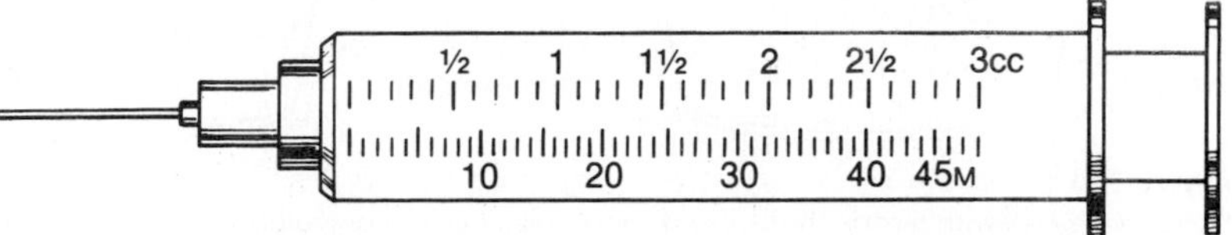

Figure 2-2
A 3-mL (cc) syringe calibrated in tenths of a milliliter and in minims.

▼ HOUSEHOLD ABBREVIATIONS

Physicians may use these common household measures to order drugs. Metric equivalents are included in the *Learning Aid* column for your information.

Household Abbreviation	Meaning	Learning Aid
pt	Pint	One pint is approximately equal to 500 milliliters (1 pt ≅ 500 mL).
qt	Quart	One quart is approximately equal to 1 liter, which is equal to 1000 milliliters (1 qt ≅ 1 L = 1000 mL). One-half a quart is approximately equal to 1 pint ($\frac{1}{2}$ qt ≅ 1 pt = 500 ml).
tbsp	Tablespoon	One tablespoon equals 15 milliliters (1 tbsp = 15 mL).
tsp	Teaspoon	One teaspoon equals 5 milliliters (1 tsp = 5 mL).
oz	Ounce	One ounce equals 30 milliliters (1 oz = 30 mL). **Example:** 6 tsp = 1 oz = 30 mL 3 tsp = $\frac{1}{2}$ oz = 15 mL 2 tbsp = 1 oz = 30 mL = 6 tsp (Fig. 2-3)

Self-Test 6

After studying household measures, write the meaning of the following terms. Answers can be found at the end of the chapter.

1. 3 tsp ______________ **3.** $\frac{1}{2}$ qt ______________ **5.** 1 pt ______________

2. 1 oz ______________ **4.** 1 tsp ______________ **6.** 2 tbsp ______________

▼ TERMS AND ABBREVIATIONS FOR DRUG PREPARATIONS

The following abbreviations and terms are used to describe selected drug preparations.

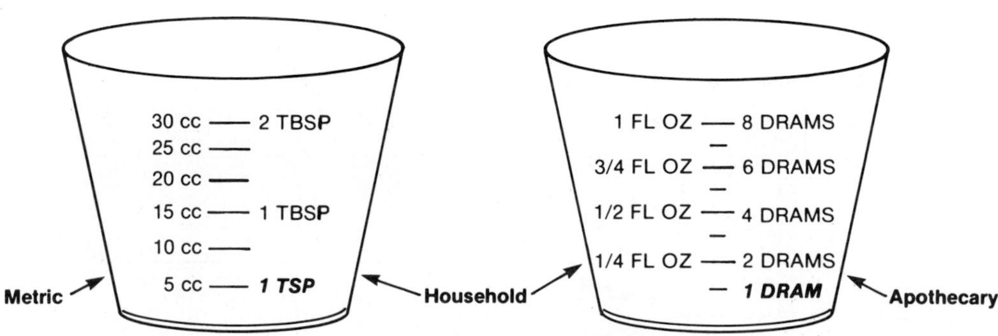

Figure 2-3
A medicine cup with metric, household, and apothecary equivalents. Two sides of the cup are shown.

Term Abbreviation	Meaning	Learning Aid
cap, caps	Capsule	Medication is encased in a gelatin shell.
CR	Controlled-release	These abbreviations indicate that the drug has been prepared in a form that allows extended action. Therefore, the drug is given less frequently.
LA	Long-acting	
SA	Sustained-action	
SR	Slow-release	
DS	Double-strength	
EC	Enteric-coated	The tablet is coated with a substance that will not dissolve in the acid secretions of the stomach; instead, it dissolves in the more alkaline secretions of the intestines.
el, elix	Elixir	A drug is dissolved in a hydroalcoholic sweetened base.
sol	Solution	The drug is contained in a clear liquid preparation.
sp	Spirit	An alcoholic solution of a volatile substance (e.g., spirit of ammonia).
sup, supp	Suppository	A solid, cylindrically shaped drug that can be inserted into a body opening (e.g., the rectum or vagina).
susp	Suspension	Small particles of drug are dispersed in a liquid base and must be shaken before pouring, Gels and magmas are also suspensions.
syr	Syrup	A sugar is dissolved in a liquid medication and flavored to disguise the taste.
tab, tabs	Tablet	Medication is compressed or molded into a solid form; additional ingredients are used to shape and color the tablet.
tr, tinct.	Tincture	This is a liquid alcoholic or hydroalcoholic solution of a drug.
ung, oint.	Ointment	This is a semisolid drug preparation that is applied to the skin (for external use only).
KVO	Keep vein open	**Example order:** 1000 mL dextrose 5% in water IVKVO. The nurse is to continue infusing this fluid.
D/C	Discontinue	**Example order:** D/C ampicillin
NKA	No known allergies	This is an important assessment that is noted on the medication record of a patient.

Self-Test 7

After studying the abbreviations for drug forms, write out the meaning of the following terms. Answers can be found at the end of the chapter.

1. elix ______
2. DS ______
3. NKA ______
4. caps ______
5. susp ______
6. tab ______
7. SR ______
8. D/C ______
9. supp ______
10. tr ______

Proficiency Test 1

Abbreviations

Aim for 90% or better on this test. There are 50 items, each worth 2 points. If you have any difficulty, study the content again. Answers may be found at the end of this chapter.

Your score ______

1. bid ______
2. hs ______
3. prn ______
4. OU ______
5. po ______
6. pr ______
7. SL ______
8. S&S ______
9. tiw ______
10. mL ______
11. q4h ______
12. cc ______
13. SC ______
14. 1 ṡṡ ______
15. g ______
16. PC ______
17. qd ______
18. stat ______
19. q12h ______
20. tid ______
21. OS ______
22. kg ______
23. ʒ ______
24. qh ______
25. OD ______
26. mEq ______
27. AC ______
28. qid ______
29. mg ______
30. IM ______
31. qod ______
32. BIW ______
33. NGT ______
34. q8h ______
35. L ______
36. mcg ______
37. q6h ______
38. μg ______
39. U ______
40. tsp ______
41. ṡṡ ______
42. gr ______
43. IV ______
44. mL ______
45. ℥ ______
46. IVPB ______
47. m ______
48. Gm ______
49. q2h ______
50. q3h ______

Proficiency Test 2

Reading Prescriptions

Now that you have studied the language of prescriptions, you are ready to interpret medication orders! Write the following orders in longhand. Give sample times. Answers are given at the end of this chapter.

1. Nembutal 100 mg hs prn po ______
2. Propranolol hydrochloride 40 mg po bid ______
3. Ampicillin 1 g IVPB q6h ______

(continued)

Proficiency Test 2 (continued)

4. Demerol 50 mg IM q4h prn for pain ______________________

5. Tylenol 325 mg tabs ii po stat ______________________

6. Pilocarpine gtt ii OU q3h ______________________

7. Scopolamine 0.8 mg SC stat ______________________

8. El Digoxin 0.25 mg po qd ______________________

9. Kaochlor 30 mEq po bid ______________________

10. Liquaemin sodium 6000 units SC q4h ______________________

11. Tobramycin 70 mg IM q8h ______________________

12. Maalox ℥ i po AC and hs ______________________

13. Humulin insulin units 15 SC qd 7:30 AM ______________________

14. Vitamin B_{12} 1000 μg IM tiw ______________________

15. Tr belladonna gtt xv and Amphojel ℥ ṡṡ qid po ______________________

16. Aspirin gr x po q4h prn for temperature over 101° ______________________

17. Neomycin ophthalmic oint 1% OS tid ______________________

18. Prednisone 10 mg po qod ______________________

19. Milk of magnesia 1 tbsp po hs qn ______________________

20. Septra DS tab i qd po ______________________

21. Morphine sulfate 15 mg SC stat and 10 mg q4h prn ______________________

ANSWERS

Self-Test 1

1. Three times a day. (**Sample times:** 10 AM, 2 PM, 6 PM)
2. Every night. (**Sample time:** 10 PM)
3. After meals. (**Sample times:** 10 AM, 2 PM, 6 PM)
4. Every other day. (**Sample times:** odd days of month at 10 AM)
5. Twice a day. (**Sample times:** 10 AM, 6 PM)
6. Hour of sleep. (**Sample time:** 10 PM)
7. Immediately. (**Sample time:** whatever the time is now)
8. Four times a day. (**Sample times:** 10 AM, 2 PM, 6 PM, 10 PM)
9. Every 4 hours. (**Sample times:** 2 AM, 6 AM, 10 AM, 2 PM, 6 PM, 10 PM)
10. Before meals. (**Sample times:** 7:30 AM, 11:30 AM, 4:30 PM)
11. Every day. (**Sample time:** 10 AM)
12. Every 8 hours. (**Sample times:** 6 AM, 2 PM, 10 PM)
13. Every hour.
14. Whenever necessary. (**Sample times:** No time routine can be written.)
15. Every 4 hours as needed. (**Sample times:** No time routine is written because we do not know when the drug will be needed.)

Self-Test 2

A.
1. 1400
2. 0900
3. 1600
4. 1200
5. 0130
6. 2115
7. 0450
8. 1820

B.
1. 1:30 AM
2. 5:45 PM
3. 11 AM
4. 8:15 PM
5. 7:10 PM
6. 6 AM
7. 12:50 PM
8. 10 AM

Self-Test 3

1. Sublingual; under the tongue
2. Both eyes
3. Nasogastric tube
4. Intravenously
5. By mouth
6. Right eye
7. Intravenous piggyback
8. Left eye
9. Intramuscularly
10. Rectally
11. Swish and swallow
12. Subcutaneously

Self-Test 4

1. Three-tenths of a gram
2. One hundred fifty micrograms
3. Eighty units
4. Five-tenths of a milliliter
5. One and seven-tenths of a cubic centimeter
6. Twenty-five hundredths of a milligram
7. Fourteen kilograms
8. Twenty milliequivalents
9. One and five-tenths liters
10. Fifty micrograms

Self-Test 5

1. Minims 10
2. Drams 2
3. Grains 5
4. Drops 10
5. Ounces 1
6. Drams 8
7. Ounces $\frac{1}{2}$ (0.5)
8. Grains 10
9. Minims 5
10. Grains $1\frac{1}{2}$ (1.5)

Self-Test 6

1. Three teaspoons
2. One ounce
3. One-half quart
4. One teaspoon
5. One pint
6. Two tablespoons

Self-Test 7

1. Elixir
2. Double-strength
3. No known allergies
4. Capsules
5. Suspension
6. Tablet
7. Slow-release
8. Discontinue
9. Suppository
10. Tincture

Proficiency Test 1—Abbreviations

1. Twice a day
2. Hour of sleep
3. When necessary
4. Both eyes
5. By mouth
6. By rectum
7. Sublingually
8. Swish and swallow
9. Three times a week
10. Milliliter
11. Every 4 hours
12. Cubic centimeters
13. Subcutaneously
14. One and a half
15. Gram
16. After meals
17. Every day
18. Immediately
19. Every 12 hours
20. Three times a day
21. Left eye
22. Kilogram
23. Dram
24. Every hour
25. Right eye
26. Milliequivalent
27. Before meals
28. Four times a day
29. Milligram
30. Intramuscularly
31. Every other day
32. Twice a week
33. Nasogastric tube
34. Every 8 hours
35. Liter
36. Microgram
37. Every 6 hours
38. Microgram
39. Unit
40. Teaspoon
41. A half
42. Grain
43. Intravenously
44. Milliliter
45. Ounce
46. Intravenous piggyback
47. Minim
48. Gram
49. Every 2 hours
50. Every 3 hours

Proficiency Test 2—Reading Prescriptions

1. Nembutal one hundred milligrams at the hour of sleep, as needed, by mouth (e.g., 10 PM)
2. Propranolol hydrochloride forty milligrams by mouth twice a day (e.g., 10 AM, 6 PM)
3. Ampicillin one gram intravenous piggyback every 6 hours (e.g., 6 AM, 12 noon, 6 PM, 12 midnight)
4. Demerol fifty milligrams intramuscularly every 4 hours as needed for pain
5. Tylenol three hundred twenty-five milligrams, two tablets by mouth immediately. (Give two tablets of Tylenol. Each tablet is 325 mg.)
6. Pilocarpine drops two in both eyes every 3 hours (e.g., 3 AM, 6 AM, 9 AM, 12 noon, 3 PM, 6 PM, 9 PM, 12 midnight)
7. Scopolamine eight-tenths milligram subcutaneously immediately
8. Elixir of digoxin twenty-five hundredths of a milligram by mouth every day (e.g., 10 AM)
9. Kaochlor thirty milliequivalents by mouth twice a day (e.g., 10 AM and 6 PM)
10. Liquaemin sodium six thousand units subcutaneously every 4 hours (e.g., 2 AM, 6 AM, 10 AM, 2 PM, 6 PM, 10 PM)
11. Tobramycin seventy milligrams intramuscularly every 8 hours (e.g., 6 AM, 2 PM, 10 PM)
12. Maalox one ounce by mouth before meals and at the hour of sleep (e.g., 7:30 AM, 11:30 AM, 4:30 PM, 10 PM)
13. Humulin insulin fifteen units subcutaneously every day at seven-thirty in the morning
14. Vitamin B_{12} one thousand micrograms intramuscularly three times a week (e.g., Monday, Wednesday, Friday at 10 AM)
15. Tincture of belladonna fifteen drops and Amphojel one-half ounce four times a day by mouth (e.g., 10 AM, 2 PM, 6 PM, 10 PM)
16. Aspirin ten grains by mouth every 4 hours as needed for temperature over one hundred one degrees
17. Neomycin ophthalmic ointment one percent left eye three times a day (e.g., 10 AM, 2 PM, 6 PM)
18. Prednisone ten milligrams by mouth every other day (e.g., even days of the month at 10 AM). You might substitute qod, "odd days of the month."
19. Milk of magnesia one tablespoon by mouth at the hour of sleep every night (e.g., 10 PM)
20. Septra one double-strength tablet every day by mouth (e.g., 10 AM)
21. Morphine sulfate fifteen milligrams subcutaneously immediately and ten milligrams every 4 hours as needed. The stat time given determines when the next dose can be administered. (Next dose must be *at least 4 hours later.*)

Drug Labels and Packaging

CONTENT TO MASTER

Information available on drug labels

Unit dose and multidose packaging

Containers for oral, parenteral, and topical application

Nurses must read and interpret label information to be able to prepare, administer, and store drugs safely. When needed information is not on the label, the nurse should consult the professional literature accompanying the drug, check reliable references, or consult the pharmacist.

In general, there are two types of drug labels, those that contain detailed information, and those that are limited to specific facts.

▼ LABELS THAT CONTAIN DETAILED INFORMATION

In the institutional setting, this type of label is found on drugs that are dispensed in a dry (powder) form and must be reconstituted, or dissolved, by the nurse before they are administered to a patient. The following information is common on this type of label:

NDC Number. The National Drug Code (NDC) is a number used by the pharmacist to identify the drug and the method of packaging.

EXAMPLE NDC 71-771-52

Total Amount of Drug in the Container. This information is usually found at the top of the label to the left.

EXAMPLE 200 tablets; 1000 mL

Trade Name. The term *trade name,* which is also referred to as a brand name or a proprietary name, may be identified by the symbol ® that follows the name. Several companies may manufacture the same drug under different trade names. Trade names may be capitalized on the labels, or they may have an initial capital only. They are always written with the first letter capitalized.

EXAMPLE Monocid® is the trade name of a drug manufactured by Smith Kline Beecham Pharmaceuticals.

Generic Name. The generic name is the official accepted name of a drug, as listed in the United States Pharmacopeia (USP) and the National Formulary (NF). A drug may have several trade names but only one official generic name. The generic name is not capitalized.

EXAMPLE ceftazidime is distributed as Ceptaz; Fortaz; Pentacef; Tazicef.

Strength of the Drug. Solid drugs are given in metric weights; liquids are stated as a solution of drug in solvent.

EXAMPLE cefonicid 5 g; dicloxacillin 100 mg/5 mL

Form of the Drug. The label specifies the type of preparation in the container.

EXAMPLE tablet, capsule, oral suspension, aqueous solution

Usual Dosage. This states how much drug is given at a single time, or over a 24-hour period, and also identifies who should receive the drug.

EXAMPLE Adults 1–2 teaspoons every 4 hours

Route of Administration. The label specifies how the drug is to be given: orally, parenterally (an injection of some type), or topically (applied to skin or mucous membranes). *When the label does not specify the route, the drug is in an oral form.*

Storage. This information describes the conditions necessary to protect the drug from losing its potency (effectiveness). Some drugs come in a dry form and must be dissolved, that is, reconstituted. The drug may be stored one way when dry and another way after reconstitution.

EXAMPLE Before reconstitution protect from light and store at controlled room temperature (59°–86°). After reconstitution, it is stable at room temperature for 18 hours or for 7 days if refrigerated.

Directions for Preparation. The drug comes as a powder and must be dissolved. The amount and type of liquid to be used in reconstituting the drug and the resulting solution will be stated by the manufacturer.

EXAMPLE Dilute powder with 2 mL sterile water for injection to make 50 mg/mL.

Expiration Date. The drug cannot be used after the last day of the month indicated.

Precautions. These are specific instructions related to safety, effectiveness, or administration that must be noted and followed.

Manufacturer's Name. Any questions about the drug should be directed to this company.

Lot Number. This number indicates the batch of drug from which this stock came.

Additives. The manufacturer may have used substances to bind the drug, to aid in dissolving the drug, to produce a specific pH, and so on. This information may be found on the label or in the literature accompanying the drug.

READ ACCOMPANYING CIRCULAR
APOTHECON®
A Bristol-Myers Squibb Company
Princeton, NJ 08540
Made in USA
727650ECL-1

To the Pharmacist: Prepare suspension at time of dispensing. Add to the bottle a total of 88 mL water. For ease in preparation, add the water in two portions. Shake well after each addition. This provides 150 mL of suspension. Each 5 mL contains amoxicillin trihydrate equivalent to 125 mg amoxicillin.

NDC 0015-7276-50
NSN 6505-01-011-1464
150 mL
EQUIVALENT TO
125 mg per 5 mL
when reconstituted according to directions.
POLYMOX®
Amoxicillin For Oral Suspension,USP
CAUTION: Federal law prohibits dispensing without prescription.
APOTHECON®
A BRISTOL-MYERS SQUIBB COMPANY

KEEP BOTTLE TIGHTLY CLOSED. SHAKE WELL BEFORE USING. Discard unused portion of reconstituted suspension after 14 days storage at either room temperature or refrigeration.

READ ACCOMPANYING CIRCULAR
APOTHECON®
A Bristol-Myers Squibb Company
Princeton, NJ 08540
Made in USA

Pharmacist: See base label for dispensing directions. Physician leaflet enclosed. Remove before dispensing.
Usual Dosage: Adults – 250 mg every 8 hours. Children – 20 to 40 mg/kg/day in divided doses every 8 hours, depending on severity of infection.

Figure 3-1
Label for ampicillin for oral suspension (Polymox). (Courtesy of Apothecon, a Bristol-Meyers Squibb Company.)

Exercise 1

Read the label in Figure 3-1 and give the information requested. Answers may be found at the end of the chapter.

1. What is the trade name? ____________
2. What is the generic or official name? ____________
3. What is the total amount of drug in the container when reconstituted? ____________
4. In what form is the drug prepared by the manufacturer? ____________
5. When reconstituted, what will be the strength of the drug? ____________
6. What is the usual dosage for an adult? ____________
7. What is the usual dosage for a child? ____________
8. What is the route of administration? ____________
9. What are the directions for preparation? ____________
10. List two ways the drug can be stored after reconstitution. For each way, give the expiration time. ____________
11. Name the pharmaceutical company dispensing the drug. ____________
12. Give five precautions listed on the label. ____________

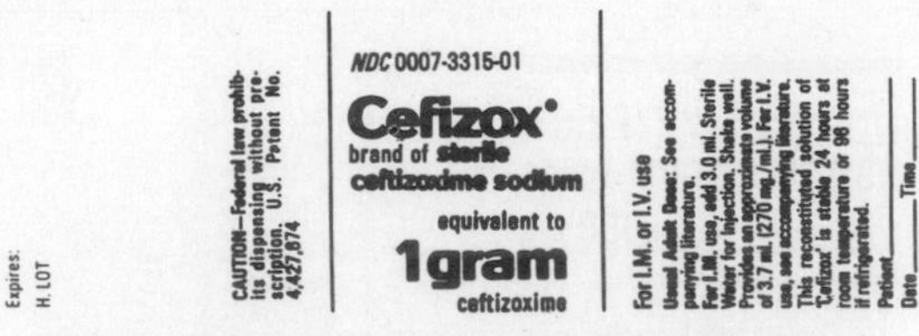

Figure 3-2
Label for ceftizoxime sodium (Cefizox). (Courtesy of Fujisawa Pharmaceutical Company.)

Exercise 2

Read the label in Figure 3-2 and give the information requested. Answers may be found at the end of the chapter.

1. What is the trade name? ______
2. What is the generic or official name? ______
3. What is the total amount of drug in the container? ______
4. In what form is the drug dispensed by the manufacturer? ______
5. By what route(s) may the drug be given? ______
6. What is the usual dose for an adult? ______
7. How should the drug be prepared for IM use? ______
8. What is the amount and strength of the solution when prepared as directed for IM use? ______
9. List two ways the drug can be stored. For each way give the expiration time. ______

▼ LABELS LIMITED TO SPECIFIC FACTS

Drugs with these types of labels are designed to be administered in the form in which they are packaged. The form may be solid or liquid. The following information is typical of this type of label:

- NDC number
- Total amount of drug in the container
- Trade and generic names
- Strength and form of the drug
- Manufacturer's name
- Expiration date and lot number

Some information, including route of administration, usual dose, and storage may not be on the label, usually because the container is too small. When the nurse needs further information, professional references should be consulted.

Labels for some combination drugs may not list any strength. Instead they give the ingredients in the combination. These drugs are ordered by the number to give if they are solid forms. Liquids are ordered in metric or household measures.

EXAMPLE Multivitamin tabs 1 po qd; Robitussin DM cough mixture 1 tsp po q4h prn

PULL DOWN TAB TO OPEN BOOKLET

NDC 0186-0360-01 6505-00-063-6197

2% Xylocaine® Viscous

(lidocaine HCl) Solution 100 mL

FOR ORAL USE ONLY

CAUTIONS: Numbness of the mouth and throat increase the risk of food aspiration and biting trauma. Do not eat or chew gum for 60 minutes following use. Keep this and all medications out of the reach of children.

COMPOSITION: Lidocaine hydrochloride 2%, sodium carboxymethylcellulose, methylparaben, propylparaben, saccharin sodium and flavoring.

USUAL ADULT DOSAGE: 15 mL (One tablespoonful). Reduce dose and use extreme caution when administering to children. Consult package insert for complete prescribing details.

CAUTION: Federal law prohibits dispensing without prescription.

ASTRA®

Astra Pharmaceutical Products, Inc.
Westborough, MA 01581

Dispense in child-resistant packaging.
Shake well before using.
Squeeze bottle to dispense contents.

072099R00

NBOOK

Figure 3-3
Label for lidocaine HCl (2% Xylocaine Viscous). (Courtesy of Astra Pharmaceuticals.)

Exercise 3

Read the label in Figure 3-3 and give the information requested. Answers may be found at the end of the chapter.

1. What is the trade name? ______
2. What is the generic name? ______
3. By what route(s) may this drug be given? ______
4. In what form is the drug dispensed? ______
5. What is the strength of the drug? ______
6. What is the total amount of drug in the container? ______
7. What is the usual adult dose? ______
8. Give seven cautions on the label regarding this drug. ______

NDC 0048-1070-03
NSN 6505-01-340-0152
Code 3P1073

SYNTHROID®

(Levothyroxine Sodium Tablets, USP)

100 mcg (0.1 mg)

100 TABLETS

CAUTION: Federal (USA) law prohibits dispensing without prescription.

See full prescribing information for dosage and administration.

Dispense in a tight, light-resistant container as described in USP

Store at controlled room temperature, 15°-30°C (59°-86°F).

Boots Pharmaceuticals, Inc.
Lincolnshire, IL 60069
USA

7885-02

Figure 3-4
Label for levothyroxine sodium (Synthroid). (Courtesy of Boots Pharmaceuticals, Inc.)

Exercise 4

Read the label in Figure 3-4 and give the information requested. Answers may be found at the end of the chapter.

1. In what form does the drug come? ______
2. What is the trade name? ______
3. What is the generic name? ______
4. What is the strength of each drug unit? ______
5. Is there literature with the drug? ______
6. Are storage directions on the label? ______
7. Is the route of administration specified on the label? Explain. ______

Exercise 5

Read the label in Figure 3-5 and give the information requested. Answers may be found at the end of the chapter.

1. What is the brand name? ______
2. What is the generic name? ______
3. Is the route specified on the label? How should the drug be administered? ______
4. What is the strength of the drug? ______
5. List three storage cautions given on the label.

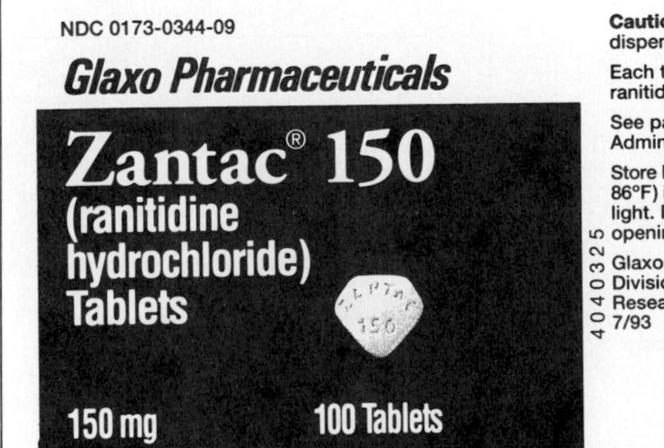

Figure 3-5
Label for ranitidine hydrochloride tablets (Zantac 150). (Courtesy of Glaxo Pharmaceuticals.)

▼ DRUG PACKAGING

In the future, innovative delivery systems will revolutionize the ways in which drugs are administered. In this chapter, however, we focus on the common types of containers that nurses handle as they prepare medications.

There are two types of packaging: *unit-dose* and *multidose.* Each type may contain a solid or liquid form of the drug for oral, parenteral, or topical use. Most institutions use a combination of unit-dose and multidose.

Unit-Dose Packaging

Each dose is individually wrapped and labeled, and a 24-hour supply is prepared by the pharmacy and dispensed. A major value of unit-dose packaging is that two professionals check the drug and the dose—the pharmacist and the nurse—thereby decreasing the possibility of error.

It should be stressed that unit-dose packaging does not relieve the nurse of the responsibility to *check the label three times* and to calculate the amount of drug needed. Unit-dose drugs come in different strengths, and there is always a chance of error when trade names are ordered instead of generic names. A dose may consist of one unit packet, two or more unit packets, or a fraction of one packet.

EXAMPLE A nurse has a unit-dose 100-mg tablet. If an order calls for 50 mg, only half the tablet would be administered.

A nurse may have an order for 75 mg. Unit packets contain 25 mg tablets. The nurse would administer 3 tablets.

For the Oral Route. For oral administration, unit-dose packaging may consist of

1. Plastic bubble, foil, or paper wrappers containing tablets or capsules (Fig. 3-6*A*).
2. Plastic or glass containers that hold a single dose of a liquid or powder. The powder is reconstituted to a liquid form by following the directions given on the label (see Fig. 3-6*B*).
3. A sealed medication cup containing one dose of a liquid. The nurse removes the cover and the dose is ready to administer (see Fig. 3-6*C*).

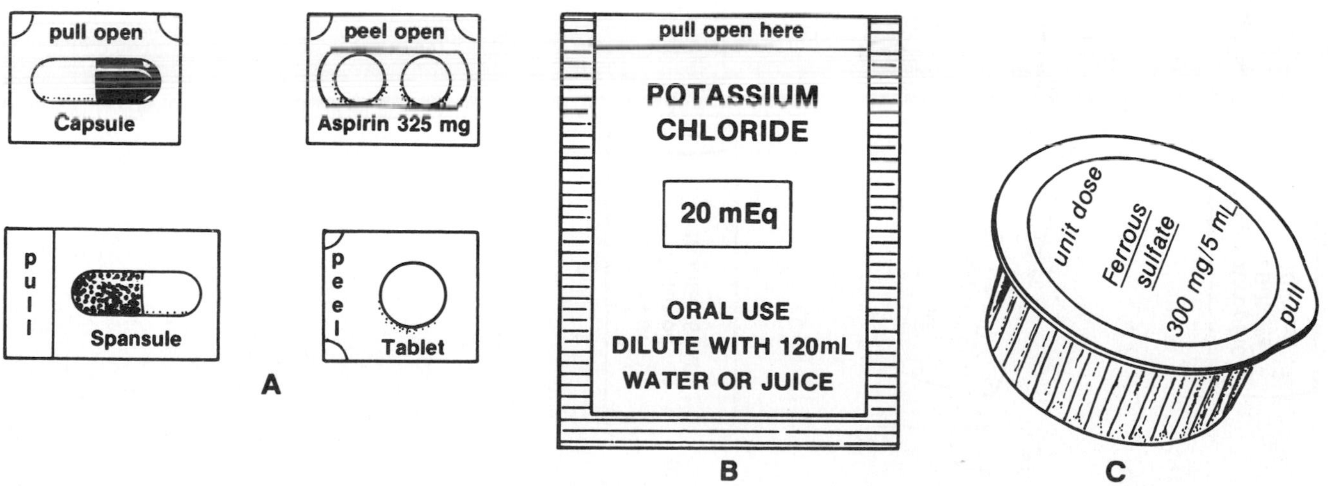

Figure 3-6
(A) Unit-dose tablets and capsules in foil wrappers. **(B)** Unit-dose powder in a sealed packet; it is diluted before giving. **(C)** Sealed cup containing one dose of a liquid medication ready to administer.

For the Parenteral Route. These drugs are given by injection. The route must be specified in the order (e.g., IM, SC, IVPB). Drugs in such containers are sterile, and sterile technique is used for their preparation and administration. The drugs may come in a solid or liquid form.

1. An *ampule* (ampoule) is a glass container that holds a single sterile dose of drug. The container has a narrow neck that must be broken to reach the drug. A sterile syringe is used to withdraw the medication (Fig. 3-7*A*). The drug in the ampule may come as a liquid, a powder, or a crystal. Directions must be followed to reconstitute the solid forms. Once the glass is broken, any portion of drug not used must be discarded because the drug cannot be kept sterile.
2. A *vial* is a glass container with a sealed rubber top. It may contain a sterile liquid or a sterile powder that must be reconstituted with a sterile diluent and syringe. Single-dose vials do not contain a preservative or a bacteriostatic agent. Therefore, any medication remaining after the dose is prepared should be discarded (see Fig. 3-7*B*).
3. Flexible *plastic bags* or *glass vials* may hold sterile medication for intravenous use. The fluid is administered with the use of IV tubing, which is connected to a needle or catheter placed in the patient's blood vessel (Fig. 3-8).

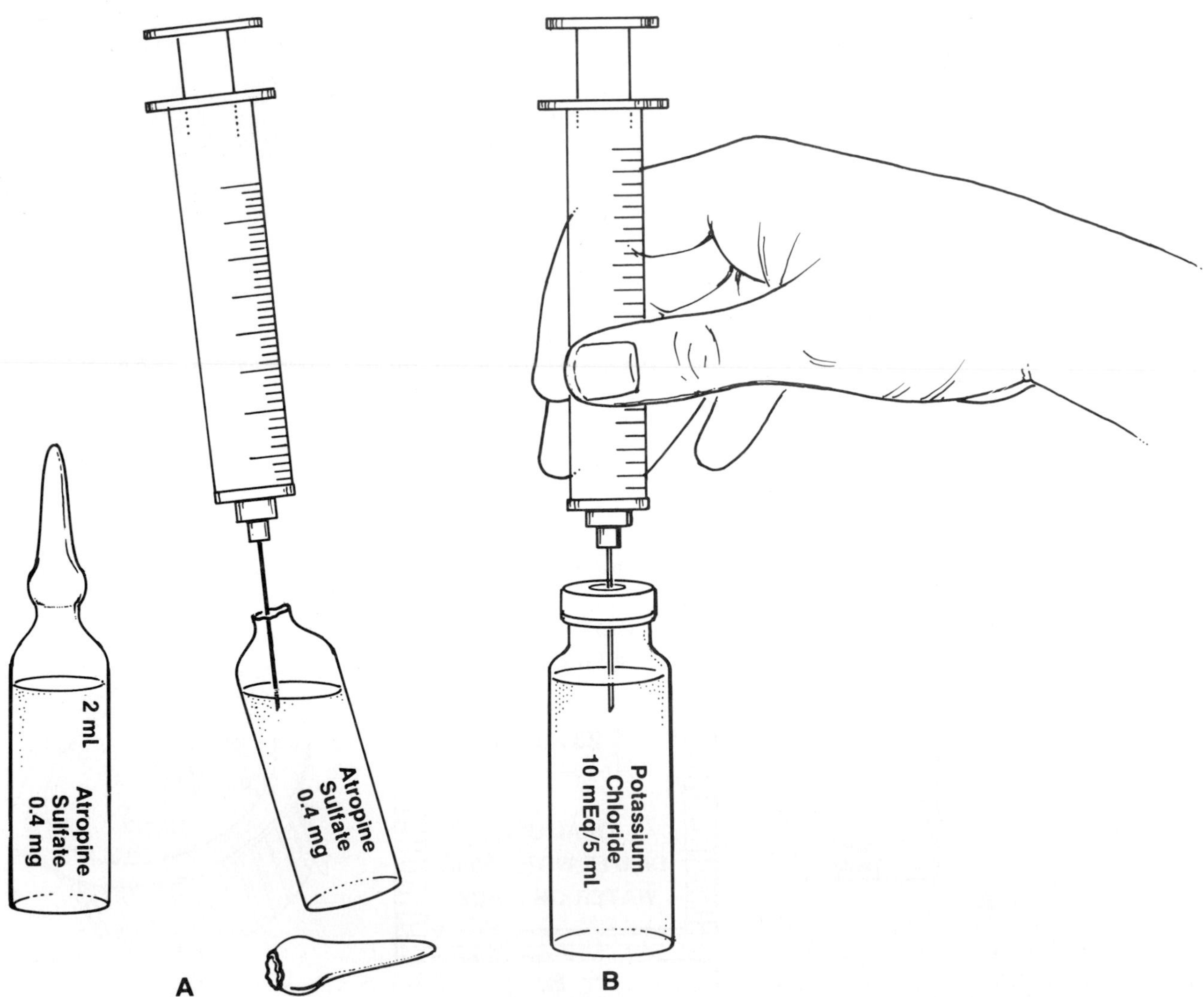

Figure 3-7
(A) Glass ampule that must be broken to reach the medication. **(B)** Vial that holds a unit dose or a multidose. The rubber top seals to keep the medication sterile.

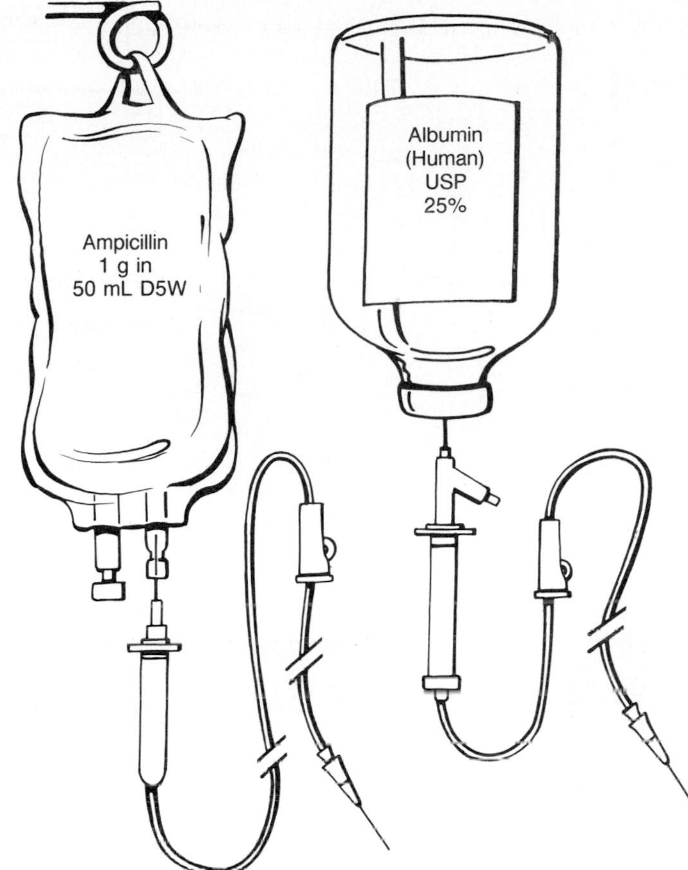

Figure 3-8
Plastic or glass containers hold medication for IV use.

4. *Prefilled syringes* contain liquid, sterile medication that is ready to administer without further preparation. This type of unit-dose packaging is expensive but lifesaving in an emergency in which speed is essential (Fig. 3-9*A*).

5. *Prefilled cartridges* are actually small vials, with a needle attached, that fit into a metal or plastic holder and eject one unit-dose of a sterile drug in liquid form (see Fig. 3-9*B*).

For Topical Administration. Drugs are applied to the skin or mucous membranes to achieve a local effect or to act systemically throughout the body.

1. *Transdermal patches or pads* are adhesive bandages placed on the skin. They hold a drug form that is slowly absorbed into the circulation, over a period ranging from hours to several days (Fig. 3-10).

2. *Lozenges and pastilles* are disklike solids that are slowly dissolved in the mouth (e.g., cough drops). Some drugs are prepared in a gum that is released by chewing (e.g., nicotine).

3. *Suppositories,* in foil or plastic wrappers, are molded forms that can be inserted into the rectum or vagina. They hold medication in a substance, such as cocoa butter, that melts at body temperature and releases the drug (Fig. 3-11).

4. *Plastic, disposable, squeezable containers* hold prepared solutions for the vagina (douches) or enema solutions that are administered rectally. The containers for enemas have a lubricated nozzle for ease in insertion. As the container is squeezed, the solution is forced out (Fig. 3-12).

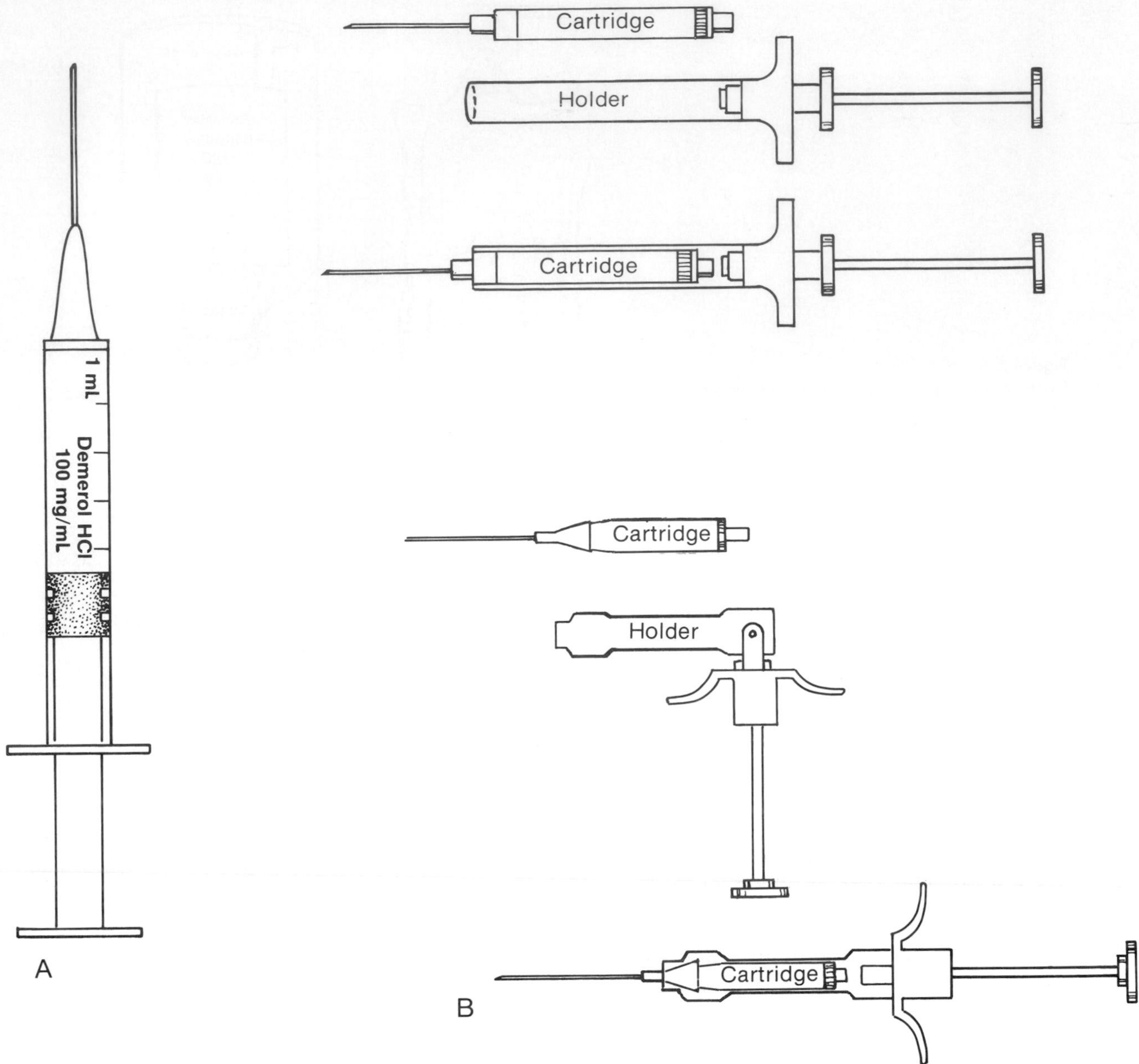

Figure 3-9
(A) Prefilled syringes are ready to administer. **(B)** Prefilled cartridges fit into a holder.

Multidose Packaging

Each patient unit receives large, stock containers of medications commonly used in that area. The nurse identifies the drug, checks the strength, and calculates and prepares the dose. This type of packaging reduces the pharmacy's workload, but it requires more nursing time. The possibility of error is increased.

For the Oral Route. Stock bottles contain a liquid or a solid form, such as tablets, capsules, powders. When powders are reconstituted, the date and time of preparation must be written on the label and storage directions and expiration carefully noted. Large stock bottles hold medication that is dispensed over a period of days (Fig. 3-13*A*).

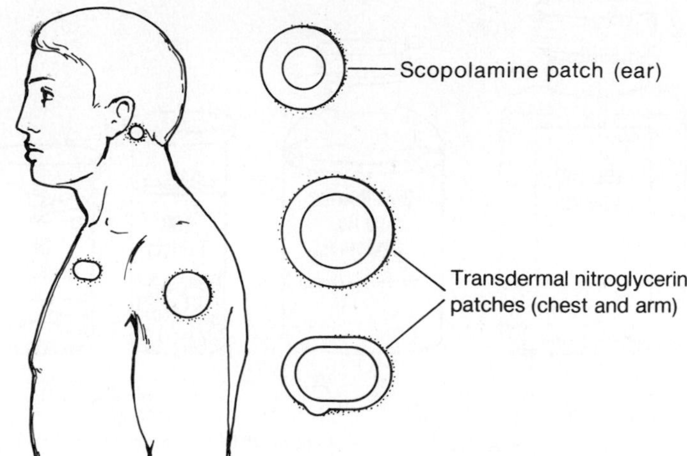

Figure 3-10
Transdermal patches or pads are placed on the skin.

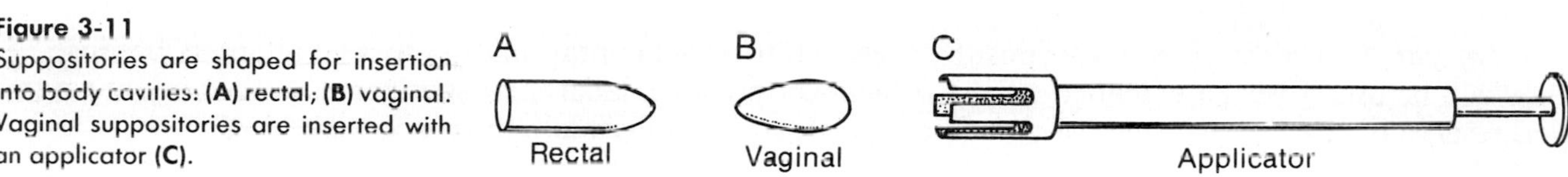

Figure 3-11
Suppositories are shaped for insertion into body cavities: **(A)** rectal; **(B)** vaginal. Vaginal suppositories are inserted with an applicator **(C)**.

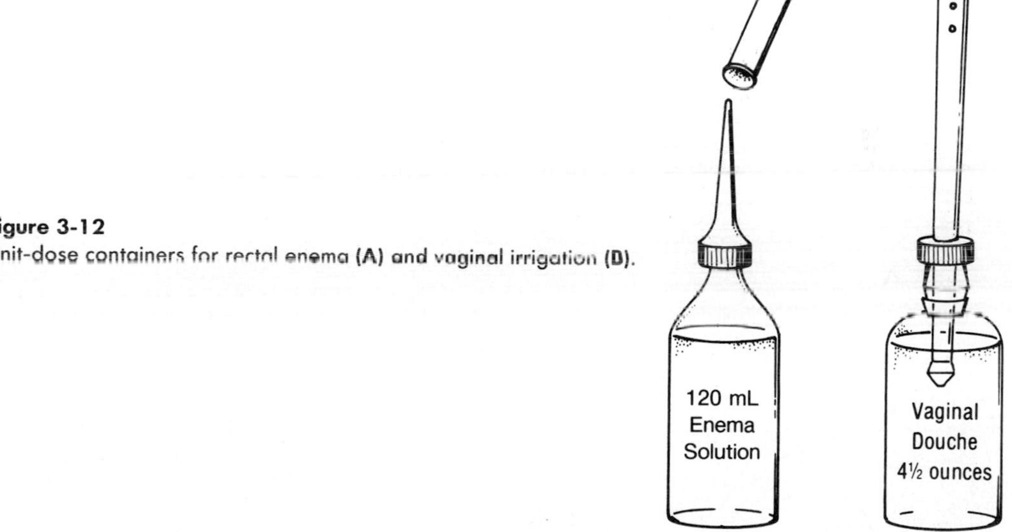

Figure 3-12
Unit-dose containers for rectal enema **(A)** and vaginal irrigation **(B)**.

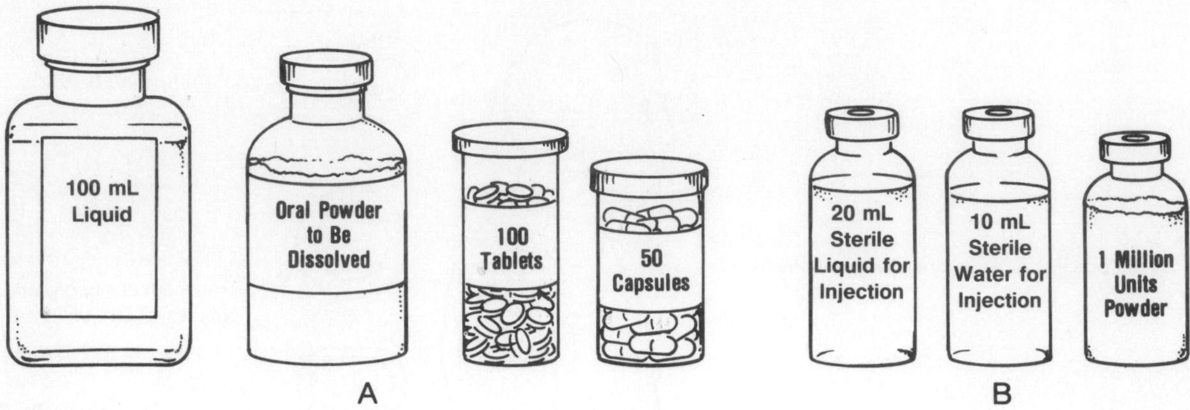

Figure 3-13
Multidose containers: **(A)** for the oral route; **(B)** for the parenteral route.

For the Parenteral Route. Large-volume vials contain a sterile liquid or powder to be reconstituted, using sterile technique. As with powders for oral use, the nurse must write the date and time of preparation on the powder label and note storage directions and expiration (see Fig. 3-13*B*).

For Topical Administration. Care must be exercised to avoid contaminating these containers because they will be used over an extended period. Whenever possible, label the container with the patient's name and reserve its use for that one patient. The following types of containers may be used:

1. *Metal or plastic tubes* that contain ointments or creams to be applied to the skin or mucous membranes are squeezed to release the medication (Fig. 3-14*A*).
2. Medication is removed from *jars for creams, ointments, and pastes* by using a sterile tongue blade or sterile glove to avoid contamination.
3. To prevent cross-contamination, *dropper bottles* for eye, ear, or nose medications should be labeled with one patient's name. The nurse must be careful to avoid touching mucous membranes with the dropper, because contamination of the dropper could result in the growth of pathogens.

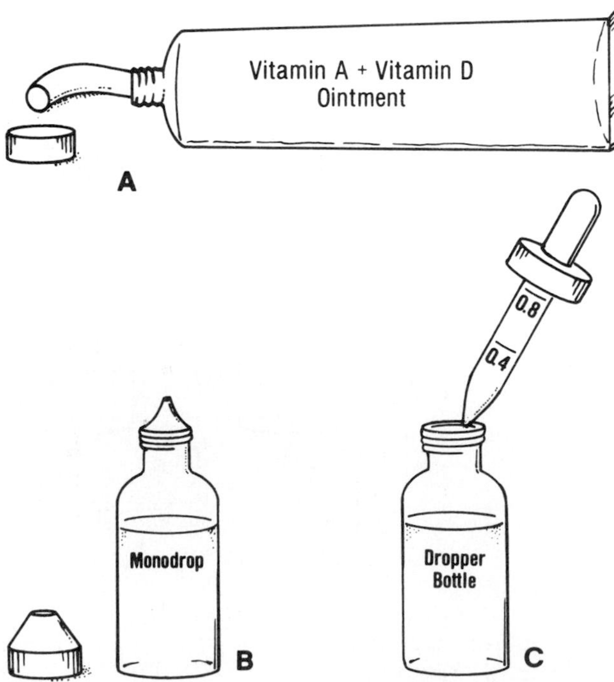

Figure 3-14
Topical multidose containers: **(A)** tubes for creams or ointments; **(B)** monodrop containers—the dropper is attached; **(C)** removable dropper is sometimes calibrated for liquid measures.

There are two kinds of droppers: monodrop containers that are squeezed to release the medication and those in which the dropper can be removed from the bottle. Separate, packaged droppers are available to administer medications. These are calibrated, that is, marked in milliliters (see Figs. 3-14*B*,*C*).

Eye medications are labeled "ophthalmic" or "for the eye." Ear drugs are labeled "otic" or "auric" or "for the ear." Drugs for nasal administration are labeled "nose drops." Routes must *never* be interchanged.

4. *Lozenges and pastilles* may be packaged in multidose as well as unit-dose containers.
5. *Metered-dose inhalers (MDI)* are aerosol devices that consist of two parts: a canister under pressure and a mouthpiece. The canister contains multiple drug doses in a liquid form or as a microfine powder or crystal. The mouthpiece fits on the canister. Finger pressure on the mouthpiece opens a valve on the canister that discharges one dose. The physician's order will state the number of inhalations or "puffs" to be taken (Fig. 3-15).

   Medications for inhalation may also be packaged as liquids in vials or bottles to be used with a hand-held nebulizer, or with an intermittent positive-pressure breathing apparatus (IPPB).

Exercise 6

Match Column A with the letters in Column B to identify the meaning of terms used in drug packaging. Answers may be found at the end of the chapter.

Column A	*Column B*
1._____ Unit dose	**a.** Dissolving a powder into a solution
2._____ Ampule	**b.** Glass container with a sealed rubber top
3._____ Parenteral	**c.** Route of administration to skin or mucous membranes
4._____ Prefilled cartridge	**d.** Individually wrapped and labeled drugs
5._____ Reconstitution	**e.** Disklike solid that dissolves in the mouth
6._____ Topical	**f.** Suppository ingredient that melts at body temperature
7._____ Transdermal patch	**g.** General term for an injection route
8._____ Vial	**h.** Adhesive bandage applied to the skin that gradually releases a drug
9._____ Lozenge	
10._____ Cocoa butter	**i.** Small vial, with a needle attached, that fits into a syringe holder
	j. Glass container that must be broken to obtain the drug

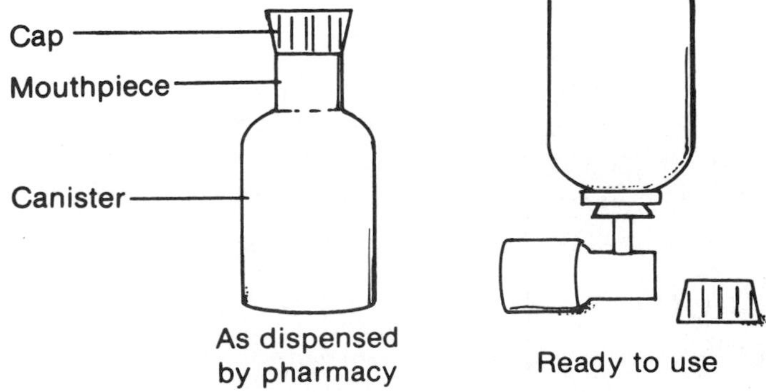

Figure 3-15
Metered-dose inhaler as dispensed by the pharmacy **(left)**, and prepared for use **(right)**.

Exercise 7

Complete these statements related to drug packaging. Answers may be found at the end of the chapter.

1. Date and time of reconstitution must be written ______________________________.

2. The best way to avoid cross-contamination of a multidose tube of ointment is to ______________________________.

3. To remove medication from a jar of paste the nurse should use ______________________________.

4. Dropper bottles for eye medications will be labeled ______________________________.

5. Doses of medication that require use of a metered-dose inhaler are ordered in ______________________________.

6. Medications for the ear will be labeled ______________________________.

7. The term "multidose" refers to ______________________________.

8. The type of drug packaging that decreases the possibility of error is termed ______________________________.

9. Drugs administered topically for a local effect may be absorbed and produce another effect that is called ______________________________.

10. The word "lozenge" describes ______________________________.

ANSWERS

Exercise 1

1. Polymox
2. amoxicillin
3. 150 mL
4. dry form
5. 125 mg per 5 mL
6. 250 mg every 8 hours
7. 20 to 40 mg/kg/day in divided doses every 8 hours depending on the severity of the infection
8. Label states "for oral suspension"
9. Add a total of 88 mL of water in two portions. Shake well after each addition.
10. Can be stored 14 days at either room temperature or refrigerated.
11. Apothecon, a Bristol Meyers Company
12. Federal law prohibits dispensing without prescription; keep bottle tightly closed; shake well before using; discard unused portion after 14 days storage at either room temperature or refrigeration; read accompanying circular.

Exercise 2

1. Cefizox
2. ceftizoxime sodium
3. 1 gram
4. dry form
5. IM or IV
6. Not given on the label. Read accompanying literature.
7. Add 3.0 mL sterile water for injection. Shake well.
8. Provides 3.7 mL (270 mg/mL).
9. Stable for 24 hours at room temperature or 96 hours if refrigerated.

Exercise 3

1. 2% Xylocaine Viscous
2. lidocaine HCl
3. oral only
4. As a solution
5. 2% = 2 grams in 100 mL
6. 100 mL
7. 15 mL (one tablespoon)
8. Numbness of the mouth and throat increases the risk of food aspiration or biting trauma; do not eat or chew gum for 60 minutes following use; keep this and all medications out of the reach of children; dispense in a child-resistant package; shake well before using; squeeze bottle to dispense contents; Federal law prohibits dispensing without a prescription.

Exercise 4

1. Tablets
2. Synthroid
3. levothyroxine sodium
4. 100 mcg (0.1 mg)
5. Yes. See full prescribing information for dosage and administration.
6. 15°–30°C (59°–86°F)
7. No. Tablets are an oral form.

Exercise 5

1. Zantac
2. ranitidine hydrochloride
3. No route is specified. Since it is a tablet administer orally.
4. 150 mg/tablet
5. Store between 15° and 30°C (59° and 86°F).
   Protect from light.
   Replace cap securely after each opening.

Exercise 6

1. d
2. j
3. g
4. i
5. a
6. c
7. h
8. b
9. e
10. f

Exercise 7

1. On the label of any powder that the nurse dissolves. Powders begin to lose their potency as soon as they are placed in solution. By writing the date and time on the label, the nurse will be able to check for expiration time.
2. Label the tube with one patient's name and restrict its use to that one patient.
3. A sterile tongue blade or sterile gloves to prevent contamination of the jar contents.
4. "Ophthalmic" or "for the eye"
5. Number of inhalations or puffs
6. "Otic" or "auric"
7. Large stock containers that hold many doses of a drug
8. Unit-dose
9. A systemic effect; the drug reaches the circulation and is carried to other parts of the body.
10. A disklike solid that is slowly dissolved in the mouth (e.g., a cough drop)

Dosage Measurement Systems

CONTENT TO MASTER

Metric solid and liquid measures

Conversions within the metric system

Household and apothecary measures

Conversions among metric, apothecary, and household systems

Three systems of measurement are discussed in this chapter: metric (SI), apothecary, and household. Most medication orders are written in metric units. Household measures such as the teaspoon and the ounce are helpful in pouring liquid doses. The apothecary system, which was brought to America from England in colonial times, is infrequently used. However, a recent survey revealed that nurses do occasionally encounter apothecary prescriptions.

METRIC SYSTEM (SI)

The metric system is a decimal system based on tens; it has three basic units of measurement: gram (weight), liter (volume), and meter (length). Measures of length will not be discussed because medication orders are written for weight and volume.

The metric system uses arabic numbers (e.g., 1, 2, 3) and decimals (e.g., 0.4, 0.008).

Measures of Weight

Solid measures in the metric system are

Gram: abbreviated g or gm

Milligram: abbreviated mg

Microgram: abbreviated μg or mcg (μg, which uses the Greek letter *mu* [μ], is printed; mcg is written)

Kilogram: abbreviated kg

Weight Equivalents

The basic weight equivalents in the metric system are

1 g = 1000 mg

1 mg = 1000 μg (mcg)

Note that the gram is larger than a milligram. It takes 1000 mg to equal the weight of 1 g. A milligram is itself larger than a microgram; it takes 1000 μg to equal the weight of 1 mg. These relationships can be indicated using the symbol >, which means "is greater than":

g > mg > μg

Read: A gram is greater than a milligram, which is greater than a microgram.

Converting Solid Equivalents

The nurse will have to calculate how much of a drug to give if the supply on hand is not in the same weight measure as the medication order.

EXAMPLE

Order: 0.25 g
Supply: tablets labeled 125 mg

We know the equivalent 1 g = 1000 mg. Therefore, we could change 0.25 g to milligrams by multiplying the number of grams by 1000.

$$\begin{array}{r} 0.25 \\ \underline{\times 1000} \\ 250.00 \end{array}$$

The order, then, is that 0.25 g = 250 mg.

There is a shortcut. In decimals, the thousandth place is three numbers after the decimal point. We can change grams to milligrams by moving the decimal point three places to the right, which produces the same answer as multiplying by 1000. We can also change milligrams to grams by moving the decimal point three places to the left, which is the same as dividing by 1000. This is the method we will learn.

RULE **CHANGING GRAMS TO MILLIGRAMS**

To multiply by 1000, move the decimal point three places to the right.

EXAMPLE

Example 1:

0.25 g = ______ mg

0.250. = 250

0.25 g = 250 mg

Example 2:

0.1 g = ______ mg

0.100. = 100

0.1 g = 100 mg

Grams to Milligrams Quick Rule: Some students have difficulty deciding whether to move decimal points to the left or the right. Here is a method that might be helpful.

1. Write the order first.
2. Write the equivalent measure needed.
3. Use an arrow to show which way the decimal point should move.
4. The open part of the arrow always faces the *larger* measure.
5. In the equivalent 1 g = 1000 mg, the gram is the larger measure. It takes 1000 mg to make 1 g.

EXAMPLE

Example 1:

Order: 0.25 g
Supply: 125 mg
You want to convert grams to milligrams
0.25 g > ______ mg
The arrow is telling you to move the decimal point three places to the right.
0.250. = 250
Hence, 0.25 g = 250 mg

Example 2:

Order: 1.5 g
Supply: 500 mg
You want to convert grams to milligrams
1.5 g > ______ mg
1.500. = 1500
Hence, 1.5 g = 1500 mg

Exercise 1

Try these conversions from grams to milligrams. Answers may be found at the end of the chapter.

1. 0.3 g = ______ mg

2. 0.001 g = ______ mg

3. 0.02 g = ______ mg

4. 1.2 g = ______ mg

5. 5 g = ______ mg

6. 0.4 g = ______ mg

7. 0.08 g = ______ mg

8. 0.275 g = ______ mg

RULE

CHANGING MILLIGRAMS TO GRAMS

To divide by 1000, move the decimal point three places to the left.

EXAMPLE

Example 1:

100 mg = ______ g

.100. = 0.1

100 mg = 0.1 g

Example 2:

8 mg = ______ g

.008. = 0.008

8 mg = 0.008 g

Milligrams to Grams Quick Rule: The arrow method also works to convert milligrams to grams. Remember the steps:

1. Write the order first.
2. Write the equivalent measure needed.
3. Use an arrow to show which way the decimal point should move.
4. The open part of the arrow always faces the *larger* measure.
5. In the equivalent 1 g = 1000 mg, the gram is the larger measure.

EXAMPLE

Example 1:

Order: 15 mg
Supply: 0.03 g
You want to convert milligrams to grams
15 mg < g
The arrow tells you to move the decimal point three places to the left.
.015. = 0.015
15 mg = 0.015 g

Example 2:

Order: 500 mg
Supply: 1 g
You want to convert mg to g
500 mg = ______ g
500 mg < g
The arrow tells you to move the decimal point three places to the left.
.500. = 0.5
500 mg = 0.5 g

Exercise 2

Try these conversions from milligrams to grams. Answers may be found at the end of the chapter.

1. 4 mg = ______________ g

2. 120 mg = ______________ g

3. 40 mg = ______________ g

4. 75 mg = ______________ g

5. 250 mg = ______________ g

6. 1 mg = ______________ g

7. 50 mg = ______________ g

8. 600 mg = ______________ g

The second major weight equivalent in the metric system is

1 mg = 1000 μg *Remember:* μg is *written* mcg.

Some medications are so powerful that minute microgram doses are sufficient to produce a therapeutic effect. It is easier to write orders in micrograms as whole numbers than to use milligrams written as decimals.

RULE

CHANGING MILLIGRAMS TO MICROGRAMS

To multiply by 1000, move the decimal point three places to the right.

EXAMPLE

Example 1:

0.1 mg = ______ μg

0.100 = 100

0.1 mg = 100 μg

Example 2:

0.25 mg = ______ μg

0.250 = 250

0.25 mg = 250 μg

Milligrams to Micrograms Quick Rule: Some students have difficulty deciding whether to move decimal points to the left or the right.

1. Write the order first.
2. Write the equivalent measure needed.
3. Use an arrow to show which way the decimal point should move.
4. The open part of the arrow always faces the *larger* measure.
5. In the equivalent 1 mg = 1000 μg, the milligram is the larger measure. It takes 1000 μg to make 1 mg.

EXAMPLE

Example 1:

Order: 0.1 mg
Supply: 200 μg
You want to convert milligrams to micrograms.
0.1 mg > ______ μg
The arrow is telling you to move the decimal point three places to the right.
0.100 = 100
Hence: 0.1 mg = 100 μg

Example 2:

Order: 0.3 mg
Supply: 600 μg
You want to convert milligrams to micrograms.
0.3 mg > ______ μg
0.300 = 300
Hence, 0.3 mg = 300 μg

Exercise 3

Try these conversions from milligrams to micrograms. Use either method. Answers may be found at the end of the chapter.

1. 0.3 mg = ______________ μg
2. 0.001 mg = ______________ μg
3. 0.02 mg = ______________ μg
4. 0.08 mg = ______________ μg
5. 1.2 mg = ______________ μg
6. 0.4 mg = ______________ μg
7. 5 mg = ______________ μg
8. 0.7 mg = ______________ μg

RULE

CHANGING MICROGRAMS TO MILLIGRAMS

To divide by 1000, move the decimal point three places to the left.

EXAMPLE

Example 1:

300 μg = ________ mg

300. = 0.3

300 μg = 0.3 mg

Example 2:

50 μg = ________ mg

050. = 0.05

50 μg = 0.05 mg

Micrograms to Milligrams Quick Rule: The arrow method also works to convert micrograms to milligrams. Remember the steps.

1. Write the order first.
2. Write the equivalent measure needed.
3. Use an arrow to show which way the decimal point should move.
4. The open part of the arrow always faces the *larger* measure.
5. In the equivalent 1 mg = 1000 μg, the milligram is the larger measure.

EXAMPLE

Example 1:

Order: 100 μg
Supply: 0.1 mg
You want to convert micrograms to milligrams.
100 μg < mg
The arrow tells you to move the decimal point three places to the left.
100. = 0.1
100 μg = 0.1 mg

Example 2:

Order: 50 µg
Supply: 0.1 mg
You want to convert micrograms to milligrams.
50 µg = ______ mg
µg $<$ mg
The arrow tells you to move the decimal point three places to the left.
050. = 0.05
50 µg = 0.05 mg

Exercise 4

Try these conversions from micrograms to milligrams. Answers may be found at the end of the chapter.

1. 800 µg = ______________ mg
2. 4 µg = ______________ mg
3. 14 µg = ______________ mg
4. 25 µg = ______________ mg
5. 1 µg = ______________ mg
6. 200 µg = ______________ mg
7. 50 µg = ______________ mg
8. 750 µg = ______________ mg

Exercise 5

Now try mixed conversions in metric weight measures. Be careful when reading and take the time to think and apply the rules you have learned. Answers may be found at the end of the chapter.

1. 0.3 mg = ______________ g
2. 0.03 g = mg
3. 15 µg = ______________ mg
4. 0.1 g = ______________ mg
5. 100 µg = ______________ mg
6. 50 mg = ______________ g
7. 0.014 g = mg
8. 200 mg = ______________ g
9. 0.2 mg = ______________ µg
10. 0.65 mg = ______________ µg

Table of Common Metric Solid Equivalents

Most practicing nurses know certain common equivalents in the metric system. Study Table 4-1 to familiarize yourself with them.

Metric Liquid Measures

Liquid measures in the metric system are

Liter: abbreviated L

Milliliter: abbreviated mL (may be written as ml)

Cubic centimeter: abbreviated cc

TABLE 4-1
Common Metric Weight Equivalents

Weight	Equivalent
1000 mg	1 g
600 mg	0.6 g
500 mg	0.5 g
300 mg	0.3 g
200 mg	0.2 g
100 mg	0.1 g
60 mg	0.06 g
30 mg	0.03 g
15 mg	0.015 g
10 mg	0.01 g
1 mg	1000 μg
0.6 mg	600 μg
0.4 mg	400 μg
0.3 mg	300 μg
0.1 mg	100 μg

Metric Liquid Equivalents

The basic liquid equivalents in the metric system are

1 mL = 1 cc

1 L = 1000 mL or 1000 cc

It is not necessary to study liquid conversions within the metric system, because orders are given and supplies are in the same measure.

▼ APOTHECARY SYSTEM

Some drug labels are printed in both apothecary and metric measures. Although the U.S. Pharmacopeia has requested doctors to stop prescribing in the apothecary system, nurses may find a medication order written in an apothecary dose.

Overview

The system is expressed in fractions (e.g., $\frac{1}{4}$; $\frac{1}{2}$) and in Roman numerals. The Roman numerals are made up of letters of the alphabet.

M = 1000 x = 10

D = 500 v = 5

C = 100 i = 1

L = 50

(x, v, and i may or may not be capitalized)

When a smaller numeral precedes a larger numeral, the smaller numeral is **subtracted** from the larger.

XL = 40 (10 from 50)

IX = 9 (1 from 10)

When the smaller numeral follows a larger numeral, the smaller numeral is **added** to the larger.

MX = 1010 (1000 plus 10)

LII = 52 (50 plus 1 plus 1)

XI = 11 (10 plus 1)

Roman numerals never use more than three of the same digit in a row. The year 1995 would be written by analyzing its component parts.

1000 = M (1000)

900 = CM (100 from 1000)

90 = XC (10 from 100)

5 = V (five)

1995 = MCMXCV

Arabic Number	Roman Number	Arabic Number	Roman Number
$\frac{1}{2}$	$\dot{s}\dot{s}$	6	vi
1	i	7	vii
$1\frac{1}{2}$	i$\dot{s}\dot{s}$	$7\frac{1}{2}$	vii$\dot{s}\dot{s}$
2	ii	8	viii
3	iii	9	ix
4	iv	10	x
5	v	20	xx
		30	xxx

Apothecary Grain

The solid measure in the apothecary system is the grain (abbreviated gr). An example of an order is gr v. Note that the Roman numeral follows the measure. Some physicians write this order using Arabic numbers, so you might see 5 gr or 10 gr. Do not confuse this symbol (gr) with the metric gram (g).

Liquid Measures

In the apothecary system, the liquid measures are

Minim: abbreviated M or Mx

Dram: abbreviated ʒ or dr

Ounce: abbreviated ℥

Drop: abbreviated gtt

Remember that an ounce is larger than a dram; hence, the symbol for an ounce has two loops.

Common Liquid Equivalents

In the apothecary system, the common liquid equivalents are

Spoken	Written
1 minim = 1 drop	m i = gtt i
1 dram = 4 mL	ʒi = 1 dr = 4 mL
8 drams = 1 ounce	ʒviii = 8 dr = ℥i

▼ HOUSEHOLD MEASURES

Although used in the home, these measures are acceptable in preparing medications in the medical setting when a standard medication receptacle is used. Household measures are

Teaspoon: abbreviated tsp

Tablespoon: abbreviated tbsp or T

Ounce: abbreviated oz

Pint: abbreviated pt

Quart: abbreviated qt

Common Equivalents in the Household System

Spoken	Written
One teaspoon = 5 milliliters	1 tsp = 5 mL
One tablespoon = 15 milliliters	1 tbsp = 15 mL
One ounce = 30 milliliters	1 oz = 30 mL
One pint = 500 milliliters	1 pt = 500 mL
One quart = 1 liter = 1000 milliliters	1 qt = 1 L = 1000 mL
2.2 pounds = 1 kilogram	2.2 lb = 1 kg

▼ CONVERSIONS AMONG METRIC, APOTHECARY, AND HOUSEHOLD SYSTEMS

Solid Equivalents

The physician's drug order may not be written in the same system as the supply. The nurse must convert either the order *or* the supply amount to calculate the dose needed. In changing from one system to another, conversions are not exact. Table 4-2 lists common equivalents the nurse should know.

Three equivalents require explanation. Look at the alternative values in Table 4-2.

gr x = 0.6 g = 600 mg *or 650 mg*

gr v = 0.3 g = 300 mg *or 325 mg*

gr i = 0.06 g = 60 mg *or 65 mg*

Equivalents between the metric and apothecary systems are not exact. Note that

gr xv = 1000 mg

TABLE 4-2
Common Solid Metric and Apothecary Equivalents

Milligram	Gram*	Grain	Microgram
1000 mg	1 g	gr xv	
(650)† 600 mg	0.6 g	gr x	
500 mg	0.5 g	gr vii ss̈	
(325)† 300 mg	0.3 g	gr v	
200 mg	0.2 g	gr iii	
100 mg	0.1 g	gr i ss̈	
(65)† 60 mg	0.06 g	gr i	
30 mg	0.03 g	gr ss̈ or gr $\frac{1}{2}$	
15 mg	0.015 g	gr $\frac{1}{4}$	
10 mg	0.01 g	gr $\frac{1}{6}$	
0.6 mg		gr $\frac{1}{100}$	600 μg
0.4 mg		gr $\frac{1}{150}$	400 μg
0.3 mg		gr $\frac{1}{200}$	300 μg

* g = gram; μg = microgram or mcg.
† Alternative values.

If you multiply 15 gr by 60 mg, the answer is 900 mg, not 1000 mg. To remedy this discrepancy, some drug companies have manufactured the grain to contain 65 mg, 5 gr to contain 325 mg, and 10 gr to contain 650 mg.

When solving dosage problems, use whichever equivalent is closer.

Order	Supply	Answer
0.3 g po	gr v tab	1 tab
325 mg po	gr v tab	1 tab
0.06 g po	gr i tab	1 tab
gr i po	65 mg tab	1 tab
gr x po	325 mg tab	2 tab
650 mg po	0.6 g tab	1 tab
gr ii po	60 mg tab	2 tab
0.3 g po	325 mg	1 tab

EXAMPLE

Exercises 6 through 17 contain drills in solid conversions between metric and apothecary measures. Answers may be found at the end of the chapter.

Exercise 6

Practice exercises in solid equivalents. Answers may be found at the end of the chapter.

1. What is the short rule for converting milligrams to grams? ______________________

____

____

2. 0.60 mg = ____________ g
3. 0.6 mg = ____________ g
4. 300 mg = ____________ g
5. 500 mg = ____________ g

Exercise 7

Fill in the blanks to convert mg to g or to μg.

1. 1000 mg = ____________ g
2. 600 mg = ____________ g
3. 500 mg = ____________ g
4. 300 mg = ____________ g
5. 200 mg = ____________ g
6. 100 mg = ____________ g
7. 60 mg = ____________ g
8. 30 mg = ____________ g
9. 15 mg = ____________ g
10. 10 mg = ____________ g
11. 0.6 mg = ____________ μg
12. 0.4 mg = ____________ μg
13. 0.3 mg = ____________ μg
14. 0.25 mg = ____________ μg

Exercise 8

1. What is the short rule for converting grams to milligrams? ______________________

____

____

2. 1 g = ____________ mg
3. 0.01 g = ____________ mg
4. 0.2 g = ____________ mg
5. 0.12 g = ____________ mg

Exercise 9

Fill in the table of grams to milligrams.

1. 1 g = ____________ mg
2. 0.6 g = ____________ mg
3. 0.5 g = ____________ mg
4. 0.3 g = ____________ mg
5. 0.2 g = ____________ mg
6. 0.1 g = ____________ mg
7. 0.06 g = ____________ mg
8. 0.03 g = ____________ mg
9. 0.015 g = ____________ mg
10. 0.01 g = ____________ mg

Exercise 10

Convert milligrams to grains.

1. 60 mg = gr ________
2. 30 mg = gr ________
3. 15 mg = gr ________
4. 0.6 mg = gr ________
5. 0.4 mg = gr ________
6. 0.3 mg = gr ________

Exercise 11

Fill in the table of grains to milligrams.

1. gr i = ________ mg
2. gr $\frac{1}{2}$ = ________ mg
3. gr $\frac{1}{4}$ = ________ mg
4. gr $\frac{1}{6}$ = ________ mg
5. gr $\frac{1}{100}$ = ________ mg
6. gr $\frac{1}{150}$ = ________ mg

Exercise 12

What is the equivalent to convert grams to grains?

1. 1 g = gr ________
2. 0.5 g = gr ________
3. 0.2 g = gr ________
4. 0.6 g = gr ________
5. 0.3 g = gr ________
6. 0.03 g = gr ________
7. 0.015 g = gr ________
8. 0.01 g = gr ________
9. 0.06 g = gr ________

Exercise 13

Fill in the table of grains to grams.

1. gr xv = ________ g
2. gr x = ________ g
3. gr viiss = ________ g
4. gr v = ________ g
5. gr iii = ________ g
6. gr i$\dot{s}\dot{s}$ = ________ g

Exercise 14 *Fill in this table.*

1. 1000 mg = ________ g = gr ________
2. 600 mg = ________ g = gr ________
3. ________ mg = 0.5 g = gr ________
4. ________ mg = ________ g = gr iii
5. ________ mg = 0.1 g = gr ________
6. 60 mg = ________ g = gr ________
7. ________ mg = 0.03 g = gr ________
8. ________ mg = ________ g = gr $\frac{1}{4}$
9. 10 mg = ________ g = gr ________
10. ________ mg = 0.0006 g = gr ________ = 600 μg
11. 0.4 mg = ________ g = gr ________ = 400 μg
12. 0.3 mg = ________ g = gr ________ = 300 μg

Exercise 15 *Practice exercise in solid equivalents. Express as milligrams.*

1. gr $\frac{1}{150}$ = ________ mg
2. 0.03 Gm = ________ mg
3. 0.5 g = ________ mg
4. 1 Gm = ________ mg
5. gr $\frac{1}{2}$ = ________ mg
6. gr i = ________ mg
7. 0.015 g = ________ mg
8. gr iss = ________ mg

Exercise 16* *Express as grams.*

1. 30 mg = ________ g
2. 100 mg = ________ g
3. gr iii = ________ g
4. gr i = ________ g
5. 500 mg = ________ g
6. gr x = ________ g
7. 0.6 mg = ________ g
8. gr xv = ________ g

Exercise 17 *Express as grains.*

1. 0.4 mg = gr ____________
2. 0.1 g = gr ____________
3. 60 mg = gr ____________
4. 15 mg = gr ____________
5. 0.3 g = gr ____________
6. 0.3 mg = gr ____________

Liquid Equivalents

The physician's order may not be written in the same system as the supply. In changing from one system to another, conversions may not be exact. Table 4-3 lists common liquid equivalents among the three systems. (See also Fig. 2-3 in Chapter 2.)

TABLE 4-3
Common Liquid Metric, Apothecary, and Household Equivalents

Metric	Apothecary	Household
	1 m = 1 gtt	
1 mL*	16 m	
4 mL	ʒi	
5 mL		1 tsp
15 mL	ʒiv	1 tbsp
30 mL	ʒviii	1 oz; 2 tbsp
500 mL		1 pt
1000 mL, 1 L		1 qt; 2 pt

* *Remember that 1 mL = 1 cc.*

Exercise 18 *Practice exercises in liquid equivalents. Answers may be found at the end of the chapter.*

1. 1 oz = dr ____________
2. 1 tbsp = ʒ ____________
3. ℥ ss̄ = ____________ cc
4. ʒii = ____________ mL
5. 1 mL = m ____________
6. 4 dr = ____________ oz
7. 1 tsp = ____________ mL
8. 1 oz = ____________ tbsp
9. 1 oz = ____________ mL
10. 1 L = ____________ mL

Exercise 19 *Express the liquid measure requested.*

1. 4 mL = ʒ ____________
2. 1 tbsp = ____________ mL
3. ℥ i ss̄ = ____________ mL
4. 5 mL = ____________ tsp
5. 30 mL = ____________ oz
6. 30 mL = ʒ ____________
7. 1 m = ____________ gtt
8. 1 pt = ____________ cc
9. 1 qt = ____________ mL
10. 1 cc = ____________ mL

Exercise 20

Fill in the measure requested.

1. ℥ i = ________ cc
2. 1 qt = ________ L
3. 15 mL = ________ tbsp
4. ʒ viii = ________ oz
5. 2 tbsp = ________ oz
6. m xvi = ________ mL
7. 1 L = ________ mL
8. ʒ iv = ________ oz
9. 500 mL = ________ pt
10. 1 kg = ________ lb

Proficiency Test

Equivalents

Aim for 90% accuracy or better on this test. There are 50 items, each worth 2 points. If you have any difficulty, reread and study Chapter 4, which explains this information. Answers may be found at the end of the chapter.

1. 100 mg = ________ gm
2. gr $\frac{1}{2}$ = ________ mg
3. ℥ i = ________ cc
4. 1 L = ________ mL
5. gr $\frac{1}{200}$ = ________ mg
6. 325 mg = gr ________
7. 1 tsp = ________ cc
8. 0.4 mg = gr ________
9. gr X = ________ mg
10. 30 mg = gr ________
11. 0.015 g = ________ mg
12. 10 mg = ________ gm
13. 1 cc = ________ mL
14. gr $\frac{1}{150}$ = ________ mg
15. gr i = ________ gm
16. 0.2 gm = ________ mg
17. gr xv = ________ gm
18. 30 mg = ________ g
19. gr III = ________ mg
20. 15 mg = gr ________
21. 500 mg = ________ g
22. gr i = ________ mg
23. 1 oz = ________ mL
24. 1 mL = ________ minims
25. gr $\frac{1}{4}$ = ________ mg
26. 1 tbsp = ________ cc
27. 1 kg = ________ lb
28. 1 g = ________ mg
29. gr i ṡṡ = ________ gm
30. 60 mg = ________ g
31. 30 mL = ________ oz
32. 1 minim = ________ gtt
33. gr V = ________ g
34. ʒ ii = ________ mL
35. 1000 mg = ________ gm
36. gr vii ṡṡ = ________ gm
37. 0.1 gm = ________ mg
38. 1 dram = ________ cc
39. 600 mg = gr ________
40. 600 mg = ________ gm
41. 10 mcg = ________ mg
42. 1 L = ________ mL
43. 0.5 μg = ________ mg
44. 0.6 mg = ________ g
45. 250 mcg = ________ mg
46. 1 mg = ________ g
47. 0.125 mg = ________ μg
48. 0.01 mg = ________ mcg
49. 0.001 mg = ________ μg
50. 1 qt = ________ mL

Your score: ________

ANSWERS

Exercise 1

1. 300
2. 1
3. 20
4. 1200
5. 5000
6. 400
7. 80
8. 275

Exercise 2

1. 0.004
2. 0.12
3. 0.04
4. 0.075
5. 0.25
6. 0.001
7. 0.05
8. 0.6

Exercise 3

1. 300
2. 1
3. 20
4. 80
5. 1200
6. 400
7. 5000
8. 700

Exercise 4

1. 0.8
2. 0.004
3. 0.014
4. 0.025
5. 0.001
6. 0.2
7. 0.05
8. 0.75

Exercise 5

1. 0.0003
2. 30
3. 0.015
4. 100
5. 0.1
6. 0.05
7. 14
8. 0.2
9. 200
10. 650

Exercise 6

1. Divide milligrams by 1000, or move decimal point three places to the left, or use an arrow with the open part facing gram to show movement of decimal point three places.

2. 0.0006 g **3.** 0.0006 g **4.** 0.3 g **5.** 0.5 g

Exercise 7

1. 1
2. 0.6
3. 0.5
4. 0.3
5. 0.2
6. 0.1
7. 0.06
8. 0.03
9. 0.015
10. 0.01
11. 600
12. 400
13. 300
14. 250

Exercise 8

1. Multiply grams by 1000, or move decimal point three places to the right, or use an arrow with the open part toward gram to show movement of decimal point three places.
2. 1000 3. 10 4. 200 5. 120

Exercise 9

1. 1000
2. 600
3. 500
4. 300
5. 200
6. 100
7. 60
8. 30
9. 15
10. 10

Exercise 10

1. i
2. ṡṡ or $\frac{1}{2}$
3. $\frac{1}{4}$
4. $\frac{1}{100}$
5. $\frac{1}{150}$
6. $\frac{1}{200}$

Exercise 11

1. 60
2. 30
3. 15
4. 10
5. 0.6
6. 0.4

Exercise 12

1. xv
2. viiṡṡ
3. iii
4. x
5. v
6. $\frac{1}{2}$
7. $\frac{1}{4}$
8. $\frac{1}{6}$
9. i

Exercise 13

1. 1
2. 0.6
3. 0.5
4. 0.3
5. 0.2
6. 0.1

Exercise 14

1. 1; xv
2. 0.6; x
3. 500; vii ṡṡ
4. 200; 0.2
5. 100; i ṡṡ
6. 0.06; i
7. 30; $\frac{1}{2}$ or ṡṡ
8. 15; 0.015
9. 0.01; $\frac{1}{6}$
10. 0.6; $\frac{1}{100}$
11. 0.0004; $\frac{1}{150}$
12. 0.0003; $\frac{1}{200}$

Exercise 15

1. 0.4
2. 30
3. 500
4. 1000
5. 30
6. 60 or 65
7. 15
8. 100 (not 90 mg!)

Exercise 16

1. 0.03
2. 0.1
3. 0.2
4. 0.06
5. 0.5
6. 0.6
7. 0.0006
8. 1

Exercise 17

1. $\frac{1}{150}$
2. i̇ṡṡ
3. i
4. $\frac{1}{4}$
5. v
6. $\frac{1}{200}$

Exercise 18

1. 8 or ʒ viii
2. iv
3. 15
4. 8
5. xvi
6. $\frac{1}{2}$
7. 5
8. 2
9. 30
10. 1000

Exercise 19

1. i
2. 15
3. 45
4. 1
5. 1
6. viii
7. 1
8. 500
9. 1000
10. 1

Exercise 20

1. 30
2. 1
3. 1
4. 1
5. 1
6. 1
7. 1000
8. $\frac{1}{2}$
9. 1
10. 2.2

Proficiency Test—Equivalents

1. 0.1
2. 30
3. 30
4. 1000
5. 0.3
6. v
7. 5
8. $\frac{1}{150}$
9. 600
10. $\frac{1}{2}$
11. 15
12. 0.01
13. 1
14. 0.4
15. 0.06
16. 200
17. 1
18. 0.03
19. 200
20. $\frac{1}{4}$
21. 0.5
22. 60
23. 30
24. 16
25. 15
26. 15
27. 2.2
28. 1000
29. 0.1
30. 0.06
31. 1
32. 1
33. 0.3
34. 8
35. 1
36. 0.5
37. 100
38. 4
39. x
40. 0.6
41. 0.01
42. 1000
43. 0.0005
44. 0.0006
45. 0.25
46. 0.001
47. 125
48. 10
49. 1
50. 1000

Drug Preparations and Equipment to Measure Doses

CONTENT TO MASTER

Drug forms for oral administration:

- Tablets
- Capsules

Types of liquids

Medicine cups

Parenteral preparations and syringes

Preparations for topical application

Rounding off dosage answers

Drugs are manufactured in different forms for oral, parenteral, and topical administration. This chapter focuses on the more common drug preparations used in the clinical area and on the equipment that nurses use to prepare accurate doses.

DRUG PREPARATIONS

Oral Route

Oral drug forms are generally the easiest for the patient to take and the most convenient for the nurse to administer.

Tablets are powdered drugs that are compressed or molded into solid shapes. Tablets may contain ingredients that bind the powder or aid in its gastrointestinal absorption (Fig. 5-1*A*). Plain tablets for oral administration may be crushed if a patient has difficulty swallowing (see Fig. 5-1*B*).

Scored tablets have a line down the center, such that the tablet can be broken into halves. Unscored tablets should not be broken because there is no certainty that the drug is evenly distributed (see Fig. 5-1*C*).

Coated tablets or film-coated tablets are smooth and easy to swallow because of their coating. If necessary, these tablets may be crushed.

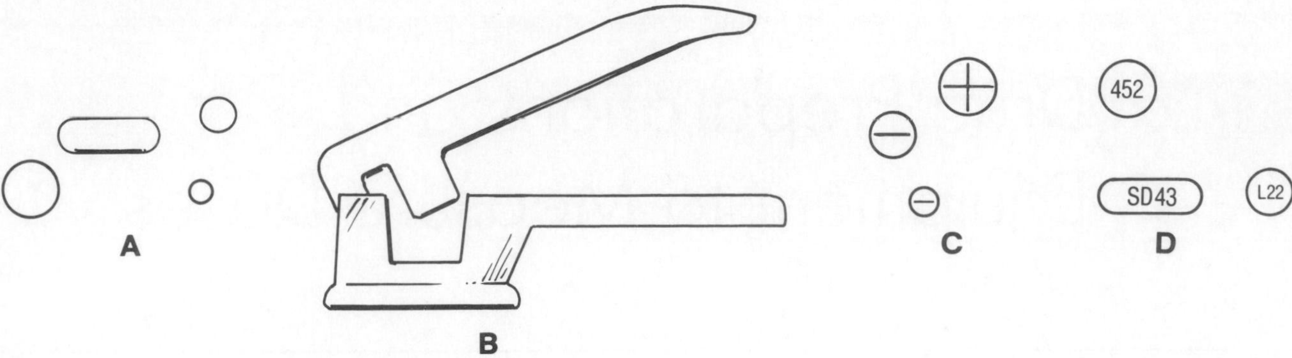

Figure 5-1
(A) Tablets that can be crushed. **(B)** Tablet crusher. The tablet is placed in a paper cup on the bottom. A second cup is placed over the pulverizer on top and the tablet is crushed between the two cups. **(C)** Scored tablets that can be broken. **(D)** Coded tablets—identification of the drug may be by number, letters, or shape.

Enteric-coated tablets dissolve in the less acidic secretions of the intestine, rather than in the highly acidic stomach juices. The enteric coating protects the drug from being inactivated in the stomach and reduces the chance that the drug will irritate the gastric mucosa. Enteric-coated tablets should *not* be crushed.

Prolonged-release or extended-release tablets disintegrate more slowly and have a longer duration of action. The use of these preparations decreases the number of doses needed to only one or two tablets each day. Prolonged-release tablets should not be crushed.

Sublingual tablets dissolve quickly under the tongue. Medication is absorbed through the capillaries and reaches the circulation without passing through the gastrointestinal tract.

Coded tablets have a number or letters, or both, that make them easily identifiable (see Fig. 5-1*D*).

Capsules are gelatin containers that hold a drug in solid or liquid form. Nurses should avoid opening capsules; the drug is encased in the capsule for a reason—possibly because contact with gastric juices will decrease its potency, or because it could irritate the stomach lining. Occasionally, however, if a patient has difficulty swallowing, the nurse may open a capsule and combine the contents with a semisolid, such as applesauce or custard. Before doing this, always check with the pharmacist to find out if the drug is available as a liquid or if there is another alternative (Fig. 5-2*A*).

Some capsules are enteric-coated. Others (called *spansule, timespan, time-release,* or *sustained-release*) contain particles of the drug that are coated to dissolve at different times. These capsules are long acting and should not be opened (see Fig. 5-2*B*).

Syrups are solutions of sugar in water, which disguise the unpleasant taste of a medication. Syrups may be contraindicated in patients with diabetes mellitus because they contain sugar.

Elixirs are clear, hydroalcoholic liquids that are sweetened. Elixirs may be contraindicated in patients with a history of alcoholism.

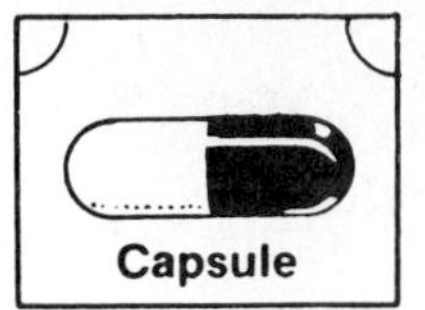

A

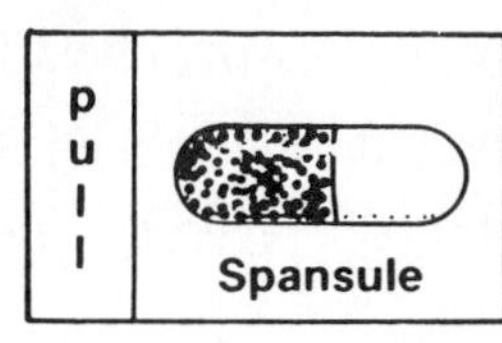

B

Figure 5-2
(A) Capsules should not be opened. **(B)** Spansules are long-acting capsules.

Fluidextracts and *tinctures* are alcoholic, liquid concentrations of a drug; they are potent and, consequently, are ordered in small amounts. Tinctures are ordered in drops. The average dose of a fluidextract is two teaspoons or less. Fluidextracts are the most concentrated of all liquids.

Solutions are clear liquids that contain a drug dissolved in water.

Suspensions are solid particles of a drug dispersed in a liquid. The particles settle to the bottom of the container upon standing and must be resuspended to obtain an accurate dose; therefore, oral preparations must be shaken before pouring.

Magmas contain large bulky particles, for example, milk of magnesia.

Gels have small particles, for example, magnesium hydroxide gel.

Emulsions are creamy, white suspensions of fats or oils in an agent that reduces surface tension and makes the oil easier to swallow, for example, emulsified castor oil.

Powders are dry, finely ground drugs that are reconstituted according to directions. Oral antibiotics are frequently supplied as powders. In liquid form these preparations become oral suspensions. Powders must be dissolved according to the manufacturer. When the nurse reconstitutes a powder, three facts should be written on the label: the date, the nurse's initials, and the solution made.

Parenteral Route

The drug forms for parenteral administration include solutions, suspensions, and powders (see definitions above). The term "parenteral" does not indicate a specific route; it is a general term that means *by injection.* Four common parenteral routes are intramuscular (IM), subcutaneous (SC), intravenous (IV), and intravenous piggyback (IVPB). Drug forms for parenteral use are sterile, and sterile technique is utilized to prepare and administer them.

Topical Route

Commonly-ordered preparations include aerosol powders or liquids, creams, ointments, pastes, suppositories, and transdermal medications. The physician's orders will indicate application to the skin, eye, ear, nose, vagina, rectum.

Aerosol powders and liquids are combined with a propellant and used for sprays on the skin, or in nebulizers and inhalers to reach the mucous membranes of the lower respiratory tract.

Powders may be applied to the skin or vagina in dry form.

Creams are semisolid drug preparations applied externally to the skin or mucous membranes. Vaginal creams require a special applicator for insertion.

Ointments are semisolid preparations in a petroleum or lanolin base for topical use. Ointments used for the eye must be labeled "ophthalmic."

Pastes are thick ointments used to protect the skin. They absorb secretions and soften the skin.

Suppositories contain medication molded with a firm base, such as cocoa butter, that melts at body temperature. Suppositories are shaped for insertion into the rectum, vagina, and, less commonly, the urethra.

Transdermal medications are drug molecules contained in a unique polymer patch that is applied to the skin, as one would an ordinary plastic bandage. The medication is thus easy to apply and is effective for hours or days at a time, as it is slowly released and absorbed through the skin.

Exercise 1

Match Column A with the letters in Column B to identify the meaning of the terms used for drug preparations. Answers can be found at the end of the chapter.

Column A	*Column B*
1. ____ Scored tablet	**a.** Coated drug particles dissolve at different times
2. ____ Enteric-coated	**b.** The most concentrated of all liquids
3. ____ Spansule	**c.** Hydroalcoholic liquid ordered in drops
4. ____ Sublingual tablet	**d.** Large particles suspended in a liquid
5. ____ Capsule	**e.** A solid which can be broken in half
6. ____ Syrup	**f.** Route applied to skin or mucous membrane
7. ____ Elixir	**g.** Small particles suspended in a liquid
8. ____ Fluidextract	**h.** Medication dissolves under the tongue
9. ____ Tincture	**i.** Gelatin containers for solid or liquid drug
10. ____ Magma	**j.** Molded solid inserted into the rectum
11. ____ Gel	**k.** Drug dissolves in the less acidic secretions of the intestine
12. ____ Topical	**l.** Sweetened, hydroalcoholic liquid
13. ____ Suppository	**m.** Solution of sugar in water to improve the taste of a drug

Exercise 2

Complete these statements related to drug preparation. Answers may be found at the end of the chapter.

1. Elixirs may be contraindicated for patients with a history of ______________________
   or ____.
2. The average dose of a fluidextract is ______________________________.
3. In giving medications parenterally, four common routes are ____________________,
   ____________________, ____________________, and ____________________.

(continued)

Exercise 2 (continued)

4. When a powder is reconstituted, what three facts must the nurse write on the label?

a. ______________________

b. ______________________

c. ______________________

5. What route(s) require(s) sterile technique in preparing and administering drugs?

______________________.

6. An example of a drug listed as a magma is ______________________.

7. What action must always be carried out before pouring an oral suspension?

______________________.

8. List six drug preparations that can be administered topically.

______________ ______________

______________ ______________

______________ ______________

9. List two advantages in using transdermal medications.

____

____

10. Define an ointment. ______________________.

▼ EQUIPMENT TO MEASURE DOSES

Nurses do not use a scale to weigh oral solid doses such as the gram and the grain. Solids for oral administration come in tablets and capsules. The nurse calculates the number to give and pours the amount needed into a paper cup, a small container that is discarded once the medication has been given.

Liquids may be prepared as unit doses ready to administer or in stock bottles which require calculation and measurement. Liquids must be measured accurately. Two practices will aid in achieving this goal:

1. *Pour liquids to a line.* Never estimate a dose between two lines.
2. *Pour liquids at eye level* (Fig. 5-3*A*). The surface of a liquid has a natural curve called the *meniscus.* At eye level the center of the curve should be on the measurement line. The fluid at the sides of the container will appear to be above the line. (Fig. 5-3*B*).

The equipment used most often by nurses to measure liquids are the medicine cup and syringes.

Medicine Cup

The medicine cup is a plastic disposable container that has equivalent measures for metric doses in cubic centimeters, for apothecary doses in drams, and for household doses in tablespoons and teaspoons (Fig. 5-4).

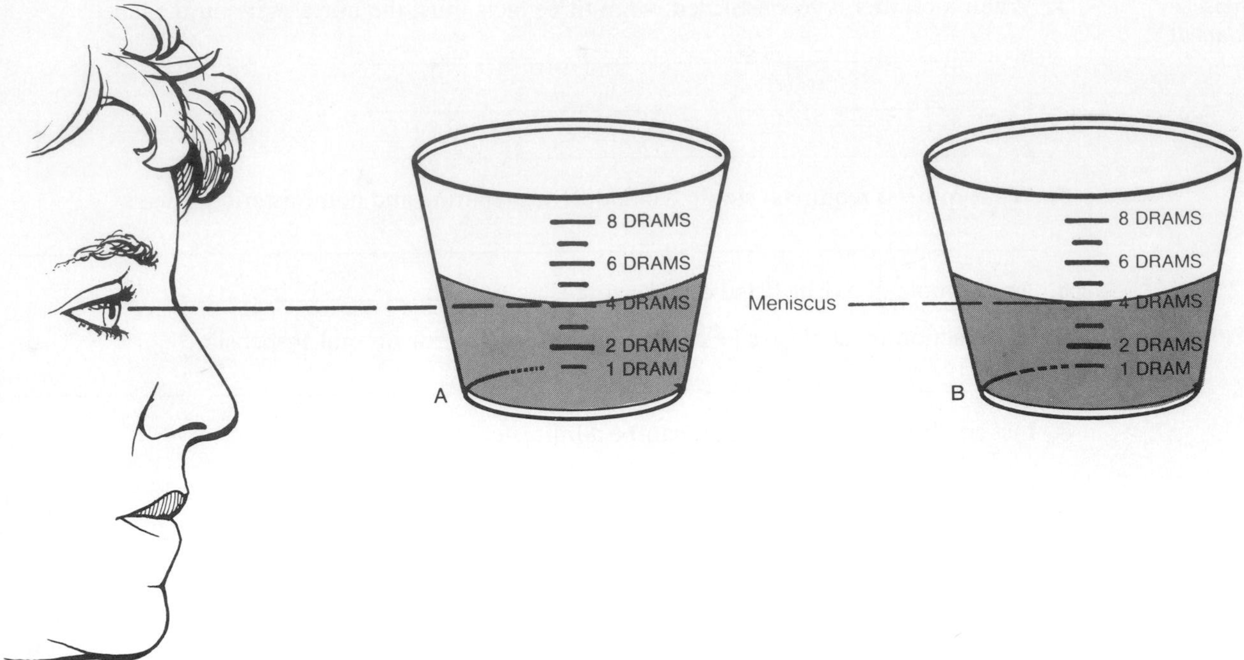

Figure 5-3
(A) Liquids are poured at eye level. The meniscus (lower curve of the fluid) should be on the line **(B)**.

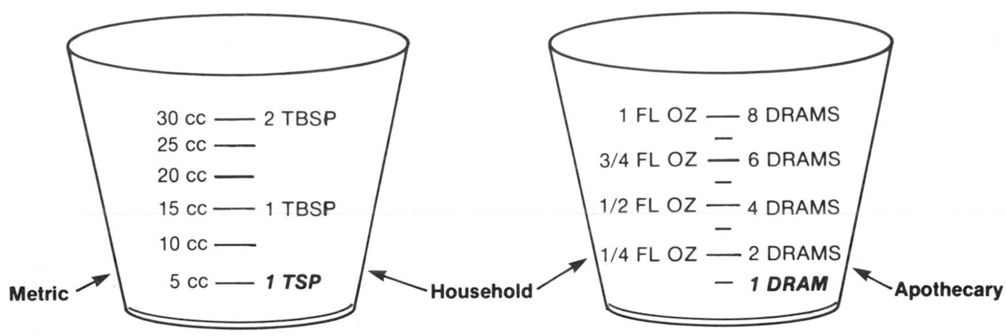

Figure 5-4
A medicine cup for measurement of metric, apothecary, or household dose units.

The following exercise will help you apply your knowledge of liquid equivalents.

Exercise 3

Look at the medicine cup in Figure 5-4. Two sides are shown. Fill in answers related to this measuring device. Check your answers at the end of the chapter.

1. Find 30 cc. What other measures are equivalent to this?

_______ _______ _______ _______

2. Find 5 cc. Hold the page of this book up so that the 5 cc line is at eye level. Is a dram equal to 5 cc? ____________________

(continued)

Exercise 3 (continued)

3. If an order reads ʒi what line would you use to pour the dose? ________

4. Find 15 cc. What other equivalents equal this?

________ ________ ________ ________

5. Consider the following answers to oral liquid dosage problems. What measurement line would you use?

   a. 8 cc Pour ________

   b. 4 tsp Pour ________

   c. $\frac{1}{2}$ oz Pour ________

6. Suppose an answer to an oral liquid problem is 2 mL. Could you pour this dose into a medicine cup?

   Explain what you would do. ________

Syringes

There are four types of syringes used by nurses to prepare routine parenteral doses. Each is different from the others; understanding these differences will help you to prepare doses. The syringes are a 3-mL (cc) syringe, a 1-cc syringe, and two insulin syringes.

3-mL Syringe. The syringe shown in Figure 5-5 is routinely used for injections. It has a 22-gauge needle, $1\frac{1}{2}$ inches long. The term "gauge" indicates the diameter (width) of the needle.

Note the following on the 3-mL syringe:

- The markings on one side are in cc (mL) to the nearest tenth. Each line indicates 0.1 mL.
- The markings on the opposite side are in minims. Each line indicates 1 minim.
- When preparing a dose, the syringe is held with the needle up. The medication is drawn down into the barrel. Suppose a dose was calculated to be 1.1 cc or 18 minims. Look at Figure 5-5, and count the lines to reach the dose.

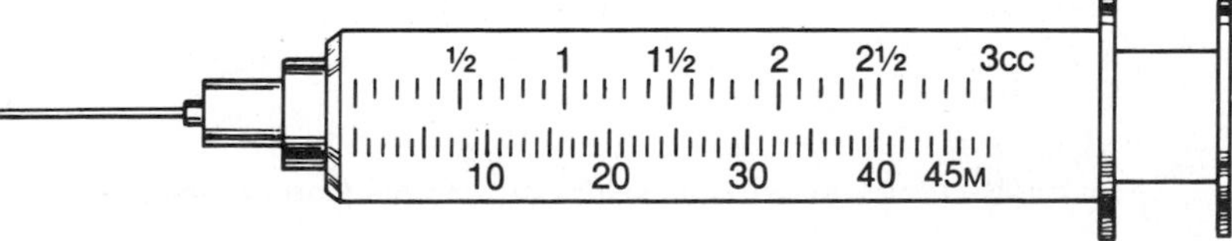

Figure 5-5
A 3-mL (cc) syringe with metric and apothecary measures.

Exercise 4 *Use an arrow to indicate these amounts on the 3-mL syringe in Figure 5-5. Check your answers at the end of this chapter.*

0.3 mL

25 m

1.2 cc

4 m

2.7 mL

The 3-mL syringe has markings for 0.7 mL and 0.8 mL. What would you do if a dosage answer were 0.75 mL? Nurses do not approximate doses between lines. There are two ways to handle this problem:

1. Round off 0.75 mL to the nearest tenth. The answer would be 0.8 mL, which can be drawn up onto a line. (Rounding off numbers was discussed in Chapter 1, and is discussed again in this chapter.)
2. Use a different syringe with markings to the nearest hundredth. There is a precision syringe that has markings to the nearest hundredth.

1-mL Precision Syringe. The 1-mL (cc) precision syringe with a 25-gauge, $\frac{5}{8}$ inch needle is the most accurate of the syringes nurses use. It is sometimes called a tuberculin syringe. The syringe is marked in hundredths of a milliliter (cubic centimeter) and in half minims (Fig. 5-6).

Note the following on the 1-mL precision syringe:

- The markings on one side are in minims. There is a short line between each half minim and a long line for a whole minim.
- The markings on the other side are in milliliters (mL; cc). There are nine lines before 0.10. Each line is 0.01 ml.
- To prepare an injection, the syringe is held with the needle up and the medication is drawn down into the barrel. Suppose a dose was calculated to be 0.13 ml or 2 minims. Look at Figure 5-6 and count the lines to reach the dose.

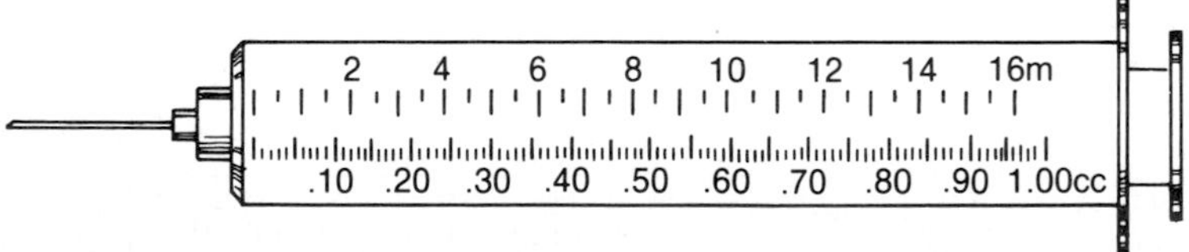

Figure 5-6
A 1-mL (cc) precision syringe with metric and apothecary measures.

◀ ***Learning Aid***
Whenever you use a syringe, check to be certain that you have chosen the correct dose. For 0.13 mL, the nurse would see the longer lines at 0.10 and 0.20. The slightly shorter line between them is 0.15 and two lines below that would be 0.13 mL.

Exercise 5

Use arrows to mark the following doses on the 1-mL (cc) precision syringe in Figure 5-6. Check your answers at the end of this chapter.

3 minims

$6\frac{1}{2}$ minims

0.66 mL

0.95 mL

Rounding Off Numbers in Liquid Dosage Answers

In solving liquid injection problems answers are in milliliters, cubic centimeters, or minims. The answer may not be an even number and the nurse must decide the degree of accuracy to be obtained. *The degree of accuracy depends on the syringe chosen to give the dose.*

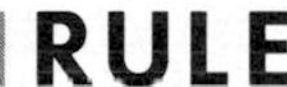

RULE

ROUNDING OFF NUMBERS

1. When the last number is 5 or more, add 1 to the previous number.
2. When the number is 4 or less, drop the number.

EXAMPLE

0.864 becomes 0.86 4.562 becomes 4.56

1.55 becomes 1.6 2.38 becomes 2.4

0.33 becomes 0.3 0.25 becomes 0.3

With the *3-mL syringe* carry out decimals two places and round off to the *nearest tenth for milliliters.* Carry out answers in *minims* to the nearest tenth and *round off to the nearest whole number.*

With the *1-mL precision syringe,* carry out decimals three places and round off to the *nearest 100th* for milliliters. Carry out answers in *minims* to the nearest 100th and *round off to the nearest tenth.*

Exercise 6

The following are possible answers to dosage problems that require use of a 3-mL syringe. Put a check (✓) next to the answer if it is acceptable. If not acceptable, change the answer to a correct form. Check your answers at the end of this chapter.

a. 0.1 mL ________

b. $1\frac{1}{2}$ cc ________

c. 0.83 cc ________

d. 0.98 minims ________

e. 0.2 mL ________

f. $8\frac{1}{2}$ minims ________

g. 1.7 mL ________

h. $\frac{1}{2}$ mL ________

i. 0.4 cc ________

j. 0.65 mL ________

k. 3 minims ________

l. 5.5 minims ________

Exercise 7

The following are possible answers to dosage problems that require the use of a 1-mL precision syringe. Put a check (✓) next to the answer if it is acceptable. If not acceptable, change the answer to a correct form. Check your answers at the end of this chapter.

a. 0.65 mL	________	d. 12.8 mg	________	g. 0.758 mL	________
b. 12.5 minims	________	e. 0.346 mL	________	h. 5 minims	________
c. 0.04 mL	________	f. 0.290 mL	________		________

1-cc Insulin Syringe. The 1-cc insulin syringe (for Unit 100 insulin) is marked in units rather than in milliliters or minims. It is used to prepare only U 100 insulins. The physician orders the type of insulin, the strength of insulin, and the number of units (Fig. 5-7).

EXAMPLE Order: 20 units NPH (U 100) insulin qd SC

Look at Figure 5-7. Note that there are four short lines between 10 units and 20 units. This indicates that each line is equal to 2 units on this syringe. Always check the markings on a syringe to be certain you understand what each line equals.

Exercise 8

Use arrows on the insulin syringe in Figure 5-7 to indicate the following amounts. Check your answers at the end of this chapter.

6 units

34 units

50 units

Odd-numbered insulin doses should not be drawn up with the syringe in Figure 5-7. Another insulin syringe is used to prepare these doses. Doses should be exact, not approximate.

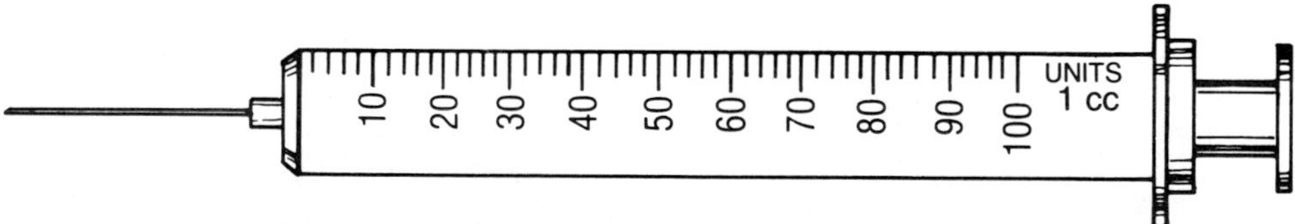

Figure 5-7
A 1-mL (cc) insulin syringe (for U 100 insulin).

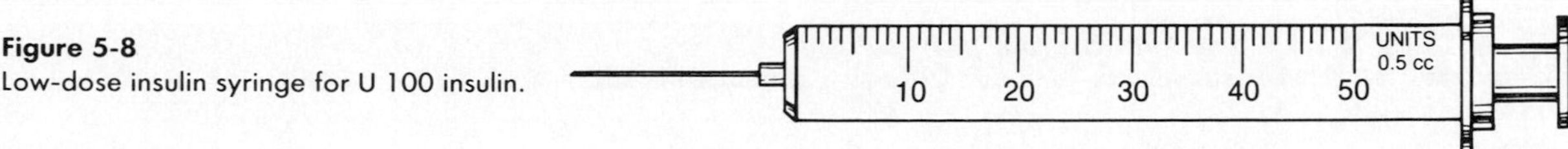

Figure 5-8
Low-dose insulin syringe for U 100 insulin.

Low-Dose Insulin Syringe. The low-dose unit 100 insulin syringe with a 28-gauge, $\frac{1}{2}$-inch needle (Fig. 5-8) has four short lines between 10 and 15. This indicates that each line is equal to 1 unit. The syringe is marked for 50 units, so any dose of insulin (U 100) up to 50 units can be drawn up with this syringe.

Exercise 9

Use arrows on the insulin syringe in Figure 5-8 to indicate the following amounts. Answers may be found at the end of this chapter.

Units 33

Units 7

Units 40

Needles for Intramuscular and Subcutaneous Injections

Each of the four syringes discussed has a different injection needle.

Syringe	Gauge	Length (inches)
3 ml	22 g	$1\frac{1}{2}$
1 mL	25 g	$\frac{5}{8}$
U 100 insulin	26 g	$\frac{1}{2}$
U 100 low-dose insulin	28 g	$\frac{1}{2}$

Gauge (g) indicates the diameter or width of the needle. *The higher the gauge number, the finer the needle.* In the gauges just given the low-dose insulin syringe has the needle with the smallest diameter (28-gauge) and, hence, is the finest needle in this group. A 15-gauge needle would be very wide and would have a wide opening. It is used to transfuse blood cells.

The *length* of the needle used depends upon the route of injection. For deep intramuscular injections, a long needle is necessary. A short needle is used for subcutaneous injections.

The nurse determines what type of needle to use for adults and children, depending upon the route of administration, the size and condition of the patient, and the amount of adipose tissue present at the site.

You have now looked at medication orders, types of drug preparations, labels, systems of dosage, and measurement equipment. The next chapters will concentrate on solving dosage problems for oral and parenteral routes.

ANSWERS

Exercise 1

1. e
2. k
3. a
4. h
5. i
6. m
7. l
8. b
9. c
10. d
11. g
12. f
13. j

Exercise 2

1. Diabetes mellitus; alcoholism
2. Two teaspoons or less
3. SC, IM, IVPB, and IV
4. a. The date; b. the nurse's initials; c. the dilution made
5. Sterile technique is required in preparing and administering drugs parenterally (IM, SC, IV, IVPB).
6. Milk of magnesia
7. Before pouring an oral suspension, the liquid must always be shaken.
8. Aerosol powders; creams; ointments; pastes; suppositories; transdermal medications
9. Ease in administering; prolonged action
10. An ointment is a semisolid preparation in a petroleum or lanolin base for topical use.

Exercise 3

1. Other equivalents are 2 tbs, 1 oz, 8 drams, 30 mL. (Remember 1 mL = 1 cc.)
2. No, a dram is slightly less than 5 mL (5 cc).
3. Use the 1-dram line!
4. 15 cc is equal to 1 tbsp, $\frac{1}{2}$ oz, 4 drams, and 15 mL.
5. **a.** Pour 2 drams
   b. 4 tsp × 5 mL = 20 mL; use the 20-cc line
   c. $\frac{1}{2}$ oz. Use the line for $\frac{1}{2}$ oz.
6. No, there is no line for 2 mL. Use a syringe to obtain the 2 mL and then pour the amount into a medicine cup.

Exercise 4

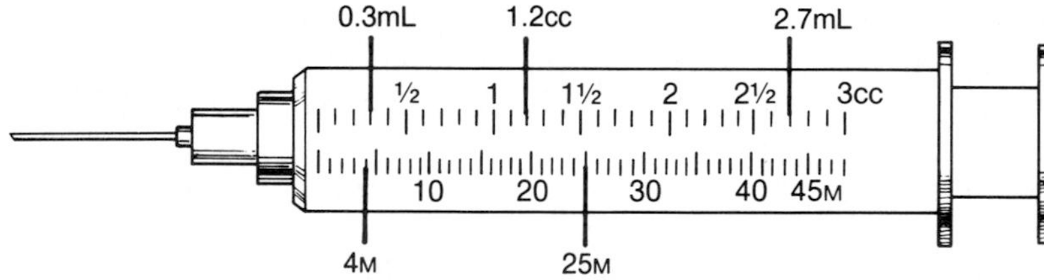

Exercise 5

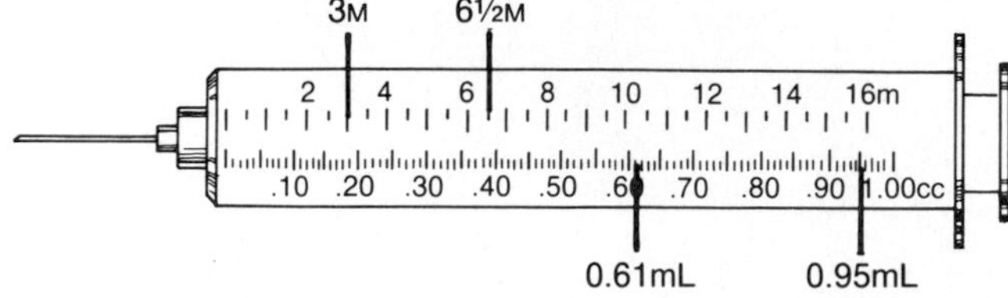

Exercise 6

a. 0.1 mL	✓	
b. $1\frac{1}{2}$ cc	✓	
c. 0.83 cc	0.8 cc	
d. 0.98 m	1 minim	
e. 0.2 mL	✓	
f. $8\frac{1}{2}$ m	9 m	
g. 1.7 mL	✓	
h. $\frac{1}{2}$ mL	✓	
i. 0.4 cc	✓	
j. 0.65 mL	0.7 mL	
k. 3 minims	✓	
l. 5.5 minims	6 minims	

Exercise 7

a. 0.65 mL	✓
b. 12.5 m	✓
c. 0.04 mL	✓
d. 12.8 m	13 minims
e. 0.346 mL	0.35 mL
f. 0.290 mL	0.29 mL
g. 0.758 mL	0.76 mL
h. 5 minims	✓

Exercise 8

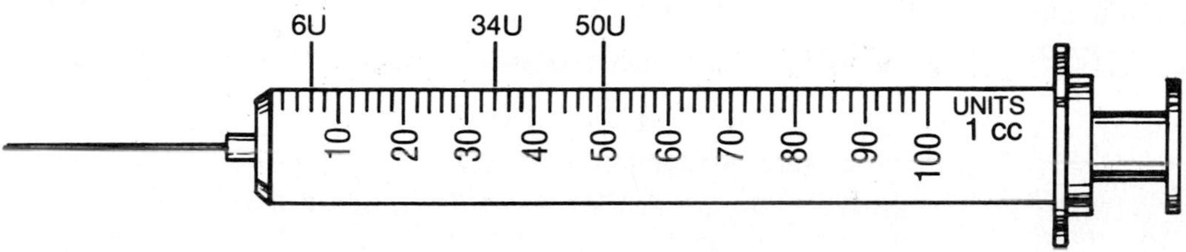

Exercise 9

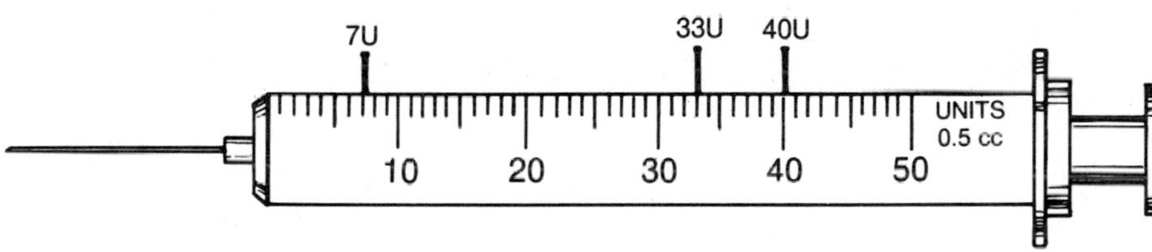

6 Calculation of Oral Medications—Solids and Liquids

CONTENT TO MASTER

Using the rule: $\frac{\text{Desire}}{\text{Have}} \times \text{Stock} = \text{Amount}$

Converting order and stock to the same weight measure

Clearing decimal points before solving a problem

Using equivalents when conversions are needed

Interpreting special types of oral solid orders: over-the-counter (OTC), multivitamins, and liquids

Drugs for oral administration are prepared by pharmaceutical companies as solids (tablets, capsules) and liquids. When the dose ordered by the physician differs from the stock the nurse calculates the amount to be given. The problems are solved using a rule derived from ratio and proportion.

RULE

CALCULATING ORAL MEDICATIONS

$$\frac{\text{Desire}}{\text{Have}} \times \text{Stock} = \text{Amount}$$

Desire is the physician's order.

Have is the strength of the drug in the container.

Stock is the form in which the drug comes.

Amount is how much of the stock to give.

◀ ***Learning Aid***
Abbreviate the rule:

$\frac{D}{H} \times S = A$

▼ ORAL SOLIDS

Application of the Rule for Oral Solids

RULE $\frac{\text{Desire}}{\text{Have}} \times \text{Stock} = \text{Amount}$

EXAMPLE Order: alprazolam 0.5 mg po bid

Stock:

See package insert for complete product information.
Keep container tightly closed.
Dispense in tight, light-resistant container.
Store at controlled room temperature 15° to 30° C (59° to 86° F).
U.S. Patent No. 3,987,052
812 006 507
The Upjohn Company
Kalamazoo, MI
49001, USA

Upjohn
NDC 0009-0029-02
500 Tablets
6505-01-197-3966
Xanax® CIV
Tablets
alprazolam tablets, USP
0.25mg
Caution: Federal law prohibits dispensing without prescription.

◀ ***Learning Aid***
Note that the doctor ordered the drug generically as alprazolam.
The trade name is Xanax.
CIV on the label indicates that this is a controlled drug.
See Chapter 11 for information about controlled drugs.

Desire: The desire is the physician's order. In the example, desired is 0.5 mg.

Have: Have is the strength of the drug supplied in the container. In the example, the label indicates that each tablet contains 0.25 mg.

Stock: The stock is the unit form in which the drug comes. Alprazolam comes in tablet form. *Since tablets and capsules are single entities, the stock for oral solid drugs is always one.*

Amount: The amount is how much of the stock to give. For oral solids the answer will be the number of tablets or capsules to administer.

To solve any problem, first check that the order and the stock are in the same weight measure. If they are not, you must convert one or the other amount to its equivalent. In this example no equivalent is needed; both the order and the stock are in mg.

EXAMPLE Order: alprazolam 0.5 mg

Stock: tablets of 0.25 mg

Rule: $\frac{D}{H} \times S = A$

$$\frac{\overset{2}{0.\cancel{50}\ \cancel{\text{mg}}}}{\underset{1}{0.\cancel{25}\ \cancel{\text{mg}}}} \times 1 \text{ tab} = 2 \text{ tabs}$$

◀ ***Learning Aid***

$$0.25\overline{)0.50}^{\ 2.}$$

This is long division. See below for an easier way to clear decimals.

Clearing Decimals

When the numerator and denominator in $\frac{D}{H}$ are decimals, add zeros to make the number of decimal places the same. Then drop the decimal points. This is a short arithmetic operation to replace long division:

added
↓

$$\frac{0.\ 50 \text{ mg}}{0.\ 25 \text{ mg}} \qquad \frac{\text{numerator}}{\text{denominator or divisor}}$$

In division the denominator is the divisor and must be cleared of decimal points before carrying out the arithmetic. The decimal point in the numerator is moved the same number of places. Refer to Chapter 1 for further help in division of decimals.

EXAMPLE Order: digoxin 0.125 mg po qd

Stock: scored tablets labeled 0.25 mg

No equivalent is needed. Both are in mg.

$$\frac{0.\overset{1}{\cancel{125}} \text{ mg}}{0.\underset{2}{\cancel{250}} \text{ mg}} \times 1 \text{ tab} = \frac{1}{2} \text{ tab}$$

◀ ***Learning Aid***
Long division

$$0.25 \overline{)0.12\,5}^{\,0.5} = \frac{5}{10} = \frac{1}{2} \text{ tab}$$

Short way

$$\frac{0.125}{0.250} = \frac{1}{2} \text{ tab}$$

EXAMPLE Order: triazolam 0.125 mg po q4h prn

Stock:

Use of bulk packaged tablets is for institutional, in-patient use.
See package insert for complete product information.
Keep container tightly closed.
Dispense in tight, light-resistant container.
Store at controlled room temperature 15° to 30° C (59° to 86° F).
U.S. Patent No. 3,987,052
812 108 205
The Upjohn Co.
Kalamazoo, MI
49001, USA

Upjohn
NDC 0009-0017-02
500 Tablets
6505-01-161-5036
Halcion® CIV
Tablets
triazolam tablets, USP
0.25mg
Caution: Federal law prohibits dispensing without prescription.

◀ ***Learning Aid***
You would check to see that the Halcion tablets are scored and can be broken in half.

$$\frac{D}{H} \times S = A$$

$$\frac{0.\overset{1}{\cancel{125}} \text{ mg}}{0.\underset{2}{\cancel{250}} \text{ mg}} = \frac{1}{2} \text{ tab}$$

Give $\frac{1}{2}$ tab.

EXAMPLE

Order: ranitidine hydrochloride 0.3 g po qn

Stock:

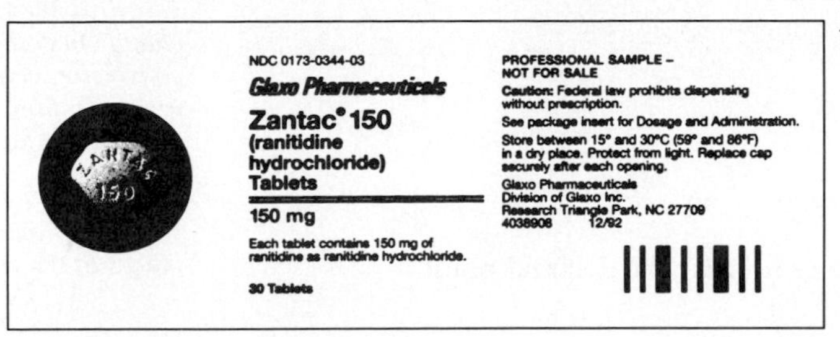

◀ ***Learning Aid***

Remember 1 g = 1000 mg. If necessary review Chapter 4.

The quick rule for converting states that you write the equivalent you wish to change first. Then write the conversion you want. The open arrow faces the larger measure.

0.3 g = ____ mg

0.3 g > mg

The arrow tells you to move the gram number three places to the right.

0.300 g = 300 mg

Equivalent 0.3 g = 300 mg

Rule: $\frac{D}{H} \times S = A$

$\frac{\overset{2}{\cancel{300}}\text{ mg}}{\underset{1}{\cancel{150}}\text{ mg}} \times 1\text{ tab} = 2\text{ tabs}$

EXAMPLE

Order: synthroid 100 mcg po qd

Stock:

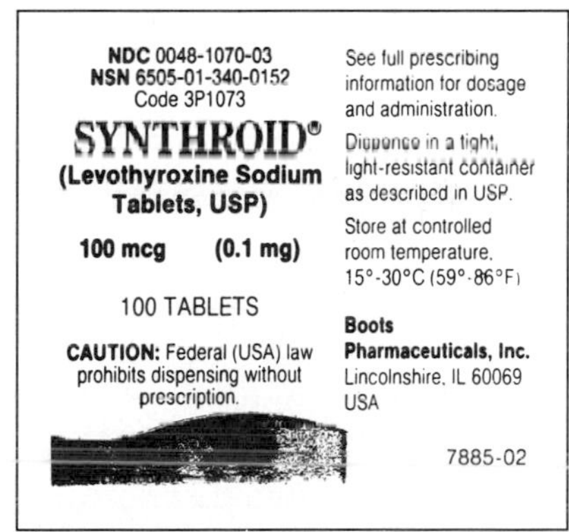

Note that the label gives the equivalent measure: 100 mcg = 0.1 mg

Since the order and the stock are in the same weight measure, no calculation is necessary.

Give 1 tablet.

EXAMPLE

Order: aspirin 0.6 g po stat

Stock:

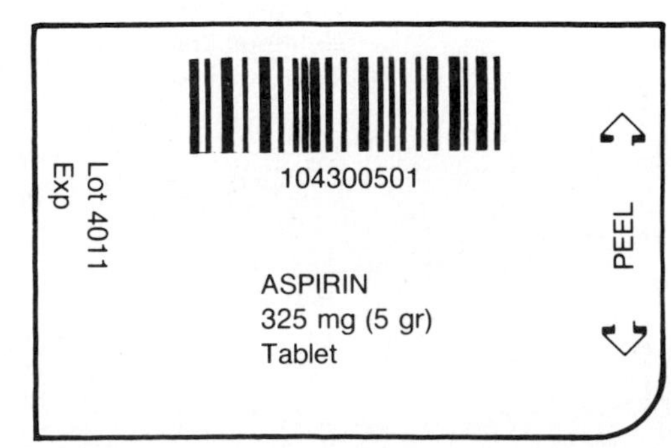

Equivalent 0.6 g = 600 mg or 650 mg

Rule: $\frac{D}{H} \times S = A$

$\frac{\overset{2}{\cancel{650}}\text{ mg}}{\underset{1}{\cancel{325}}\text{ mg}} \times 1\text{ tab} = 2\text{ tabs}$

EXAMPLE

Order: levothyroxine sodium 37.5 μg po qd

Stock: scored tablets of 0.025 mg

Equivalent 0.025 mg = 25 μg

Rule: $\frac{D}{H} \times S = A$

$\frac{37.5\ \mu g}{25\ \mu g} \times 1 = A$

Use the quick way to clear the decimal point.

$\frac{\overset{3}{\cancel{37.5}}}{\underset{2}{\cancel{25.0}}} \times 1 \text{ tab} = \frac{3}{2}$

(Divided by 125)

$\frac{3}{2} = 1\frac{1}{2}$ tabs

You can administer $1\frac{1}{2}$ tablets because the stock is scored.

◀ ***Learning Aid***
Remember 1 mg = 1000 μg. The quick rule for converting states that you write the equivalent you want to change first. Then write the conversion you want. Change the mg to μg. To find the equivalent, the open arrow faces the larger measure.

mg > μg

The arrow tells you to move mg three places to the right.

0.025 mg = 25 μg

EXAMPLE

Example 1:

Order: pentobarbital 0.1 g po hs prn

Stock: capsules labeled 100 mg

Equivalent 0.1 g = 100 mg

Rule: $\frac{D}{H} \times S = A$

$\frac{\overset{1}{\cancel{100\ mg}}}{\underset{1}{\cancel{100\ mg}}} \times 1 \text{ cap} = 1 \text{ cap}$

Example 2:

Order: Mycostatin 1 million units po tid

Stock: scored tablets labeled 500,000 units

No equivalent needed.

Rule: $\frac{D}{H} \times S = A$

$\frac{\overset{2}{\cancel{1,000,000\ units}}}{\underset{1}{\cancel{500,000\ units}}} \times 1 \text{ tab} = 2 \text{ tabs}$

Self-Test 1

Solve these practice problems. Answers may be found at the end of the chapter. Remember the rule:

$$\frac{D}{H} \times S = A$$

1. Order: Decadron 1.5 mg po bid
   Stock: tablets labeled 0.75 mg
2. Order: digoxin 0.25 mg po qd
   Stock: scored tablets labeled 0.5 mg
3. Order: ampicillin 0.5 Gm po q6h
   Stock: capsules labeled 250 mg
4. Order: prednisone 10 mg po tid
   Stock: tablets labeled 2.5 mg
5. Order: aspirin 650 mg po stat
   Stock: tablets labeled 325 mg
6. Order: digitoxin 200 mcg po qd
   Stock: scored tablets labeled 0.1 mg
7. Order: Equanil 0.2 g po q4h
   Stock: scored tablets labeled 400 mg
8. Order: penicillin G potassium 200,000 units po q8h
   Stock: scored tablets labeled 400,000 units
9. Order: digoxin 0.5 mg po qd
   Stock: scored tablets labeled 0.25 mg
10. Order: Lasix 60 mg po qd
    Stock: scored tablets labeled 40 mg

Special Types of Oral Solid Orders

Drugs that contain a number of active ingredients are ordered by the number to be administered and do not require calculation. These include over-the-counter (OTC) preparations and multivitamins.

EXAMPLE Multivitamin tabs i po qd

Gelusil tabs i po q4h prn

Physicians occasionally specify the weight measure of the drug and the number of tablets to be given. These orders do not require calculation.

EXAMPLE *Example 1:*

Darvon 65 mg caps ii po hs prn

This is interpreted: Give two capsules of Darvon 65 mg by mouth at the hour of sleep if needed.

Example 2:

aspirin 325 mg ii po stat

This is interpreted: Give two tablets of aspirin 325 mg by mouth immediately.

▼ ORAL LIQUIDS

Application of the Rule for Oral Liquids

RULE

$$\frac{\text{Desire}}{\text{Have}} \times \text{Stock} = \text{Amount}$$

◀ ***Learning Aid***
Abbreviate the rule:

$$\frac{D}{H} \times S = A$$

EXAMPLE Order: cloxacillin sodium 0.25 g po q6h
Stock:

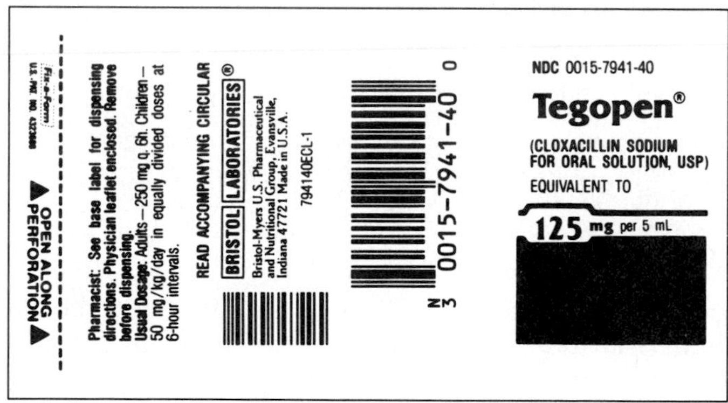

Desire: The desire is the physician's order. In the example, desire is 0.25 g.

Have: Have is the strength of the drug supplied in the container. In the example, the label indicates the strength is 125 mg.

Stock: The stock is the unit form of the drug. In the label above 5 mL contains 125 mg. The unit form is 5 mL. Other examples of liquid stock are:

250 mg per 5 mL: the unit form is 5 mL
1 g/mL: the unit form is 1 mL
100 mg in 2 mL: the unit form is 2 mL

Amount: The amount is how much of the stock to give. Because the stock is a liquid, the *answer* will be a liquid measure (mL; cc; tsp; tbsp).

Before solving each problem, check to be certain that the order and your supply are in the same measure. If they are not, you must convert one or the other to its equivalent. Convert whichever one is easier for you to solve.

EXAMPLE

Order: cloxacillin sodium 0.25 g

Stock: 125 mg per 5 mL

Equivalent: 0.25 g = 250 mg

Rule: $\frac{D}{H} \times S = A$

$$\frac{\overset{2}{\cancel{250}\ \cancel{mg}}}{\underset{1}{\cancel{125}\ \cancel{mg}}} \times 5\ mL = 10\ mL$$

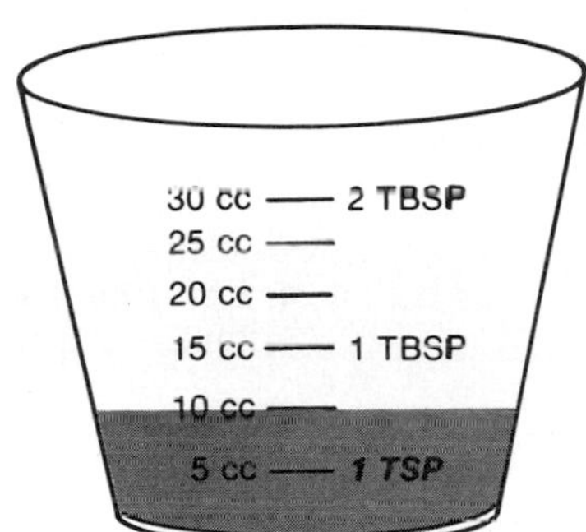

◀ ***Learning Aid***
There are many ways to solve the math.

$$\frac{\overset{10}{\cancel{250}}}{\underset{\underset{1}{\cancel{25}}}{\cancel{125}}} \times \overset{1}{\cancel{5}} = 10\ mL$$

$$250 \times 5 = \frac{\overset{10}{\cancel{1250}}}{\underset{1}{\cancel{125}}} = 10\ mL$$

EXAMPLE

Order: furosemide 34 mg po qd.

Stock:

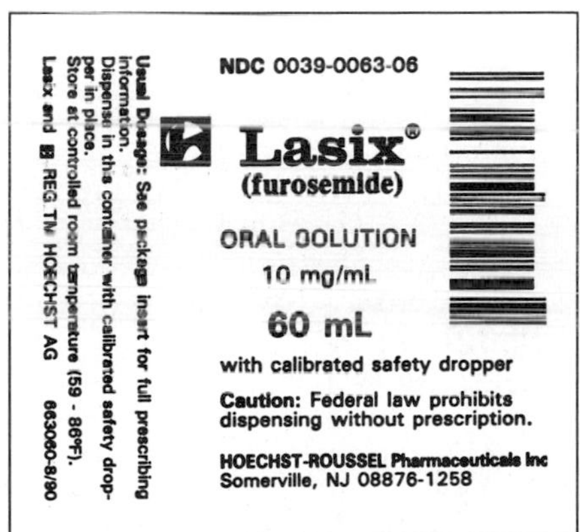

◀ ***Learning Aid***
Because the drug comes with a calibrated dropper, you are alerted that your answer will be a small amount.

No equivalent is needed

$\frac{D}{H} \times S = A$

$$\frac{34\ \cancel{mg}}{10\ \cancel{mg}} \times 1\ mL = \frac{34}{10} \quad 10\overline{)34.0}^{\,3.4}$$

Give 3.4 mL

EXAMPLE

Order: penicillin V potassium 0.4 g po q6h

Stock:

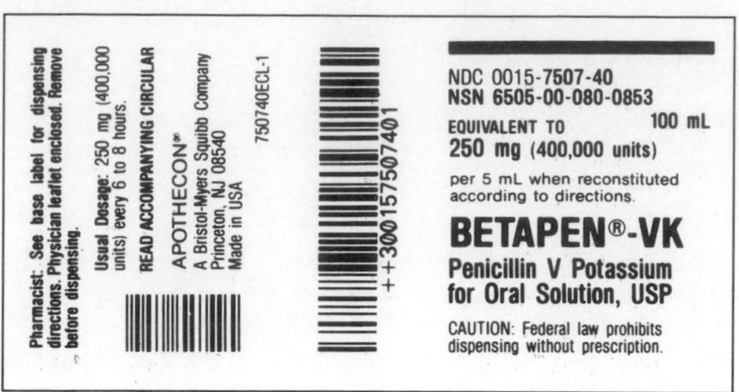

◀ ***Learning Aid***
This drug comes as a powder. When reconstituted, the bottle will contain 100 mL. The solution will be 250 mg (400,000 units) per 5 mL.

Equivalent: 0.4 g = 400 mg

$\frac{D}{H} \times S = A$

$\frac{\overset{8}{\cancel{400}}\ \cancel{\text{mg}}}{\underset{\underset{1}{\cancel{50}}}{\cancel{250}}\ \cancel{\text{mg}}} \times \overset{1}{\cancel{5}}\ \text{mL} = 8\ \text{mL}$

◀ ***Learning Aid***
8 mL = 2 drams

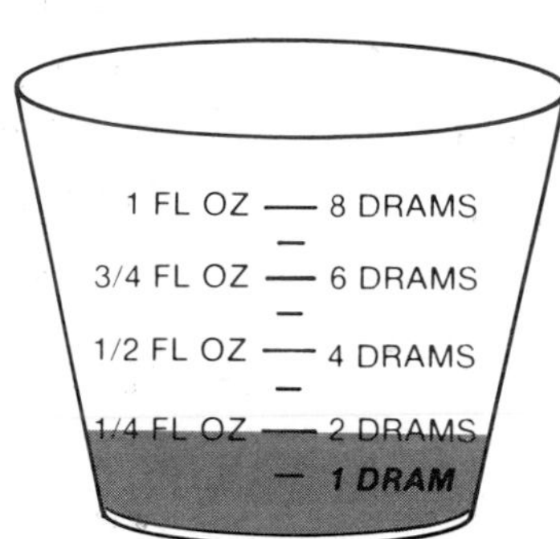

EXAMPLE

Order: amoxicillin oral suspension 500 mg po q8h

Stock:

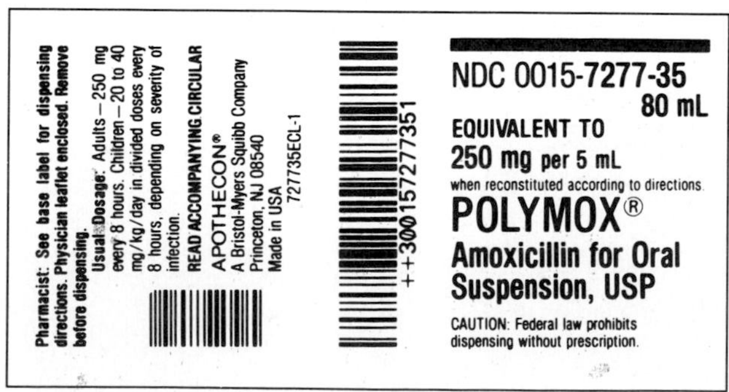

$\frac{D}{H} \times S = A$

$\frac{\overset{2}{\cancel{500}}\ \cancel{\text{mg}}}{\underset{1}{\cancel{250}}\ \cancel{\text{mg}}} \times 5\ \text{mL} = 10\ \text{mL}$

Self-Test 2

Solve these oral liquid problems. Answers may be found at the end of the chapter.

1. Order: erythromycin susp. 0.75 g po qid
   Stock: liquid labeled 250 mg/5 mL
2. Order: ampicillin susp. 500 mg po q8h
   Stock: liquid labeled 250 mg/5 mL
3. Order: Cephalex in oral suspension 0.35 Gm po q6h
   Stock: liquid labeled 125 mg/5 mL
4. Order: cyclosporine 150 mg po stat and qd
   Stock: liquid labeled 100 mg/mL in a bottle with a calibrated dropper
5. Order: sulfasoxizole susp. 300 mg po qid
   Stock: liquid labeled 250 mg/5 mL
6. Order: digoxin 0.02 mg po qd
   Stock: pediatric elixir 0.05 mg/mL in a bottle with a dropper marked in tenths of a milliliter
7. Order: potassium chloride 30 mEq po qd
   Stock: liquid labeled 20 mEq/15 mL
8. Order: elixir digoxin 0.25 mg via nasogastric tube qd
   Stock: liquid labeled 0.5 mg/10 mL
9. Order: hydrocortisone cypionate oral susp. 30 mg po q6h
   Stock: liquid labeled 10 mg/5 mL
10. Order: promethazine HCl syrup 12.5 mg po tid
    Stock: liquid labeled 6.25 mg/5 mL

Special Types of Oral Liquid Orders

Some liquids, including OTC preparations and multivitamins, are ordered in the amount to be poured and administered. No calculation is required.

EXAMPLE

Example 1:

Order: terpin hydrate elixir 2 tsp q 4 h prn po

Stock: liquid labeled terpin hydrate elixir

No calculation is needed. Pour 2 teaspoons every 4 hours by mouth if necessary.

Example 2:

Order: milk of magnesia 30 cc hs tonight po

Stock: liquid labeled milk of magnesia

No calculation is required. Pour 30 cc of milk of magnesia and give tonight by mouth.

▼ MENTAL DRILL FOR ORAL SOLID AND LIQUID PROBLEMS

As you develop proficiency in solving problems, you will be able to calculate many answers without written work. This drill combines your knowledge of equivalents and dosage.

Self-Test 3

Solve the problems mentally and write only the amount to be given. Answers will be found at the end of the chapter. Keep the rule in mind as you solve each problem.

Order	*Stock (Scored Tablets)*	*Answer*
1. 20 mg	10 mg	
2. 0.125 mg	0.25 mg	
3. 0.25 mg	0.125 mg	
4. 200,000 units	100,000 units	
5. 0.5 mg	0.25 mg	
6. 0.2 Gm	400 mg	
7. 1 Gm	gr xv	
8. 0.1 Gm	100 mg	
9. 0.01 Gm	20 mg	
10. gr x	325 mg	
11. grs vii ṡṡ	250 mg	
12. gr i	60 mg	
13. 50 mg	0.1 Gm	
14. 4 mg	2 mg	

Self-Test 4

	Order	*Stock*	*Answer*
1.	20 mg	10 mg per 5 mL	__________
2.	10 mg	2 mg/5 cc	__________
3.	0.5 Gm	250 mg/5 mL	__________
4.	0.1 Gm	200 mg per 10 mL	__________
5.	250 mg	0.1 g per 6 mL	__________
6.	100 mg	50 mg/10 cc	__________
7.	12 mg	4 mg/5 mL	__________
8.	15 mg	30 mg/10 mL	__________
9.	15 mg	10 mg per 4 mL	__________
10.	0.25 mg	0.5 mg/5 mL	__________

Proficiency Test 1

For liquid answers draw a line on the medicine cup indicating the amount you would pour. Answers may be found at the end of the chapter.

1. Order: KCl elixir 20 mEq po bid
Stock: liquid labeled 30 mEq/15 mL

Answer __________

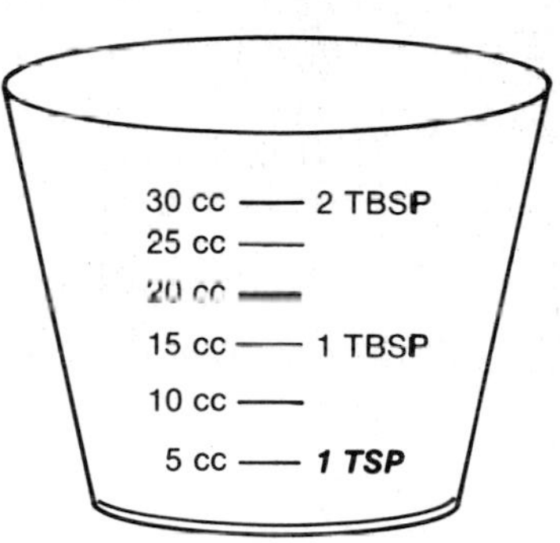

2. Order: Dilantin Susp. 150 mg po tid
Stock: liquid labeled 75 mg/7.5 mL

Answer __________

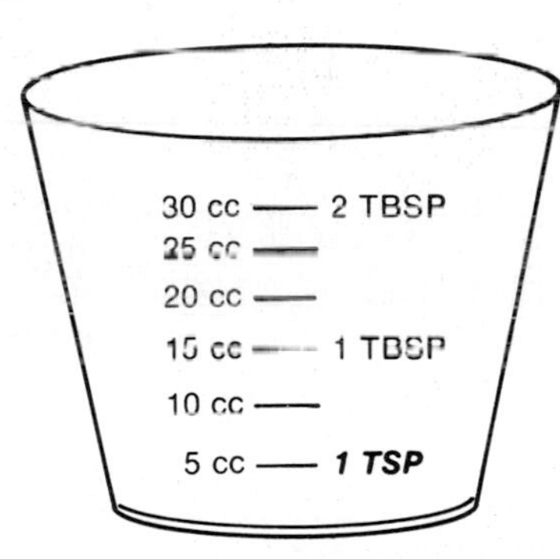

3. Order: elixir digoxin 0.125 mg po qd
Stock: liquid labeled 0.25 mg/10 mL

Answer __________

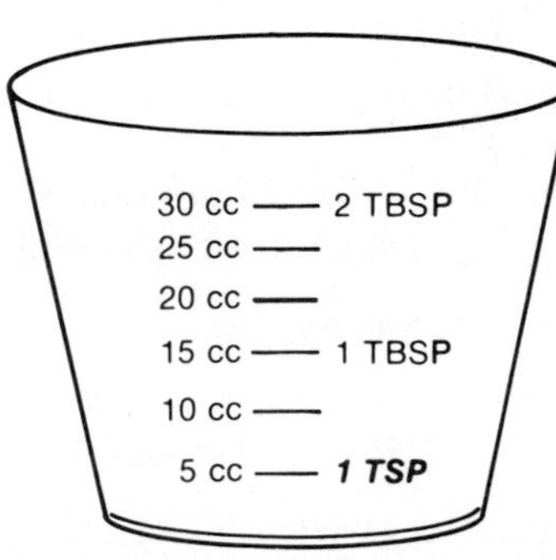

(continued)

Proficiency Test 1 (continued)

4. Order: Dilantin oral suspension 150 mg po tid
Stock: liquid labeled 75 mg/6 mL

Answer ______________

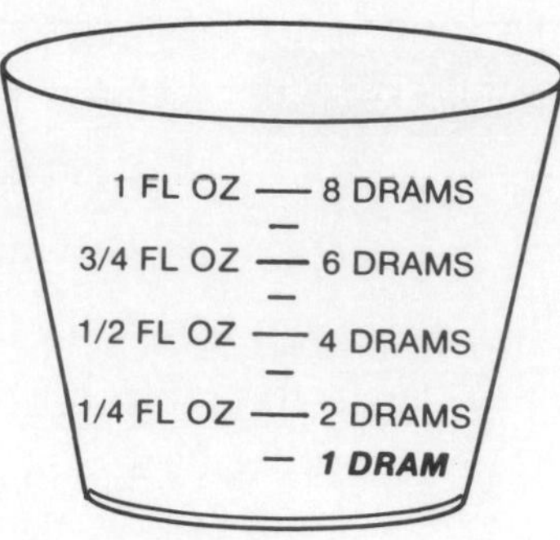

5. Order: Proximyl 10 mg po bid
Stock: liquid labeled 2 mg/5 mL

Answer ______________

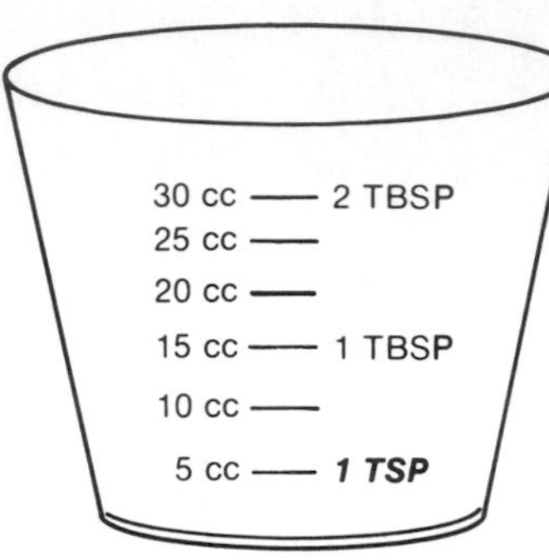

6. Order: digoxin 0.5 mg po qd
Stock: tablets labeled 0.25 mg

Answer ______________

7. Order: Lanoxin 10 μg qd po
Stock: 0.02 mg scored tablets

Answer ______________

8. Order: Zyloprim 250 mg po qd
Stock: scored tablets 100 mg

Answer ______________

9. Order: ampicillin 0.5 g po q6h
Stock: capsules labeled 250 mg

Answer ______________

10. Order: Synthroid 0.3 mg po qd
Stock: tablets labeled 300 μg scored

Answer ______________

Proficiency Test 2

For liquid answers draw a line on the medicine cup indicating the amount you would pour. Answers may be found at the end of the chapter.

1. Order: ibuprofen 0.8 gm po tid
Stock: tablets labeled 400 mg

Answer ______________

2. Order: isoniazid 0.3 Gm po qd
Stock: tablets labeled 300 mg

Answer ______________

Proficiency Test 2 (continued)

3. Order: ethambutal HCl 600 mg po qd
   Stock: tablets scored and labeled 400 mg
   Answer ______________

4. Order: acetaminophen 0.65 Gm po q4h
   Stock: tablets labeled 325 mg
   Answer ______________

5. Order: ascorbic acid 250 mg po bid
   Stock: tablets scored and labeled 500 mg
   Answer ______________

6. Order: colistin sulfate oral suspension 80 mg po tid
   Stock: liquid labeled 25 mg/tsp
   Answer ______________

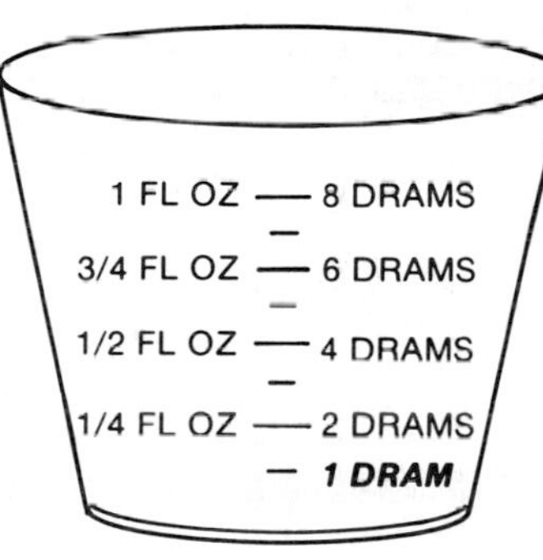

7. Order: oxacillin sodium 0.75 Gm po q6h
   Stock: liquid labeled 250 mg/5 mL
   Answer ______________

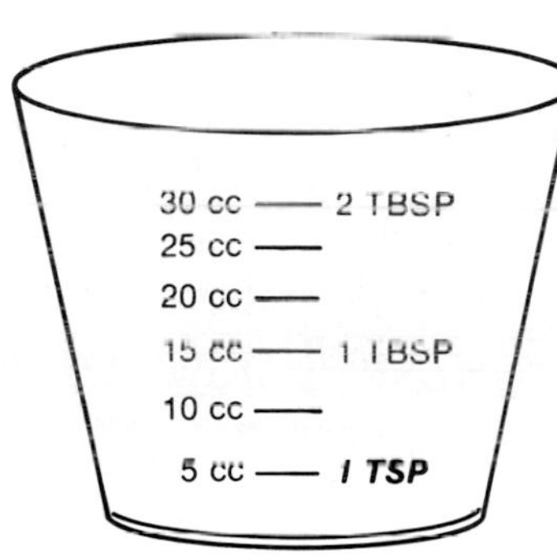

8. Order: penicillin V potassium 600 mg po q6h
   Stock: liquid labeled 250 mg/5 mL
   Answer ______________

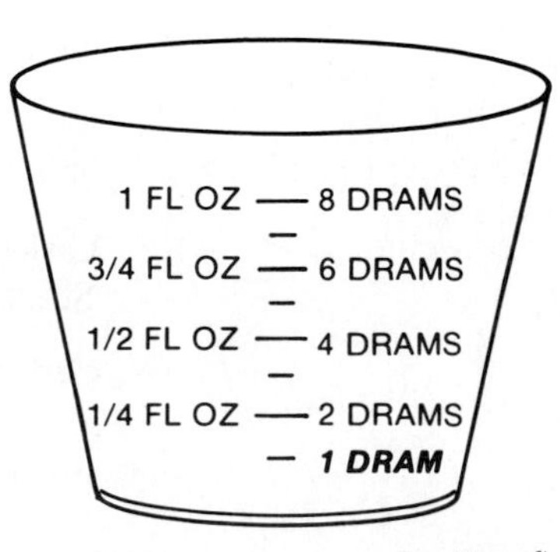

(continued)

Proficiency Test 2 (continued)

9. Order: Mylanta II 30 ml q4h prn
Stock: liquid labeled Mylanta II

Answer ______________

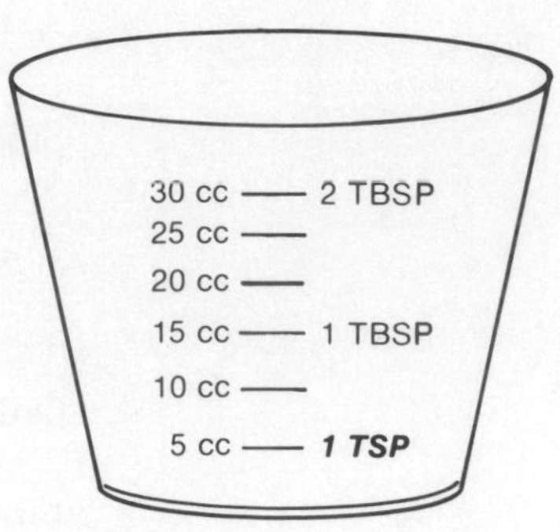

10. Order: Elixophyllin 160 mg po q6h
Stock: liquid labeled 80 mg/15 mL

Answer ______________

Proficiency Test 3

Aim for 90% or better on this test. There are 20 questions, each worth 5 points. Determine the amount to be given. If you have any difficulty, reread Chapter 6, which explains this information. Answers may be found at the end of the chapter.

1. Order: el of potassium chloride 20 mEq po in juice
Stock: liquid in a bottle labeled 30 mEq/15 mL

2. Order: syrup of tetracycline hydrochloride 80 mg po q6h
Stock: liquid in a dropper bottle labeled 125 mg/5 mL

3. Order: propranolol 0.02 g po bid
Stock: scored tablets labeled 10 mg

4. Order: ampicillin sodium 0.5 g po q6h
Stock: capsules of 250 mg

5. Order: digoxin 0.5 mg po qd
Stock: scored tablets of 0.25 mg

6. Order: Levothroid Susp. 100 mcg qd po
Stock: liquid in a bottle labeled 0.2 mg/10 mL

(continued)

Proficiency Test 3 (continued)

7. Order: hydrochlorothiazide 75 mg po qd
   Stock: scored tablets 50 mg
8. Order: furosemide 40 mg po qd
   Stock: scored tablets of 80 mg
9. Order: el digoxin 0.125 mg po
   Stock: liquid in a dropper bottle labeled 500 μg/10 mL
10. Order: Dilantin Susp 75 mg po tid
    Stock: liquid in a bottle labeled 50 mg/10 mL
11. Order: diazepam 5 mg po q4h prn
    Stock: scored tablets 2 mg
12. Order: Synthroid 0.15 mg po qd
    Stock: scored tablets 300 μg
13. Order: Antabuse 375 mg po today
    Stock: scored tablets 250 mg
14. Order: ibuprofen 0.6 g po q4h prn
    Stock: Film-coated tablets 300 mg
15. Order: chlorpheniramine maleate syr 1.5 mg po bid
    Stock: liquid in a bottle 1 mg/8 mL
16. Order: diphenhydramine maleate syrup 25 mg po q4h while awake
    Stock: liquid labeled 12.5 mg/5 mL
17. Order: simethicone liq 60 mg po in $\frac{1}{2}$ glass H_2O
    Stock: liquid in a dropper bottle labeled 40 mg/0.6 mL
18. Order: chlorothiazide oral susp 0.5 g via NGT po qd
    Stock: liquid labeled 250 mg/5 mL
19. Order: meperidine HCl syrup 150 mg po q4h prn
    Stock: liquid labeled 50 mg/5 mL
20. Order: hydroxyzine syrup 7.5 mg po q6h
    Stock: liquid labeled 10 mg/5 mL

ANSWERS

Self-Test 1

1. Rule: $\frac{D}{H} \times S = A$.

No equivalent needed

$$\frac{\overset{2}{\cancel{1.50\text{ mg}}}}{\underset{1}{\cancel{0.75\text{ mg}}}} \times 1 \text{ tab} = 2 \text{ tablets}$$

◀ ***Learning Aid***

$0.75\overline{)1.50}$ = 2.; 1 50; 0

2. No equivalent necessary

$$\frac{\overset{1}{\cancel{0.25\text{ mg}}}}{\underset{2}{\cancel{0.50}\text{ mg}}} \times 1 \text{ tab} = \frac{1}{2} \text{ tablet}$$

◀ ***Learning Aid***

$0.5\overline{)0.2.5}$ = 0.5 or $\frac{1}{2}$; 25; 0

3. Equivalent 0.5 Gm = 500 mg

$$\frac{\overset{2}{\cancel{500\text{ mg}}}}{\underset{1}{\cancel{250\text{ mg}}}} \times 1 \text{ tab} = 2 \text{ tablets}$$

◀ ***Learning Aid***

$250\overline{)500.}$ = 2.; 500; 0

4. No equivalent necessary

$$\frac{\overset{4}{\cancel{10.0\text{ mg}}}}{\underset{1}{\cancel{2.5\text{ mg}}}} \times 1 \text{ tab} = 4 \text{ tablets}$$

◀ ***Learning Aid***

$2.5\overline{)10.0}$ = 4.

5. No equivalent necessary

$$\frac{\overset{2}{\cancel{650\text{ mg}}}}{\underset{1}{\cancel{325\text{ mg}}}} \times 1 \text{ tab} = 2 \text{ tablets}$$

◀ ***Learning Aid***

$325\overline{)650.}$ = 2.; 650; 0

6. Equivalent 1 mg = 1000 mcg
mg > mcg
0.1 mg = 100 mcg

$$\frac{\overset{2}{\cancel{200\text{ mcg}}}}{\underset{1}{\cancel{100\text{ mcg}}}} \times 1 \text{ tab} = 2 \text{ tablets}$$

◀ ***Learning Aid***
Move decimal three places to the right.

0.100 = 100 mcg

7. Equivalent 0.2 g = 200 mg
g > mg

$$\frac{\overset{1}{\cancel{200\text{ mg}}}}{\underset{2}{\cancel{400\text{ mg}}}} \times 1 \text{ tab} = \frac{1}{2} \text{ tablet}$$

◀ ***Learning Aid***
Move decimal point three places to the right.

0.200 = 200 mg

Important! Do not *invert the numbers in the answer. The answer is*

$\frac{1}{2}$ tablet, *not* 2 tablets.

8. No equivalent necessary

$$\frac{\overset{1}{\cancel{200{,}000\text{ units}}}}{\underset{2}{\cancel{400{,}000\text{ units}}}} = \frac{1}{2} \text{ tablet}$$

9. No equivalent necessary

$$\frac{\overset{2}{0.5\cancel{0}\text{ mg}}}{\underset{1}{0.2\cancel{5}\text{ mg}}} \times 1 \text{ tab} = 2 \text{ tablets}$$

◀ ***Learning Aid***

$$0.25\overline{)0.50} = 2.$$
50
0

10. No equivalent necessary

$$\frac{\overset{3}{\cancel{60}\text{ mg}}}{\underset{2}{\cancel{40}\text{ mg}}} \times 1 \text{ tab} = 1\frac{1}{2} \text{ tablets}$$

◀ ***Learning Aid***

$$40\overline{)60.0} = 1.5$$
40
200
200
0

Self-Test 2

1. Rule: $\frac{D}{H} \times S = A$

Equivalent 0.75 g = 750 mg

$$\frac{\overset{3}{\cancel{750}\text{ mg}}}{\underset{1}{\cancel{250}\text{ mg}}} \times 5 \text{ mL} = 15 \text{ mL}$$

◀ ***Learning Aid***
Calculations may be done in different ways. Answers should be the same regardless of the method chosen to solve the problem.

2. No equivalent necessary

$$\frac{\overset{2}{\cancel{500}\text{ mg}}}{\underset{1}{\cancel{250}\text{ mg}}} \times 5 \text{ mL} = 10 \text{ mL}$$

◀ ***Learning Aid***
Alternate arithmetic

500 × 5 = 2500

$$250\overline{)2500.} = 10.$$
250
0

3. Equivalent 0.35 Gm = 350 mg

$$\frac{\overset{14}{\cancel{350}\text{ mg}}}{\underset{\underset{1}{\cancel{25}}}{\cancel{125}\text{ mg}}} \times \overset{1}{\cancel{5}}\text{ mL} = 14 \text{ mL}$$

◀ ***Learning Aid***
Alternate arithmetic

350 × 5 = 1750

$$125\overline{)1750.} = 14.$$
125
500
500
0

4. No equivalent necessary

$$\frac{\overset{3}{\cancel{150}\text{ mg}}}{\underset{2}{\cancel{100}\text{ mg}}} \times 1 \text{ mL} = \frac{3}{2} = 1.5 \text{ mL}$$

◀ ***Learning Aid***
Alternate arithmetic

$$100\overline{)150.0} = 1.5$$
100
500
500

5. No equivalent necessary

$$\frac{\overset{6}{\cancel{300}\text{ mg}}}{\underset{\underset{1}{\cancel{50}}}{\cancel{250}\text{ mg}}} \times \overset{1}{\cancel{5}}\text{ mL} = 6 \text{ mL}$$

◀ ***Learning Aid***
Alternate arithmetic

300 × 5 = 1500

$$250\overline{)1500.} = 6.$$
1500
0

6. No equivalent necessary

$$\frac{0.02\ \text{mg}}{0.05\ \text{mg}} \times 1\ \text{mL} = \frac{2}{5} = 0.4\ \text{mL}$$

◀ ***Learning Aid***

$0.05\overline{)0.020}$ = 0.4; 20; 0

7. No equivalent necessary

$$\frac{30\ \text{mEq}}{20\ \text{mEq}} \times 15\ \text{mL} = \frac{45}{2} \quad 2\overline{)45.0} = 22.5 = 22.5\ \text{mL}$$

8. No equivalent necessary

$$\frac{\overset{1}{0.25\ \text{mg}}}{\underset{1}{\underset{2}{0.50\ \text{mg}}}} \times \overset{5}{10}\ \text{mL} = 5\ \text{mL}$$

◀ ***Learning Aid***

0.25 × 10 = 2.5

$0.5\overline{)2.5}$ = 5.; 25

9. No equivalent necessary

$$\frac{30\ \text{mg}}{10\ \text{mg}} \times 5\ \text{mL} = 15\ \text{mL}$$

◀ ***Learning Aid***
Alternate arithmetic

30 × 5 = 150

$10\overline{)150.}$ = 15.; 10; 50; 50

10. No equivalent necessary

$$\frac{\overset{10}{12.5\ \text{mg}}}{\underset{1}{\underset{1.25}{6.25\ \text{mg}}}} \times \overset{1}{5}\ \text{mL} = 10\ \text{mL}$$

◀ ***Learning Aid***
Alternate arithmetic

12.5 × 5 = 62.5

$6.25\overline{)62.50}$ = 10.; 625; 0

Self-Test 3

1. 2 tablets
2. $\frac{1}{2}$ tablet
3. 2 tablets
4. 2 tablets
5. 2 tablets
6. $\frac{1}{2}$ tablet
7. 1 tablet
8. 1 tablet
9. $\frac{1}{2}$ tablet
10. 2 tablets
11. 2 tablets
12. 1 tablet
13. $\frac{1}{2}$ tablet
14. 2 tablets

Self-Test 4

1. 10 mL
2. 25 cc
3. 10 mL
4. 5 mL
5. 15 mL
6. 20 cc
7. 15 mL
8. 5 mL
9. 6 mL
10. 2.5 mL

Proficiency Test 1

1. $\dfrac{\overset{10}{\cancel{20}}\text{ mEq}}{\underset{\underset{1}{\cancel{2}}}{\cancel{30}}\text{ mEq}} \times \overset{1}{\cancel{15}}\text{ mL} = 10\text{ mL}$

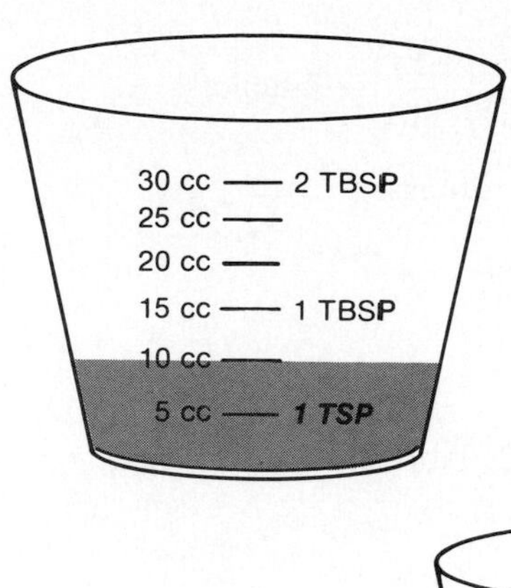

2. $\dfrac{\overset{2}{\cancel{150}}\text{ mg}}{\underset{1}{\cancel{75}}\text{ mg}} \times 7.5\text{ mL} = 15\text{ mL}$

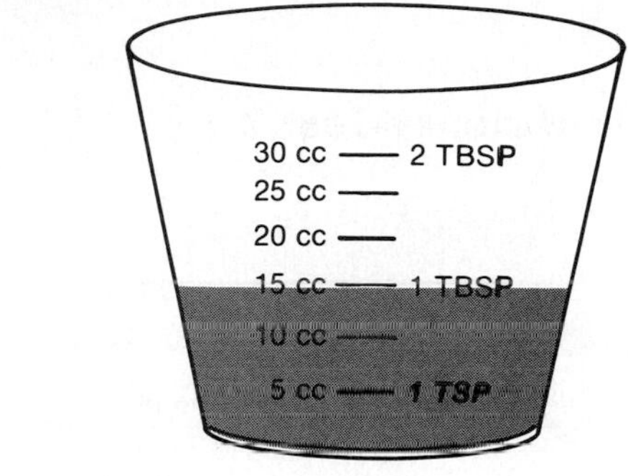

3. $\dfrac{\overset{1}{0.125}\text{ mg}}{\underset{\underset{1}{\cancel{2}}}{0.250}\text{ mg}} \times \overset{5}{\cancel{10}} = 5\text{ mL}$

Alternate arithmetic

$0.25\overline{)0.12\,5}^{\;.5} \times 10\text{ mL} = 5\text{ mL}$
$\quad\quad 12\,5$

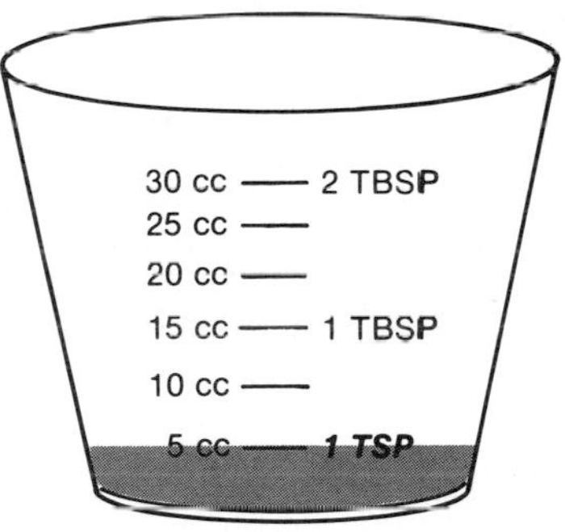

4. $\dfrac{\overset{2}{\cancel{150}}\text{ mg}}{\underset{1}{\cancel{75}}\text{ mg}} \times 6\text{ mL} = 12\text{ mL} = 3\text{ drams}$

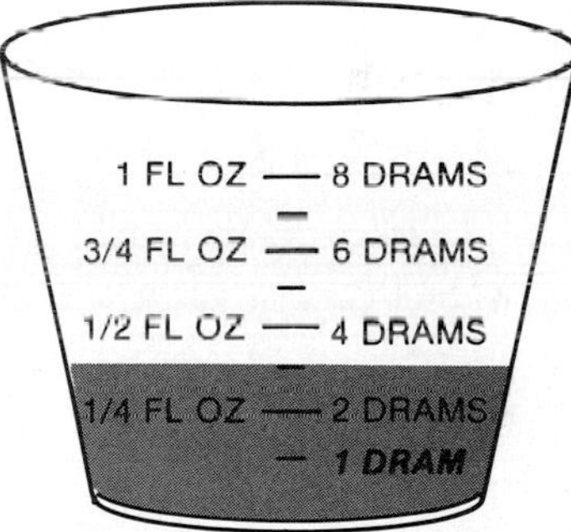

5. $\dfrac{\overset{5}{\cancel{10}}\text{ mg}}{\underset{1}{\cancel{2}}\text{ mg}} \times 5\text{ mL} = 25\text{ mL}$

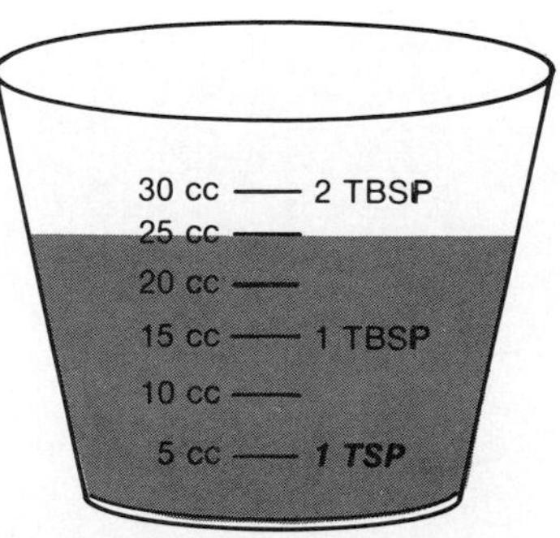

6. Rule: $\frac{D}{H} \times S = A$

$\frac{0.50 \text{ mg}}{0.25 \text{ mg}} \times 1 \text{ tab} = 0.25\overline{)0.50}$ = 2. 2 tablets

7. Equivalent 0.02 mg = 20 μg

$\frac{\overset{1}{10\ \mu g}}{\underset{2}{20\ \mu g}} \times 1 \text{ tab} = \frac{1}{2} \text{ tablet}$

8. $\frac{\overset{5}{250 \text{ mg}}}{\underset{2}{100 \text{ mg}}} \times 1 \text{ tab} = \frac{5}{2} = 2\frac{1}{2}$ tablets.

9. Equivalent 0.5 g = 500 mg

$\frac{\overset{2}{500 \text{ mg}}}{\underset{1}{250 \text{ mg}}} \times 1 \text{ tab} = 2 \text{ tablets}$

10. Equivalent 0.3 mg = 300 μg

$\frac{\overset{1}{300\ \mu g}}{\underset{1}{300\ \mu g}} \times 1 \text{ tab} = 1 \text{ tablet}$

Proficiency Test 2

1. Rule: $\frac{D}{H} \times S = A$

Equivalent 0.8 gm = 800 mg

$\frac{\overset{2}{800 \text{ mg}}}{\underset{1}{400 \text{ mg}}} \times 1 \text{ tab} = 2 \text{ tablets}$

2. Equivalent 0.3 Gm = 300 mg

$\frac{\overset{1}{300 \text{ mg}}}{\underset{1}{300 \text{ mg}}} \times 1 \text{ tab} = 1 \text{ tablet}$

3. $\frac{\overset{3}{600 \text{ mg}}}{\underset{2}{400 \text{ mg}}} \times 1 \text{ tablet} = \frac{3}{2} = 1.5 \text{ or } 1\frac{1}{2} \text{ tablets}$

4. 0.65 Gm = 650 mg

$\frac{\overset{2}{650 \text{ mg}}}{\underset{1}{325 \text{ mg}}} \times 1 \text{ tablet} = 2 \text{ tablets}$

5. $\frac{\overset{1}{250 \text{ mg}}}{\underset{2}{500 \text{ mg}}} \times 1 \text{ tablet} = \frac{1}{2} \text{ tablet}$

6. Equivalent 1 tsp = 5 mL

$\frac{\overset{16}{80 \text{ mg}}}{\underset{1}{25 \text{ mg}}} \times \overset{1}{5} \text{ mL} = 16 \text{ ml} = 4 \text{ drams}$

Alternate arithmetic

80 × 5 = 400

$$\begin{array}{r} 16. \\ 25\overline{)400.} \\ 25 \\ \hline 150 \\ 150 \\ \hline 0 \end{array}$$

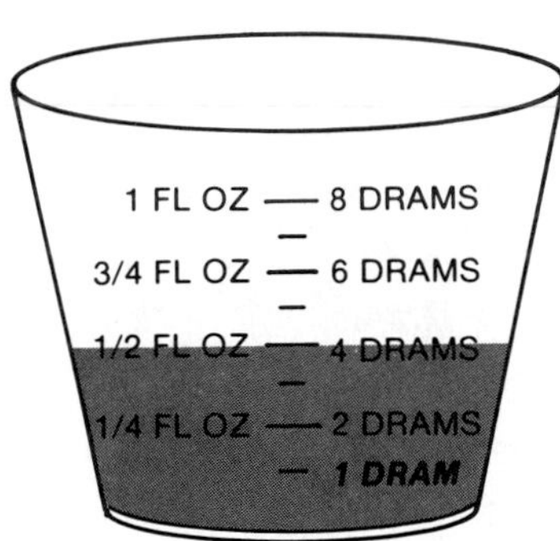

7. Equivalent 0.75 Gm = 750 mg

$\frac{\overset{3}{750 \text{ mg}}}{\underset{1}{250 \text{ mg}}} \times 5 \text{ ml} = 15 \text{ mL}$

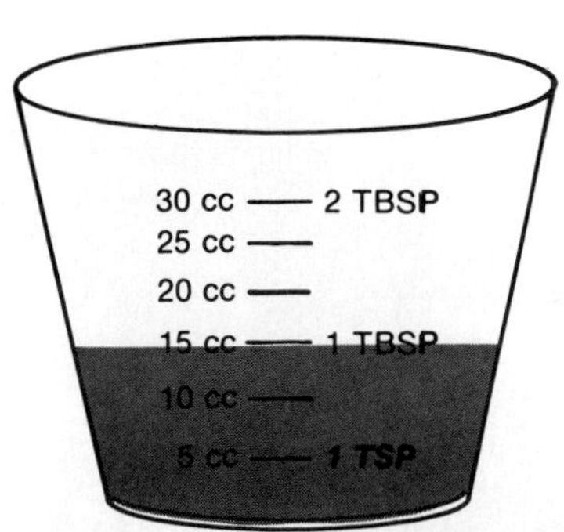

8. $\frac{\overset{12}{\cancel{600}} \text{ mg}}{\underset{1}{\cancel{250}} \text{ mg}} \times \overset{1}{\cancel{5}} \text{mL} = 12 \text{ mL}$

Alternate arithmetic

600 × 5 = 3000

$$\begin{array}{r} 12. \\ 250\overline{)3000.} \\ \underline{250} \\ 500 \\ \underline{500} \\ 0 \end{array}$$

12 ml = 3 drams

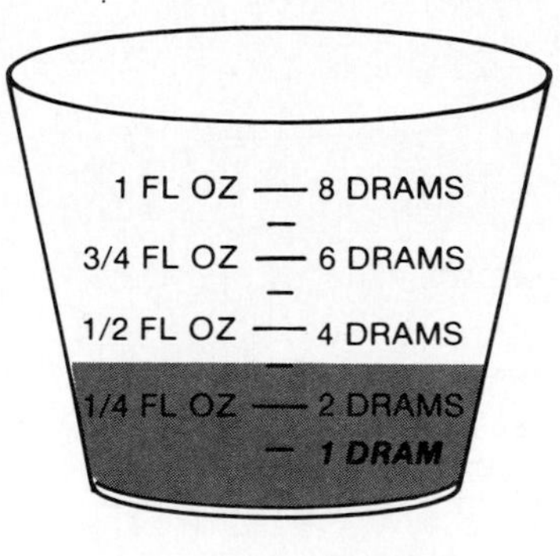

9. No arithmetic necessary Compounded drug. Pour 30 mL.

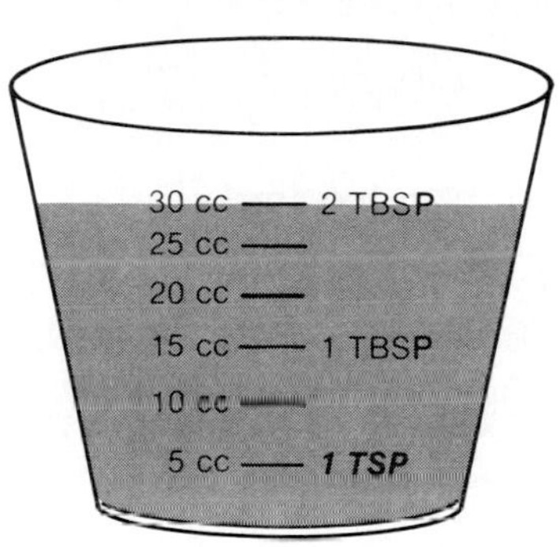

10. $\frac{\overset{2}{\cancel{160}} \text{ mg}}{\underset{1}{\cancel{80}} \text{ mg}} \times 15 \text{ mL} = 30 \text{ mL}$

Proficiency Test 3

1. $\frac{\overset{10}{\cancel{20}} \text{ mEq}}{\underset{1}{\cancel{30}} \text{ mEq}} \times \overset{1}{\cancel{15}} \text{ mL} = 10 \text{ mL}$

2. $\frac{80 \text{ mg}}{\underset{25}{\cancel{125}} \text{ mg}} \times \overset{1}{\cancel{5}} \text{mL} = \frac{\overset{16}{\cancel{80}}}{\underset{5}{\cancel{25}}} = \frac{\cancel{16}}{5} \; 5\overline{)16.0}^{\,3.2} = 3.2 \text{ mL}$

If you do not have a dropper bottle, you could use a syringe without the needle to obtain the dose.

3. 0.02 g = 20 mg

$\frac{\cancel{20} \text{ mg}}{\cancel{10} \text{ mg}} \times 1 \text{ tab} = 2 \text{ tablets}$

4. 0.5 g = 500 mg

$\frac{\overset{2}{\cancel{500}} \text{ mg}}{\underset{1}{\cancel{250}} \text{ mg}} \times 1 \text{ cap} = 2 \text{ capsules}$

5. $\frac{\overset{2}{0.\cancel{50}} \text{ mg}}{\underset{1}{0.\cancel{25}} \text{ mg}} \times 1 \text{ tab} = 2 \text{ tablets}$

6. 100 mcg = 0.1 mg

$\frac{0.1 \text{ mg}}{0.\cancel{2} \text{ mg}} \times \overset{5}{\cancel{10}} \text{ mL} = 5 \text{ mL}$

7. $\frac{\overset{1}{\cancel{3}}\;\cancel{75} \text{ mg}}{\underset{2}{\cancel{50}} \text{ mg}} \times 1 \text{ tab} = \frac{\cancel{3}}{2} \; 2\overline{)3.0}^{\,1.5} = 1\frac{1}{2} \text{ tablets}$

8. $\frac{\overset{1}{\cancel{40}} \text{ mg}}{\underset{2}{\cancel{80}} \text{ mg}} \times 1 \text{ tab} = \frac{1}{2} \text{ tablet}$

9. 0.125 mg = 125 μg

$\frac{\overset{1}{\cancel{125}} \; \mu g}{\underset{2}{\cancel{4}}\;\cancel{500} \; \mu g} \times \overset{5}{\cancel{10}} \text{ mL} = \frac{\cancel{5}}{2} \; 2\overline{)5.0}^{\,2.5} = 2.5 \text{ mL}$

10. $\frac{\overset{3}{\cancel{75}} \text{ mg}}{\underset{1}{\cancel{2}}\;\cancel{50} \text{ mg}} \times \overset{5}{\cancel{10}} \text{ mL} = 15 \text{ mL}$

11. $\frac{5\ \text{mg}}{2\ \text{mg}} \times 1\ \text{tab} = \frac{\cancel{5}\ \ 2.5}{2\ )5.0} = 2\frac{1}{2}$ tablets

12. 0.15 mg = 150 μg

$\frac{\overset{1}{\cancel{150}}\ \mu\text{g}}{\underset{2}{\cancel{300}}\ \mu\text{g}} \times 1\ \text{tab} = \frac{1}{2}$ tablet

13. $\frac{\overset{3}{\cancel{375}}\ \text{mg}}{\underset{2}{\cancel{250}}\ \text{mg}} \times 1\ \text{tab} = \frac{\cancel{3}\ \ 1.5}{2\ )3.0} = 1\frac{1}{2}$ tablets

14. 0.6 g = 600 mg

$\frac{\overset{2}{\cancel{600}}\ \text{mg}}{\underset{1}{\cancel{300}}\ \text{mg}} \times 1\ \text{tab} = 2$ tablets

15. $\frac{\overset{3}{\cancel{1.5}}\ \text{mg}}{\underset{1}{\cancel{\underset{2}{1.0}}}\ \text{mg}} \times \overset{4}{\cancel{8}}\ \text{mL} = 12$ mL; pour 3 drams!

16. $\frac{\overset{2}{\cancel{25.0}}\ \text{mg}}{\underset{1}{\cancel{12.5}}\ \text{mg}} \times 5\ \text{mL} = 10\ \text{mL}$

17. $\frac{\overset{3}{\cancel{60}}\ \text{mg}}{\underset{2}{\cancel{40}}\ \text{mg}} \times 0.6\ \text{mL} = \frac{1.8}{2} = 0.9\ \text{mL}$

18. 0.5 g = 500 mg

$\frac{\overset{2}{\cancel{500}}\ \text{mg}}{\underset{1}{\cancel{250}}\ \text{mg}} \times 5\ \text{mL} = 10\ \text{mL}$

19. $\frac{\overset{3}{\cancel{150}}\ \text{mg}}{\underset{1}{\cancel{50}}\ \text{mg}} \times 5\ \text{mL} = 15\ \text{mL}$

20. $\frac{\overset{3}{\cancel{7.5}}\ \text{mg}}{\underset{4}{\cancel{10.0}}\ \text{mg}} \times 5\ \text{mL} = \frac{\cancel{15}\ \ 3.75}{4\ )15.00} = 3.8\ \text{mL}$

If you do not have a dropper, use a syringe minus the needle to get the dose.

7 Liquids for Injection

CONTENT TO MASTER

The rule for solving injection-from-liquid problems is

$$\frac{\text{Desire}}{\text{Have}} \times \text{Stock} = \text{Amount}$$

The marks on the syringe determine the accuracy of calculations.

- 3 cc syringe—nearest tenth
- 1 cc precision syringe—nearest hundredth
- insulin syringes—units

Mixing two insulins requires special technique

Liquids for injection may be labeled:

- solutions of g or mg per mL
- as ratio
- as percent

Liquid drugs for injection are prepared by pharmaceutical companies as sterile solutions or suspensions. Sterile techniques are used to prepare and administer them. As with oral medications, the nurse may be required to calculate the correct dosage.

RULE

CALCULATING LIQUID INJECTIONS

The rule used to solve liquid injection problems is the same as that for oral solids and liquids.

$$\frac{\text{Desire}}{\text{Have}} \times \text{Stock} = \text{Amount}$$

EXAMPLE Order: Demerol HCl 75 mg IM q4h prn

Label:

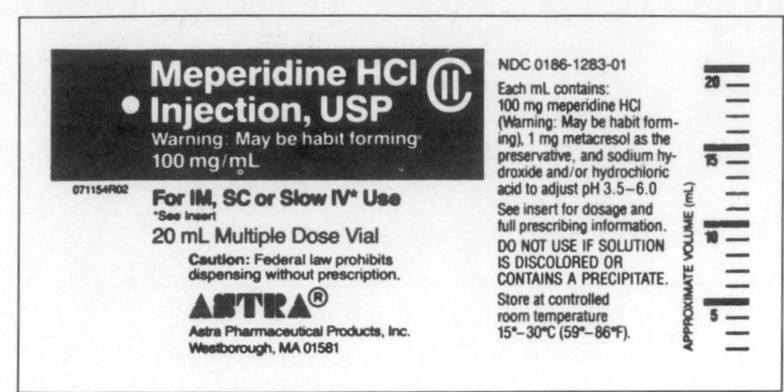

Desire is the order—75 mg

Have is the strength of the drug supplied—100 mg

Stock is the unit form of the drug—1 mL

Answer is how much liquid to give by injection in mL.

▼ CALCULATING INJECTION PROBLEMS

3-cc Syringe

The degree of accuracy in calculating injection answers depends on the syringe used. Figure 7-1 shows a 3-cc (3-mL) syringe marked in milliliters to the nearest tenth and in minims to the nearest whole number. *To calculate milliliter answers for this 3-mL syringe, the arithmetic is carried out to the hundredth place and the answer is rounded off to the nearest tenth.*

1.25 mL becomes 1.3 mL

To calculate minims on the 3-mL syringe, the arithmetic is carried out to the tenth place and the answer is rounded off to the nearest whole number.

19.7 minims becomes 20 minims

1-cc Precision Syringe

Figure 7-2 shows a 1-cc (1-mL) precision syringe marked in milliliters to the nearest hundredth and in minims to the nearest half-minim. *To calculate milliliters when the 1-mL syringe is used, the arithmetic is carried out to the thousandth place and the answer is rounded off to the nearest hundredth.*

0.978 mL becomes 0.98 mL

To calculate minims for the 1-mL syringe, the arithmetic is carried out to the nearest hundredth and the answer is reported as the closest half minim.

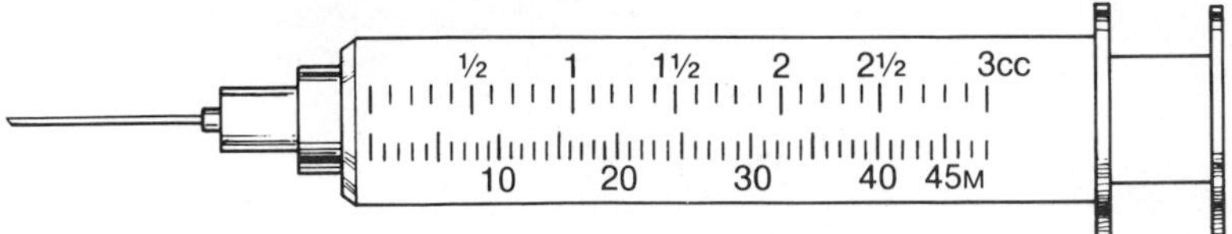

Figure 7-1
A 3-cc (3-mL) syringe.

◀ ***Learning Aid***
Rules for round-off numbers can be reviewed in Chapter 1.

Figure 7-2
A 1-cc (1-mL) syringe.

EXAMPLE 14.28 minims becomes 14 minims. (The answer 14.28 rounds off to 14.3. Because 0.3 is less than 0.5, it is dropped.)

A syringe is provided for each of the examples that follow. Calculate milliliters to the degree of accuracy required by the syringe markings. Calculation of minims is not provided because this is an apothecary measure. *Draw a line on the syringe indicating the answer for milliliters only.*

EXAMPLE Order: Demerol HCl 75 mg IM q4h prn

Label:

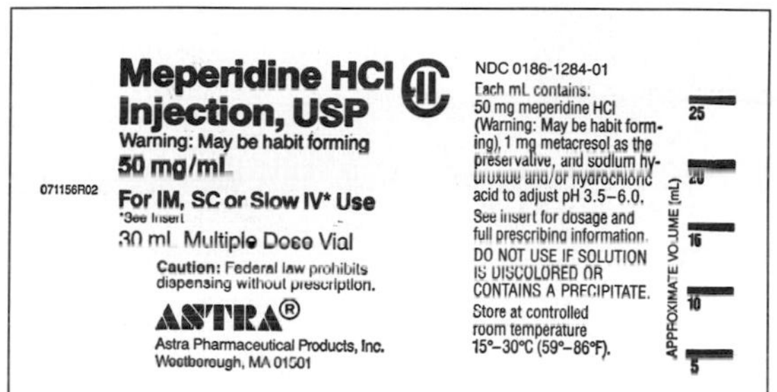

Learning Aid
Calculate answers in milliliters (mL). Avoid minims, an apothecary measure.

Rule: $\frac{D}{H} \times S = A$

$$\frac{\overset{3}{\cancel{75}\ \cancel{mg}}}{\underset{2}{\cancel{50}\ \cancel{mg}}} \times 1\ mL = \frac{3}{2} = 1.5\ mL$$

Give 1.5 mL IM.

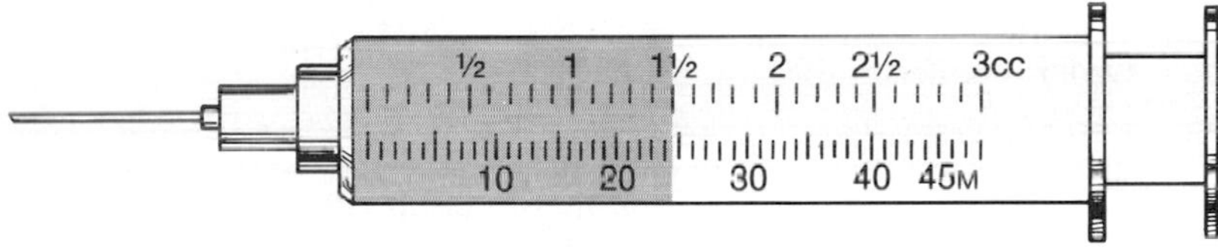

EXAMPLE Order: heparin sodium 1500 units SC bid

Label:

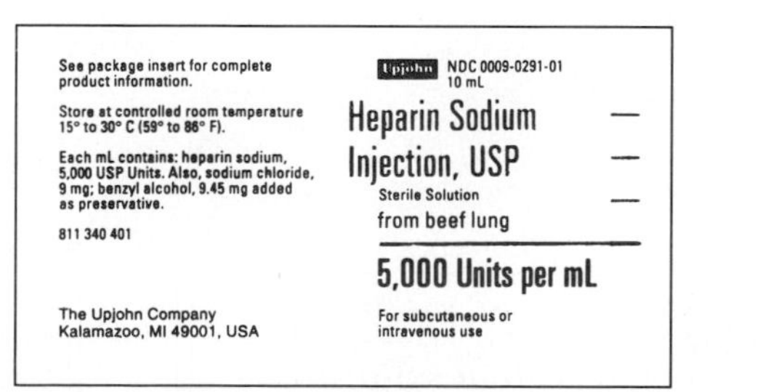

Learning Aid

$$10\overline{)3.0} = .3$$

Rule: $\frac{D}{H} \times S = A$

$$\frac{\overset{3}{\cancel{1500 \text{ units}}}}{\underset{10}{\cancel{5000 \text{ units}}}} \times 1 \text{ mL} = \frac{3}{10} = 0.3 \text{ mL}$$

Give 0.3 mL.

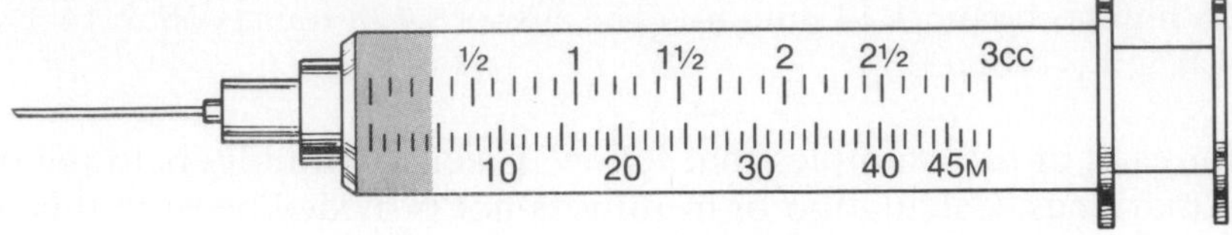

EXAMPLE

Order: Lanoxin 120 mcg IM qd

Label:

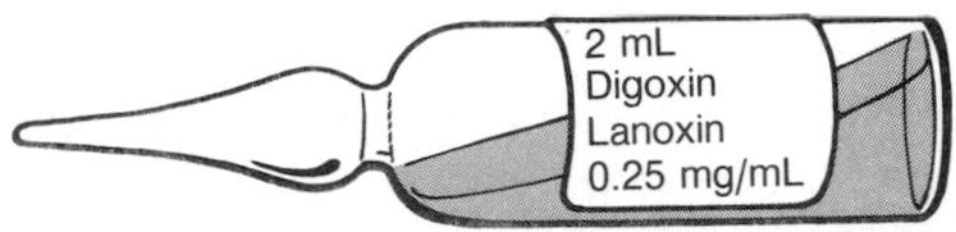

◀ ***Learning Aid***
Since you are using a 1-mL precision syringe, you can draw the medication up to the nearest 100th.

Rule: $\frac{D}{H} \times S = A$

Equivalent: 0.25 mg = 250 mcg

$$\frac{12\cancel{0} \text{ mcg}}{25\cancel{0} \text{ mcg}} \times 1 \text{ mL} = \frac{12}{25} \qquad 25\overline{)12.00} = .48$$

100
200
200

Give 0.48 mL IM.

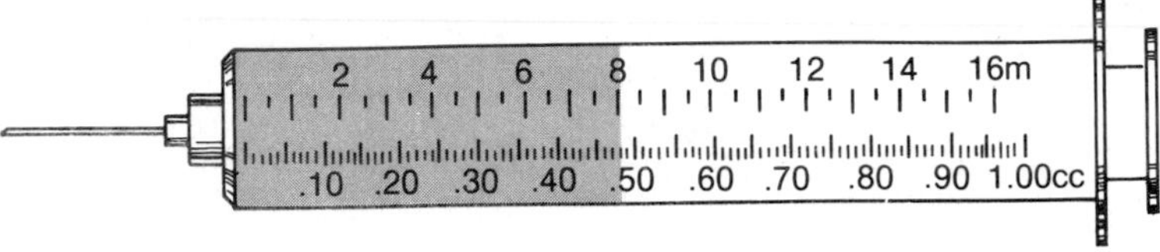

EXAMPLE

Order: Gantrisin 400 mg IM q12h

Label: vial labeled 2 g/5 mL

Logic: You have milligrams in the order and grams in the stock.
Use an equivalent (2 g = 2000 mg).

Rule: $\frac{D}{H} \times S = A$

◀ ***Learning Aid***
Note that the stock contains 2 g in 5 mL.

$$\frac{\overset{1}{\cancel{400 \text{ mg}}}}{\underset{\underset{1}{\cancel{5}}}{\cancel{2000 \text{ mg}}}} \times \overset{1}{\cancel{5}} \text{ mL} = 1 \text{ mL}$$

Give: 1 mL IM.

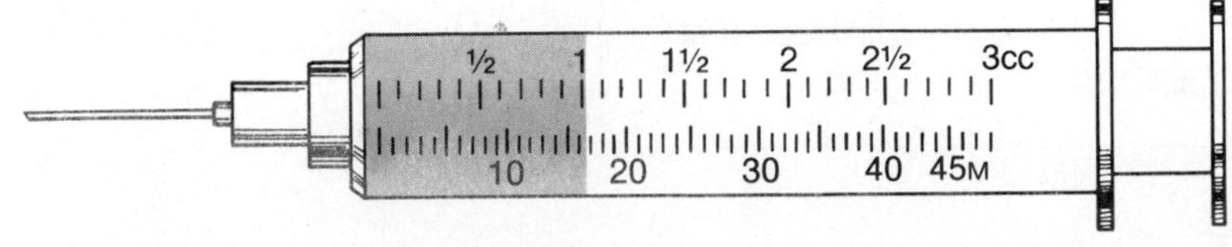

Self-Test 1

Practice calculations of injections from a liquid. Report your answer in milliliters; mark the syringe in milliliters. Answers may be found at the end of the chapter.

1. Order: Cleocin 0.3 Gm IM q6h
   Stock: liquid in a vial labeled 300 mg/2 mL

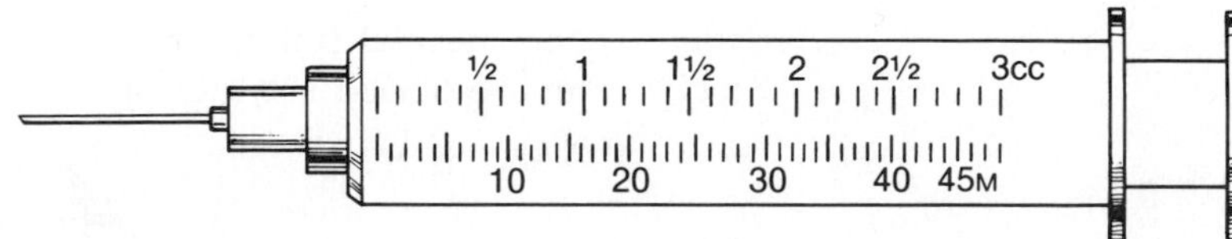

2. Order: morphine SO_4 12 mg SC stat
   Stock: vial of liquid labeled 15 mg/mL

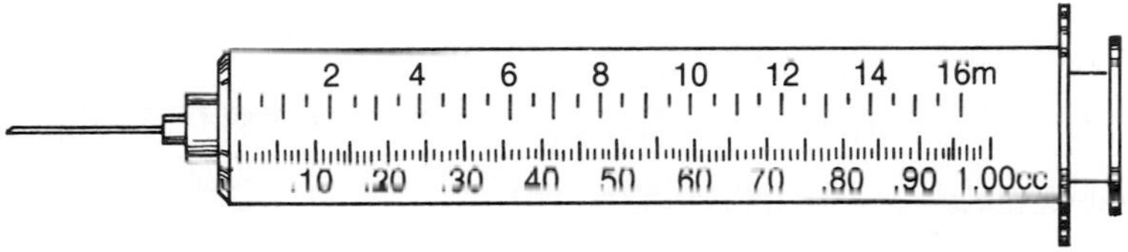

3. Order: vitamin B_{12} 1 mg IM qd
   Stock: vial of liquid labeled 1000 μg/mL

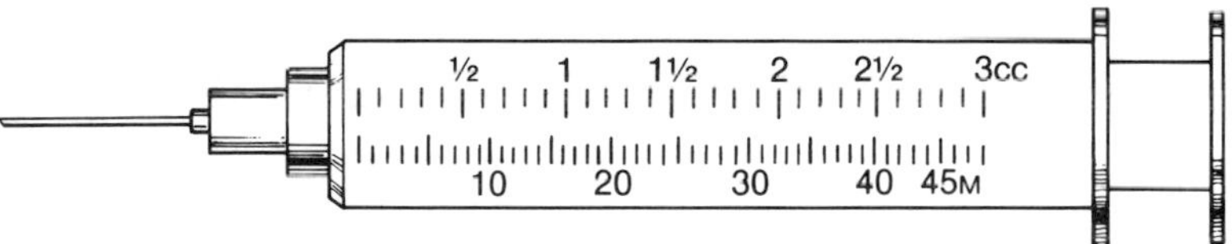

4. Order: gentamicin 9 mg IM q8h
   Stock: pediatric ampule labeled 20 mg/2 mL

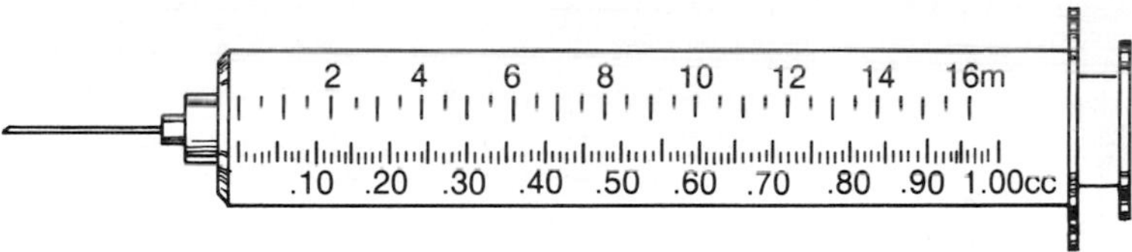

5. Order: digoxin 0.5 mg IM qd
   Stock: vial labeled 0.25 mg/mL

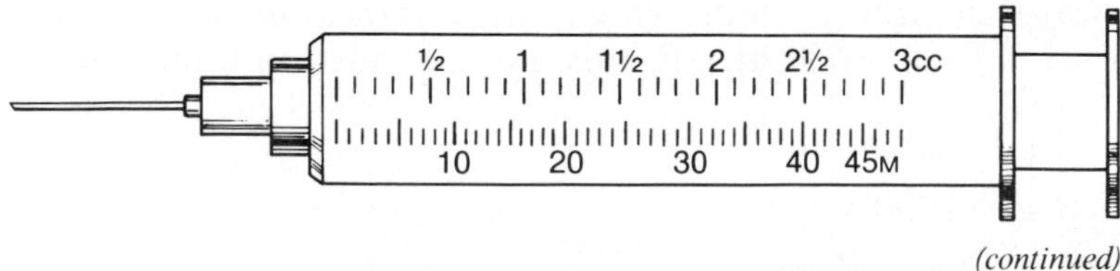

(continued)

Self-Test 1 (continued)

6. Order: gentamicin 50 mg IM q8h
   Stock: vial labeled 40 mg/mL

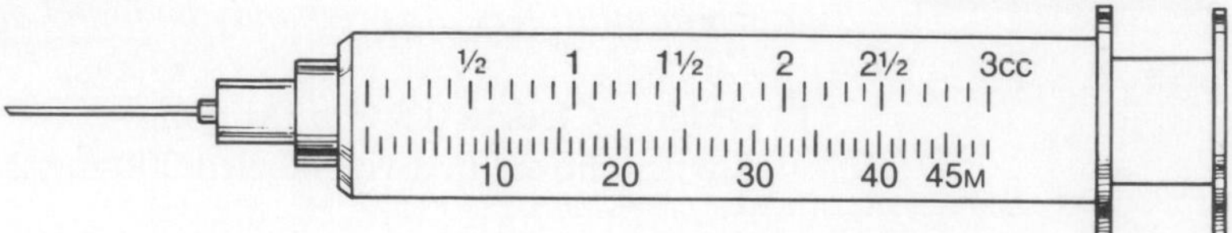

7. Order: phenobarbital 100 mg IM stat
   Stock: ampule labeled 130 mg/mL

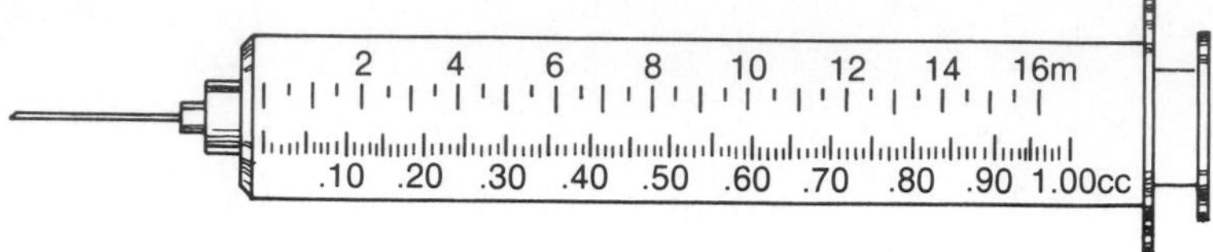

8. Order: Lanoxin 0.25 mg IM stat
   Stock: ampule labeled 0.5 mg/2 mL

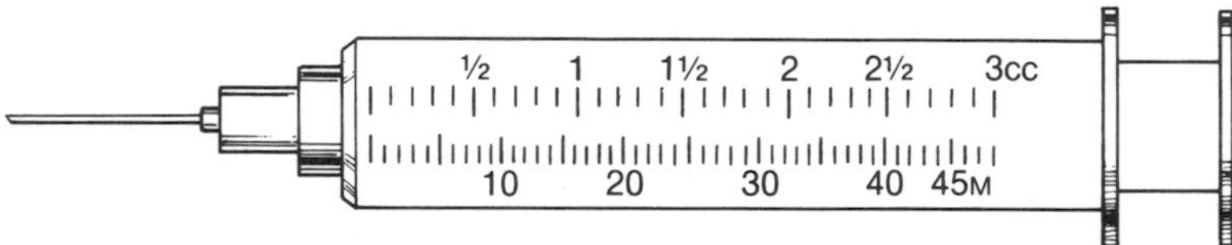

9. Order: heparin 6000 units SC q4h
   Stock: vial labeled 10,000 U/cc

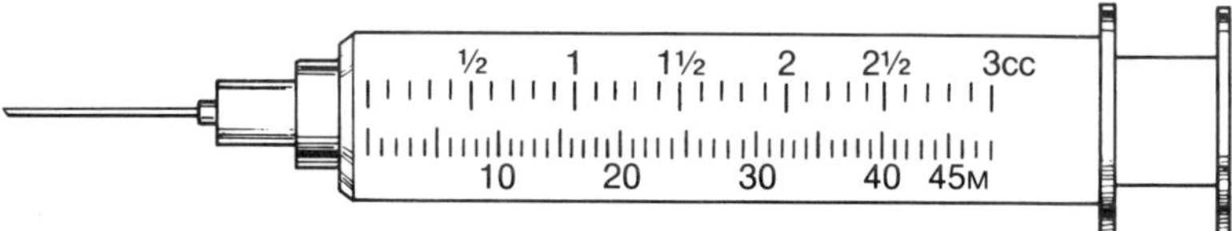

10. Order: tobramycin 70 mg IM q8h
    Stock: ampule labeled 80 mg/2 mL

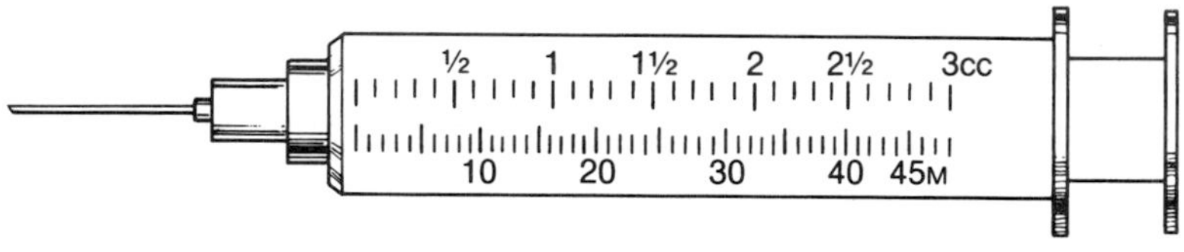

▼ SPECIAL TYPES OF PROBLEMS IN INJECTIONS FROM A LIQUID

When Stock Is a Ratio

Labels may state the strength of a drug as a ratio.

EXAMPLE Adrenalin 1:1000

Ratios are always interpreted in the metric system as grams per milliliters. In the example given, 1:1000 means 1 g in 1000 mL. Ratios may be stated in three ways:

1 g per 1000 mL

1 g = 1000 mL

1 g/1000 mL

Exercise 1 *Write the following ratios in three ways. Answers may be found at the end of the chapter.*

1. 1:20 __________ __________ __________

2. 2:15 __________ __________ __________

3. 1:500 __________ __________ __________

Some nurses have difficulty understanding the meaning of ratio in relation to drugs. A deductive line of reasoning may help to make this clear.

Figure 7-3 shows an ampule of epinephrine that is labeled 2 mL and is a 1:1000 solution. You know that 1:1000 means 1 g in 1000 mL. You also know that 1 g is equivalent to 1000 mg. Therefore, the solution can be interpreted as 1000 mg = 1000 mL. Logic tells you that if there are 1000 mg in 1000 mL, then there is 1 mg in 1 mL.

$$\frac{\cancel{1000}\text{ mg}}{\cancel{1000}\text{ mL}} = \frac{1\text{ mg}}{1\text{ mL}}$$

Because the ampule contains 2 mL, the ampule contains 2 mg of the drug. Be careful reading and writing milligram (mg) and milliliter (mL). Milligram is the solid measure; milliliter is the liquid measure.

EXAMPLE

Example 1:

Order: epinephrine 1 mg SC stat

Label: ampule labeled 1:1000

Equivalent: 1:1000 means
1 g in 1000 mL
1 g = 1000 mg, therefore
stock is 1000 mg = 1000 mL

Rule: $\frac{D}{H} \times S = A$

$$\frac{1\ \cancel{\text{mg}}}{\underset{1}{\cancel{1000}}\ \cancel{\text{mg}}} \times \overset{1}{\cancel{1000}}\text{ mL} = 1\text{ mL}$$

Give: 1 mL SC.

Example 2:

Order: isoproterenol HCl 0.2 mg IM stat

Label: ampule labeled 1:5000

Equivalents: 1:5000 means
1 g in 5000 mL
1 g = 1000 mg

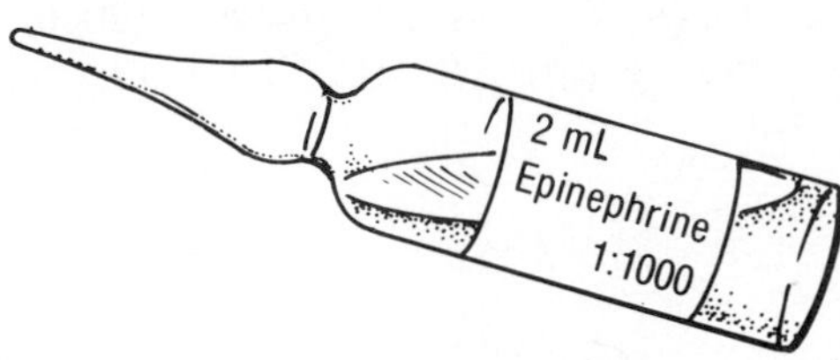

Figure 7-3
A 2-mL ampule of epinephrine 1:1000.

Therefore, the solution is 1000 mg/5000 mL.

Rule: $\frac{D}{H} \times S = A$

$$\frac{0.2\ \cancel{mg}}{\cancel{1000}\ \cancel{mg}} \times \overset{5}{\cancel{5000}}\ mL = \begin{array}{r} 5 \\ \times\ 0.2 \\ \hline 1.0\ mL \end{array}$$

Give: 1 mL IM.

Exercise 2 *Solve these problems involving ratios. Answers may be found at the end of the chapter.*

1. Order: neostigmine 0.5 mg SC
   Stock: ampule labeled 1:2000

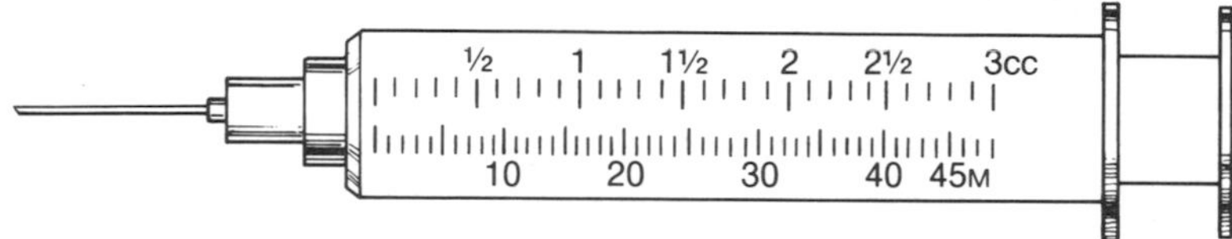

2. Order: Isuprel 1 mg; add to IV
   Stock: vial labeled 1:5000
   A 10-mL syringe is available.

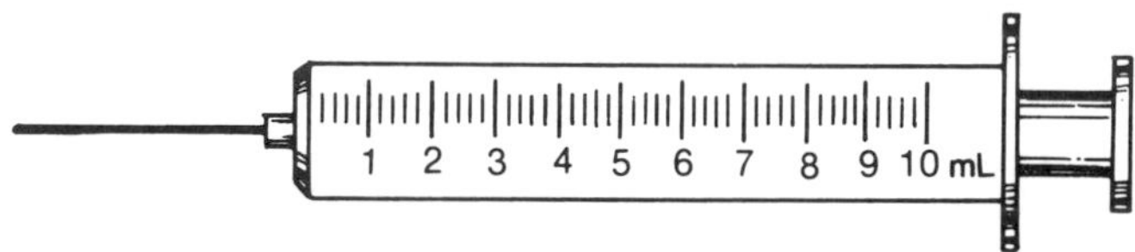

3. Order: neostigmine methylsulfate 0.75 mg SC
   Stock: ampule labeled 1:1000

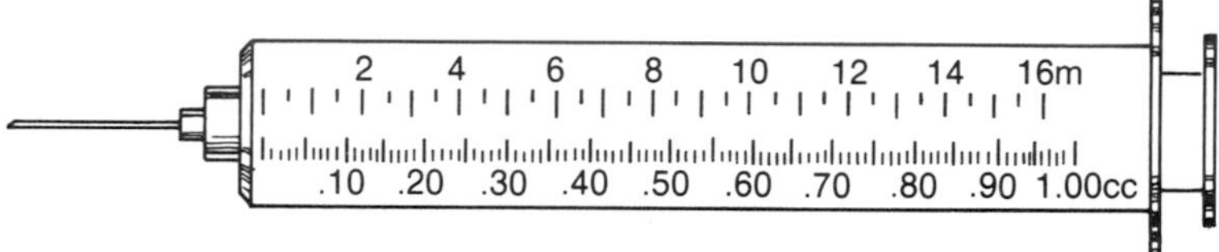

4. Order: ponthaline 50 mg IM
   Stock: ampule labeled 1:20

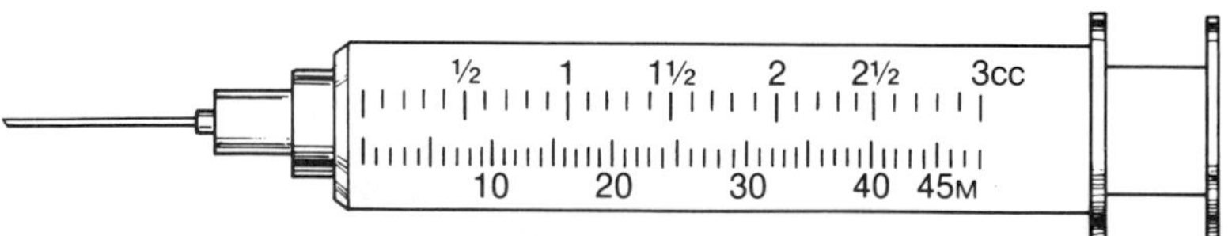

5. Order: neostigmine methylsulfate 1.5 mg IM tid
   Stock: 1:2000

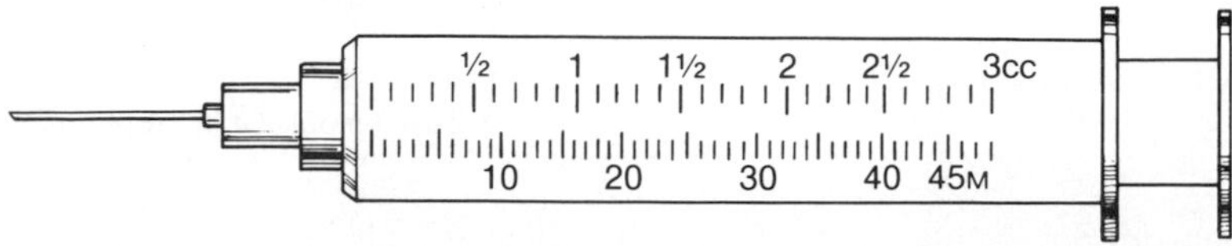

When Stock Is a Percent

Labels may state the strength of a drug as a percent. Percent means parts per hundred. *Percentages are always interpreted in the metric system as grams per 100 mL.*

EXAMPLE Lidocaine 2% (2 g in 100 mL)

Percents may be stated in three ways:

2 g per 100 mL
2 g = 100 mL
2 g/100 mL

Exercise 3 *Write the following percentages in three ways. Answers may be found at the end of the chapter.*

1. 0.9% __________ __________ __________
2. 10% __________ __________ __________
3. 0.45% __________ __________ __________

Percent problems can be solved by applying the meaning of ratio.

EXAMPLE ***Example 1:***

Order: lidocaine 30 mg for injection before suturing wound

Stock: ampule labeled 2%

Equivalents: 2% means
2 g in 100 mL
1 g = 1000 mg
2 g = 2000 mg

Stock is 2000 mg in 100 mL.

Rule: $\frac{D}{H} \times S = A$

$$\frac{\not{3}\!\not{0} \text{ mg}}{\not{2}\not{0}\not{0}\not{0} \text{ mg}} \times \overset{1}{\not{1}\not{0}\not{0}} \text{ mL} = \frac{3}{2} \qquad 2\overline{)3.0}^{\,1.5}$$

Prepare 1.5 mL for physician.

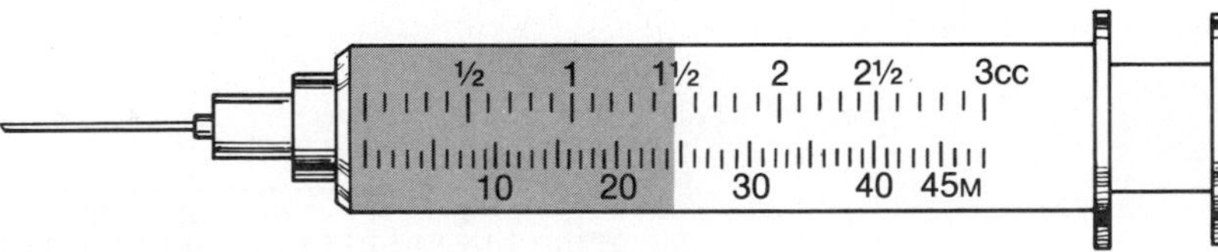

Example 2:

Order: calcium gluconate 1 g; add to IV stat

Stock: vial of liquid labeled 10%

Equivalents: 10% means 10 g in 100 mL

Rule: $\frac{D}{H} \times S = A$

$$\frac{1\ \cancel{g}}{\cancelto{1}{10}\ \cancel{g}} \times \cancelto{10}{100}\ \text{mL} = 10\ \text{mL}$$

Add: 10 mL to IV (Amount is correct. The route is IV, not IM.)

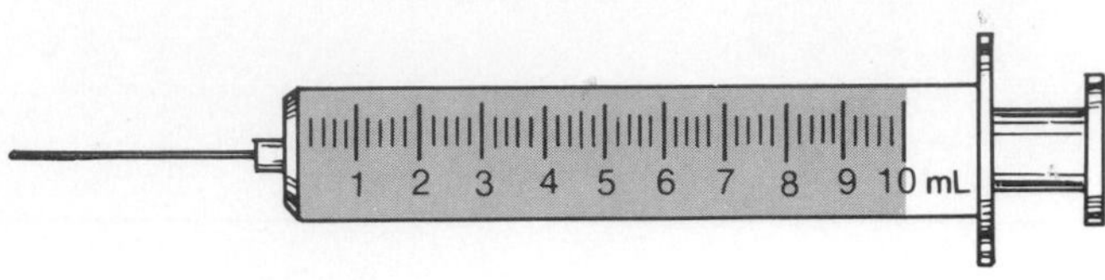

Exercise 4

Solve these problems involving percentages. Answers may be found at the end of the chapter. Answers in milliliters (mL).

1. Order: epinephrine 5 mg SC stat
   Stock: ampule labeled 1%

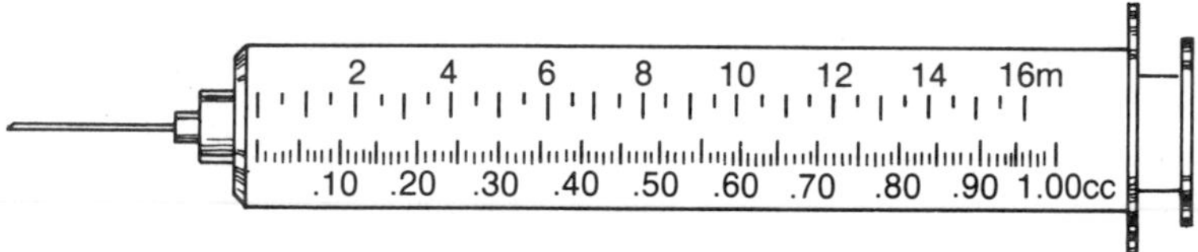

2. Order: Mesterin 2.5 mg IM
   Stock: ampule labeled 0.5%

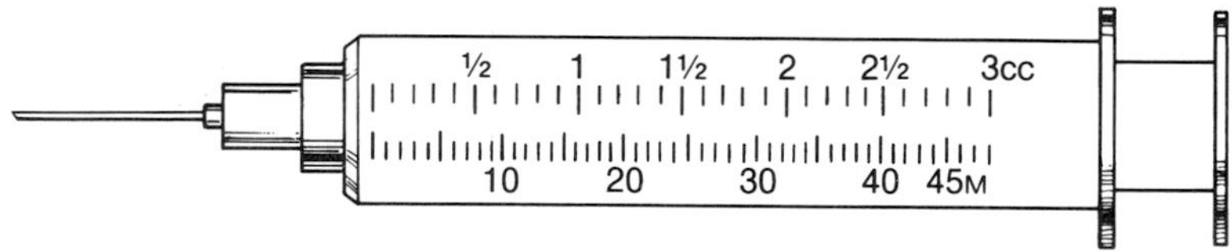

3. Order: phenylephrine HCl 3 mg SC stat
   Stock: ampule labeled 1%

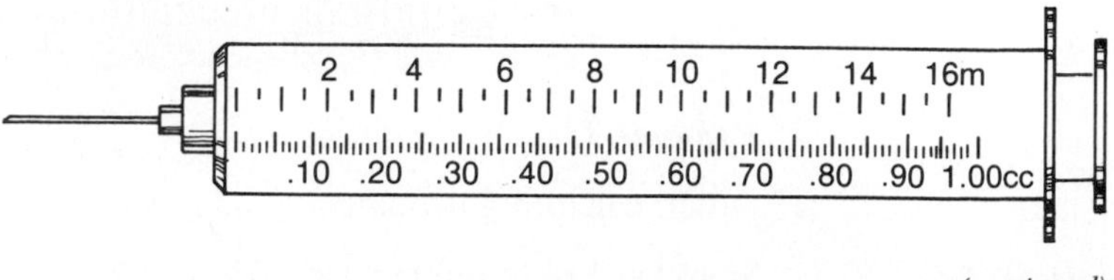

(continued)

Exercise 4 (continued)

4. Order: Prepare for IV use calcium gluconate 0.3 g
   Stock: ampule labeled 10%

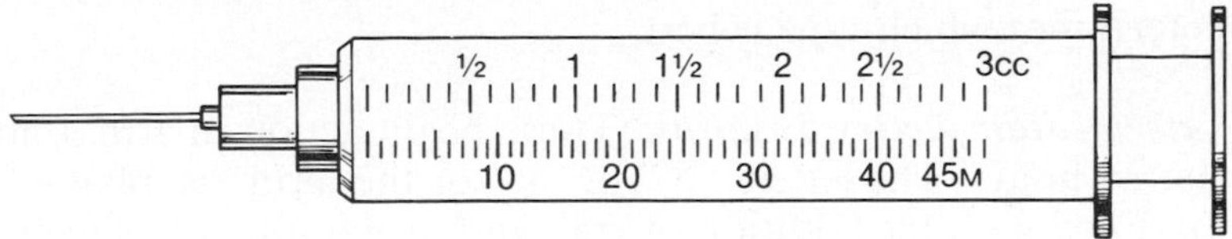

5. Order: Prepare for IV use sodium tetradecyl sulfate 0.015 g
   Stock: ampule labeled 3%

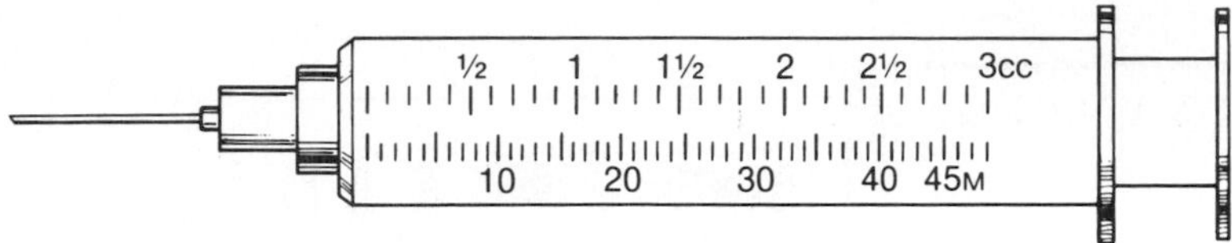

▼ INSULIN INJECTIONS

Types of Insulin

Insulin is a hormone that regulates glucose metabolism. It is measured in units and is administered by injection. Insulin is supplied in 10-mL vials containing 100 units per milliliter. There are many types of insulin currently available. Insulins may be prepared from animal tissue or semisynthetically from human recombinant DNA. Insulins are classified as rapid, intermediate, or long acting. Because onset of action, time of peak activity, and duration of action vary, *nurses must be careful to choose the correct insulin.*

Rapid Acting Insulins. These begin acting within 1 hour and peak in 2 to 4 hours; actions may last 5 to 7 hours. Insulins are administered subcutaneously, except for regular insulin, which can be given IV.

Note the large "R" on the label for quick identification as regular insulin. Regular insulin is prepared from the pancreas of beef or pork or by using recombinant DNA technology.

EXAMPLES

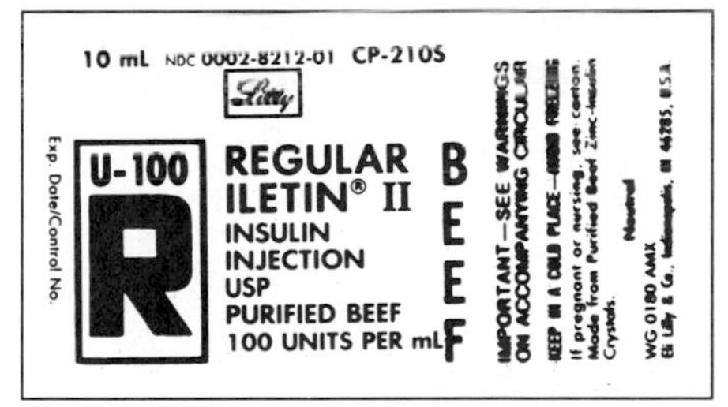

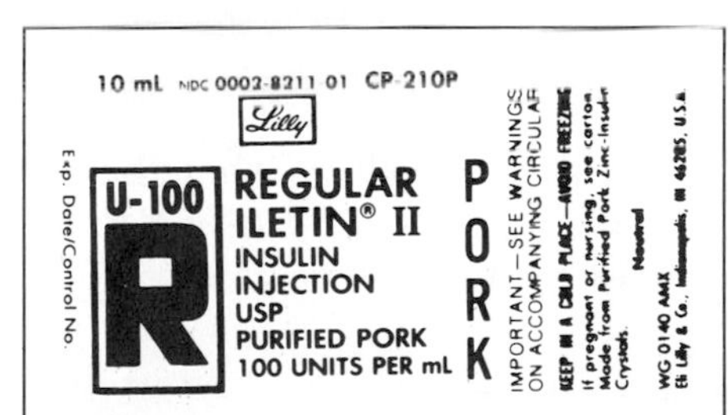

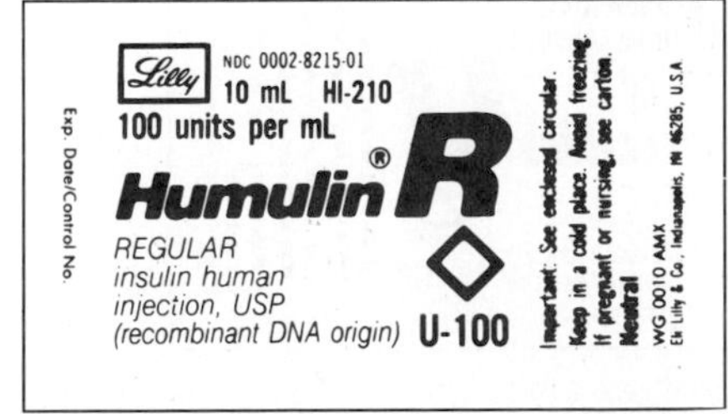

Beef insulins are ordered for patients who are allergic to pork or who avoid pork for religious reasons. Pork insulin can be used for patients with allergies or who develop insulin resistance. These insulins are less expensive than Humulin R, which is a human insulin synthesized in the laboratory. The physician determines which type is best.

Intermediate Acting Insulins. These begin action in 1 to 3 hours, peak around 6 to 12 hours, and may last 24 hours. The letters "N" or "L" or the term "isophane" indicate that regular insulin has been modified with the addition of zinc and protamine to delay absorption and prolong the time of action. These intermediate insulins can be prepared from beef, pork, or Humulin R. The letters NPH are also used to denote an intermediate action. These letters mean the following: N = the solution is neutral pH; P = the protamine content; H = Hagedorn, the laboratory which first prepared this type of insulin.

EXAMPLES

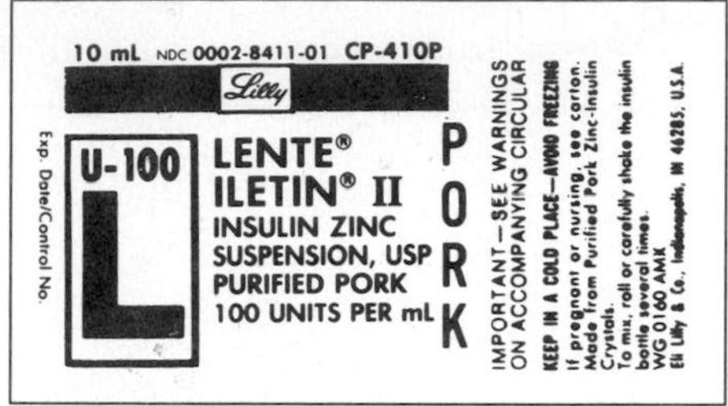

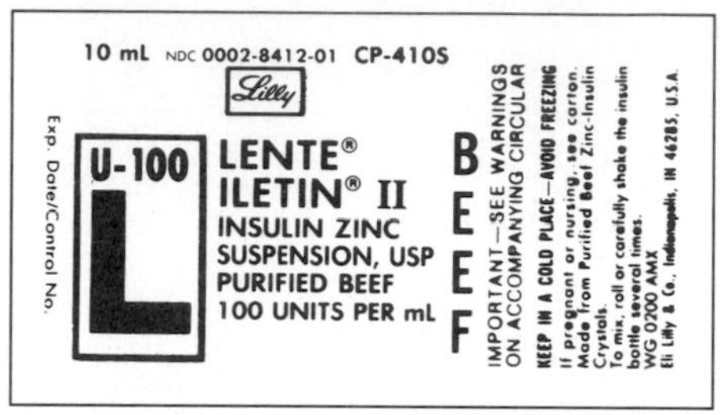

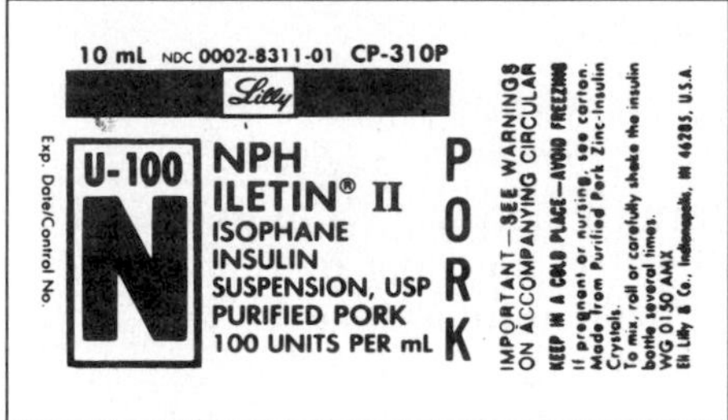

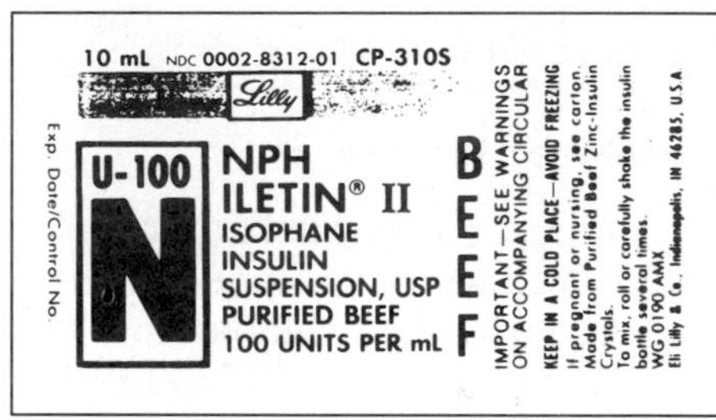

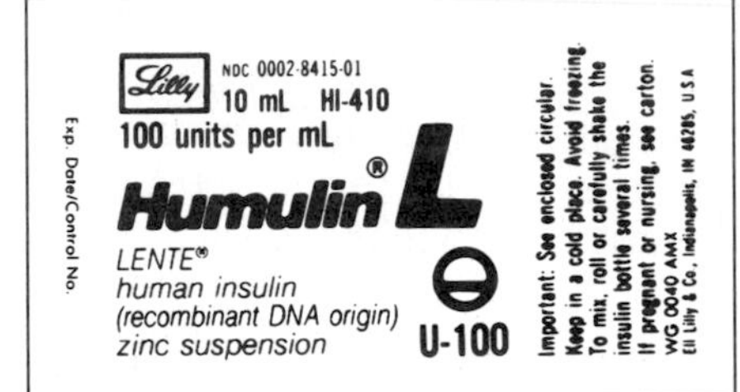

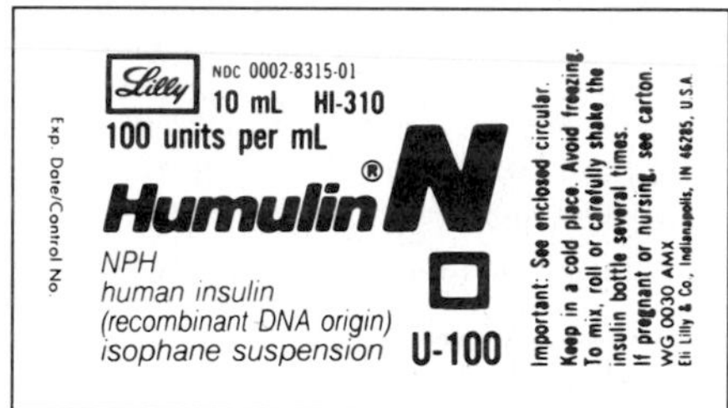

Long Acting Insulins. These have also been modified with the addition of zinc and protamine, a basic protein. These insulins take 4 to 8 hours to act, peak in 12 to 20 hours; duration of action can last as long as 36 hours.

EXAMPLE

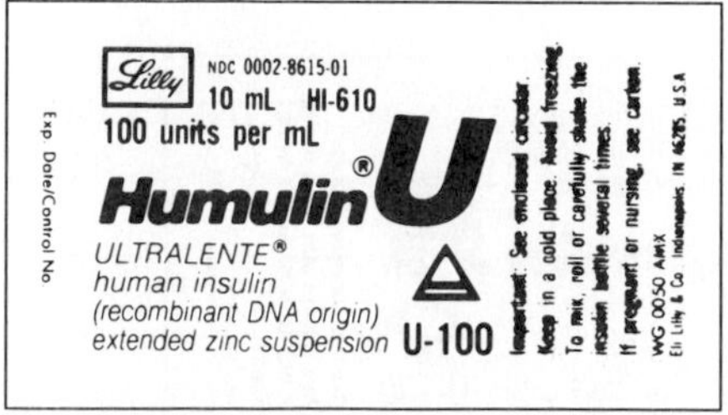

Mixed Insulins. An order may require that two insulins be mixed in one syringe and administered together. Mixed insulins combine rapid and intermediate insulin. They save nursing time in preparation and are more convenient for the patient, who must learn to draw up and self-administer an injection.

EXAMPLES

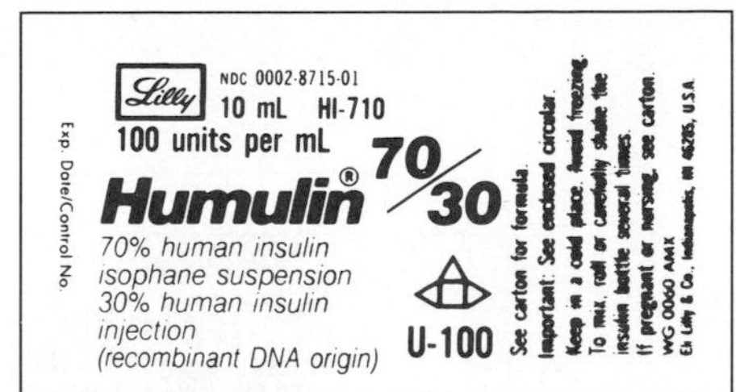

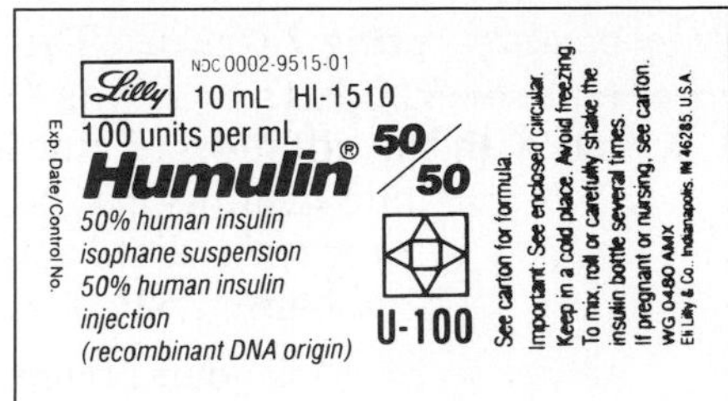

High Potency Insulins. These are manufactured for some patients who require large doses and for emergency situations. These insulins should be carefully stored away from the usual Units-100/mL insulins to protect against error.

EXAMPLE

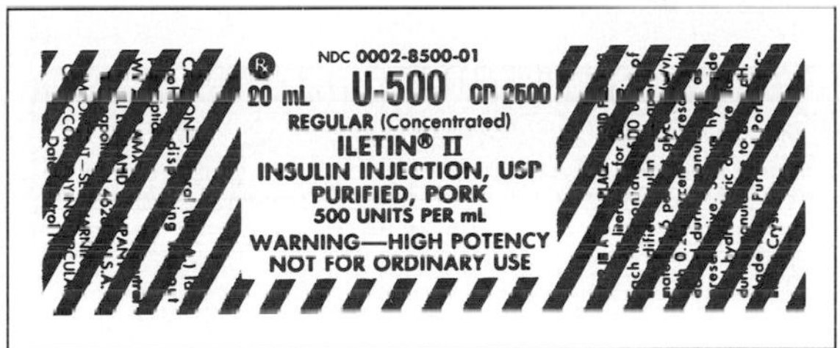

Regular insulin should appear clear and colorless; it is the only insulin that may be given IV. Other insulins appear cloudy. Insulin vials should be gently rotated between the hands to resuspend the particles. *Never shake insulin vials.* This may result in the formation of bubbles or froth and interfere with accurate measurement of the dose ordered.

Types of Insulin Syringes

Insulin doses are administered subcutaneously with an insulin syringe. Two standard syringes are available to measure U 100 insulin. The first measures doses up to 100 units (Fig. 7-4). The second, called a low-dose insulin syringe can be used when the dose is 50 units or less (Fig. 7-5).

Preparing an Injection Using an Insulin Syringe

No calculation is required to prepare an insulin dose. The physician's order is in units; the stock comes in 100 units/mL, and both syringes are calibrated (lined) for 100 units/mL.

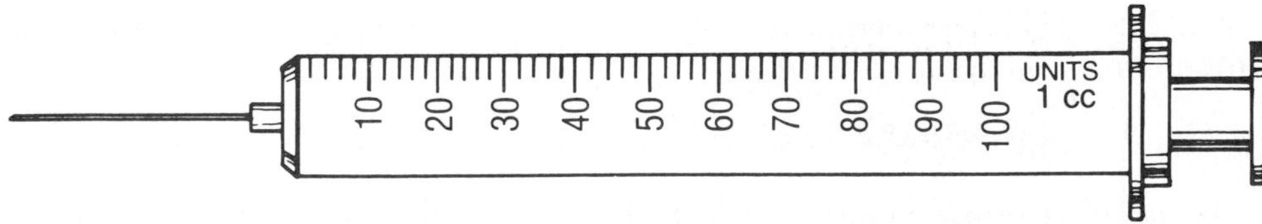

Figure 7-4
1-cc insulin syringe marked in units. Each line equals 2 units.

Figure 7-5
½-cc low dose insulin syringe. Each line equals 1 unit.

EXAMPLE

Example 1:

Order: Units 60 NPH SC qd

Label:

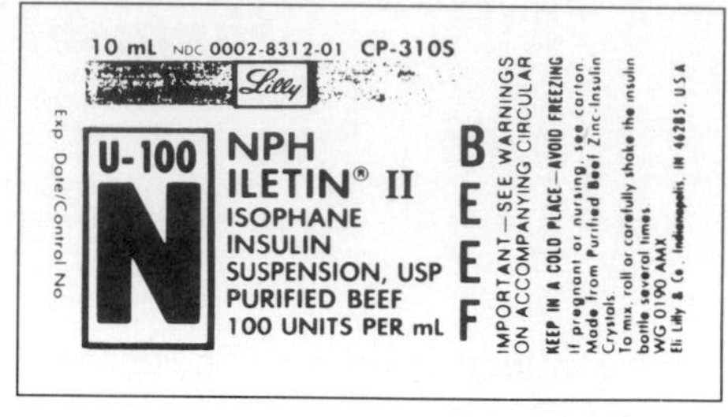

Ask yourself three questions:

1. What is the order? NPH Units 60
2. What is the stock? NPH U 100/mL
3. Is a U 100 insulin syringe available? Yes.

Draw up the amount required into the syringe using sterile technique.

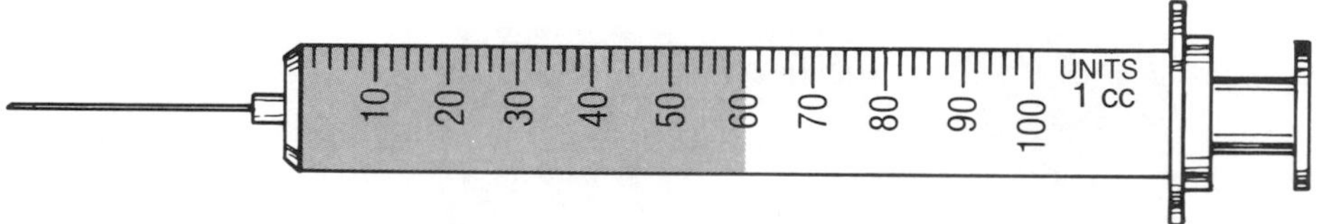

Example 2:

Order: U 35 Regular Insulin SC stat

Label:

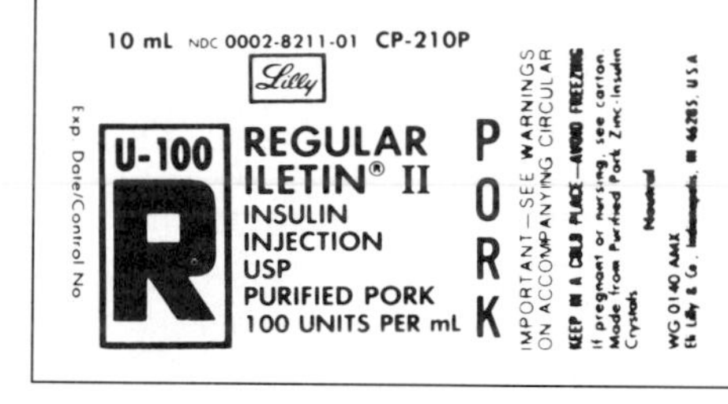

Ask yourself three questions:

1. What is the order? Regular Insulin U 35
2. What is the stock? U 100/mL Regular Insulin
3. What syringe should be used? Low-dose insulin syringe

Draw up the amount required into the syringe using sterile technique.

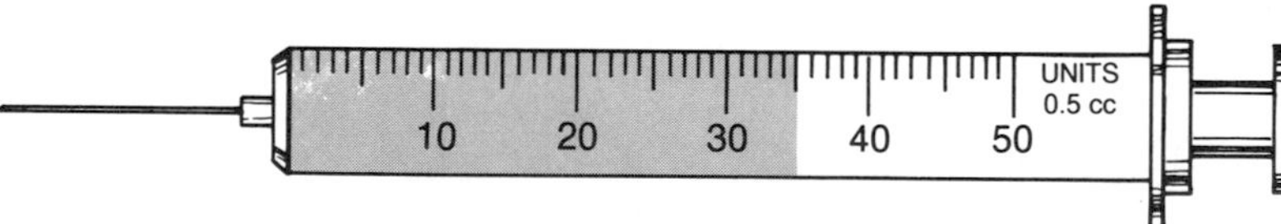

Mixing Two Insulins in One Syringe

Sometimes the physician will order regular insulin to be mixed with another insulin and injected together at the same site. The method of preparing two medications in one syringe is handled later in this book. For now, remember two facts:

1. The regular insulin is always drawn up first into the syringe.
2. The total number of units in the syringe will be the addition of the two insulin orders.

EXAMPLE

Order: Regular Humulin Insulin Units 15 } qd SC
NPH Humulin Insulin Units 10 }

Label: Regular Humulin Insulin U 100/mL
NPH Humulin insulin U 100/mL

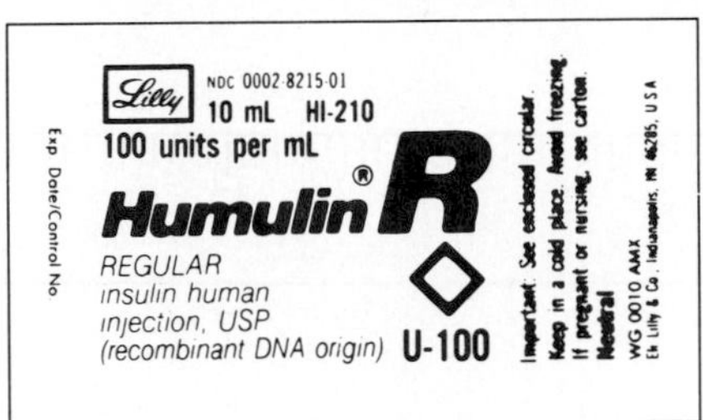

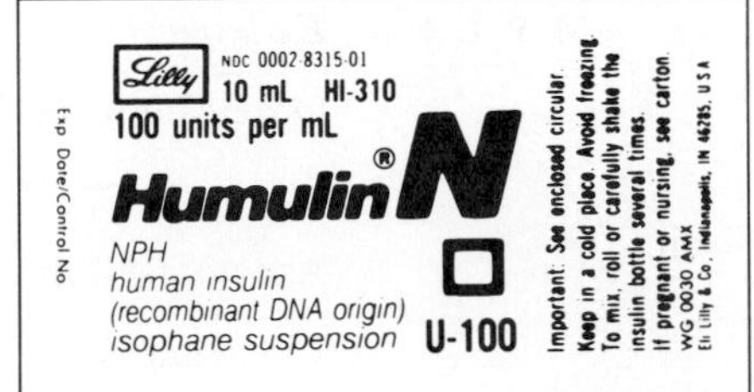

1. What are the orders? Regular (Humulin) Insulin Units 15; NPH Insulin Units 10 (Humulin)
2. What is the stock? Regular (Humulin) Insulin Units 100/mL. NPH (Humulini) Insulin Units 100/mL
3. Is there an insulin syringe? Yes.
4. What will be the total units in the syringe? 25 units

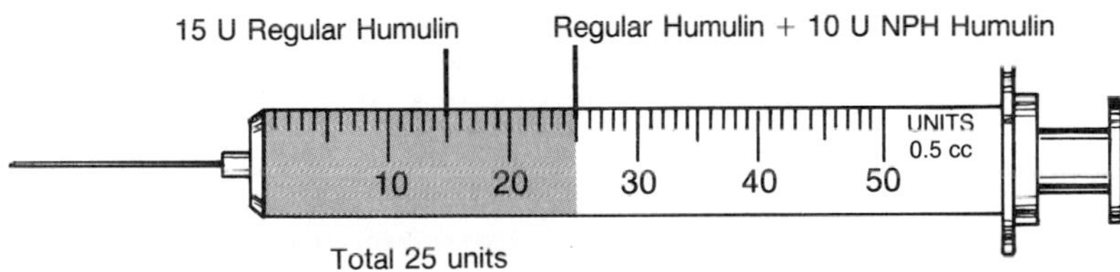

Preparing an Insulin Injection When No Insulin Syringe Is Available

When an insulin syringe is not available, it is possible to calculate and administer an insulin dose. Handle the order as an injection from a liquid and use a 1-mL precision syringe.

EXAMPLE

Order: Lente Insulin Units 40 SC qd

Label: Lente Insulin U 100/mL

No insulin syringe is available.

Rule: $\frac{D}{H} \times S = A$

$$\frac{\overset{2}{\cancel{40}}\ \cancel{\text{Units}}}{\underset{5}{\cancel{100}}\ \cancel{\text{Units}}} \times 1\text{ mL} \quad \frac{2}{5} \quad 5\overline{)2.0}^{\,0.4}$$

Give: 0.4 mL SC

Exercise 5

Solve these insulin problems. Draw a line on the syringe to indicate the dose you would prepare. Answers may be found at the end of the chapter.

1. Order: NPH Insulin 56 Units SC qd
   Stock: vial of NPH Iletin Isophane Insulin Suspension U 100/mL

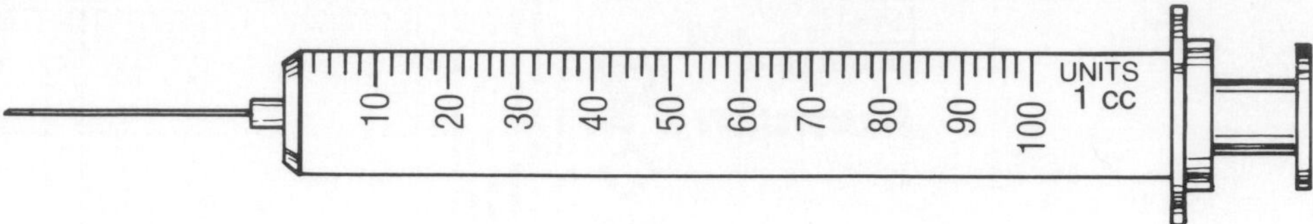

2. Order: 7 Units Regular Insulin U 100 and 20 Units NPH Insulin U 100 SC qd 7 AM
   Stock: vial of Regular Insulin U 100/mL (pork) and NPH Iletin I Isophane Insulin Suspension U 100/mL

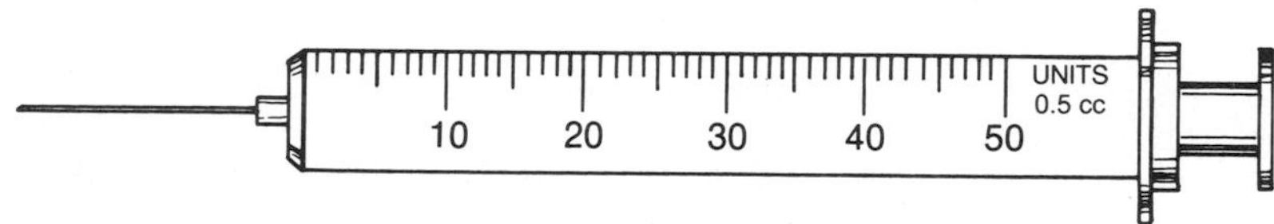

3. Order: Regular Humulin Insulin 4 Units SC stat
   Stock: vial of Novolin R Regular Insulin U 100/mL

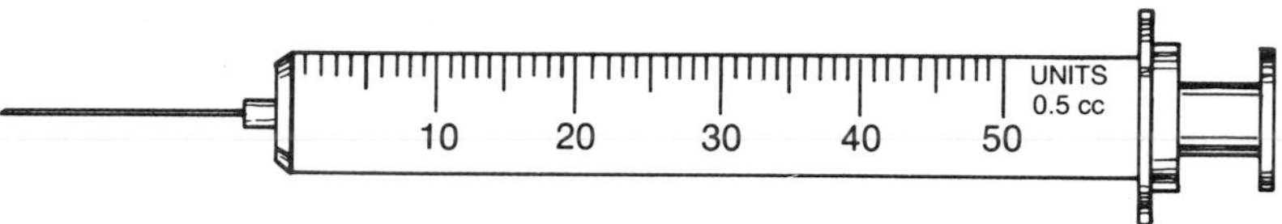

4. Order: Semilente Insulin Units 28 SC
   Stock: Semilente Insulin Prompt Insulin Zinc Suspension U 100/mL

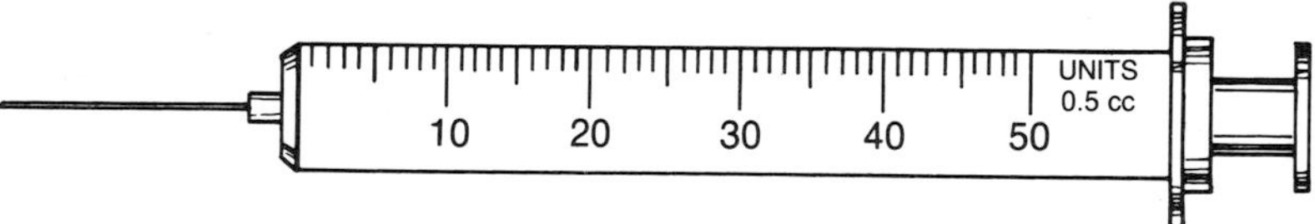

5. Order: 20 Units of NPH 100 SC qd
   Stock: vial of NPH Iletin I Isophane Insulin Suspension U 100/mL

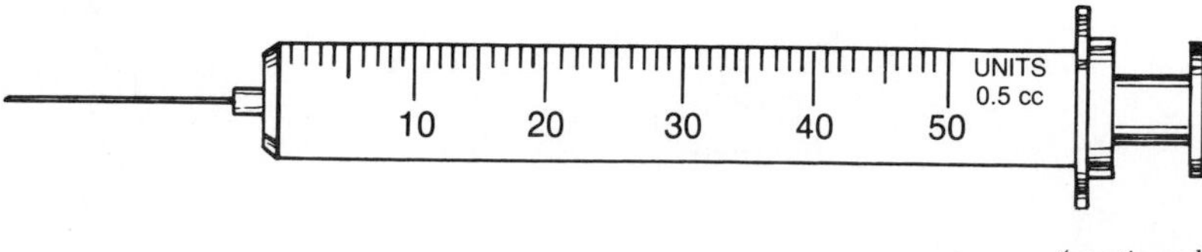

(continued)

Exercise 5 (continued)

6. Order: Regular Insulin Units 16 } SC qd
NPH Insulin Units 64
Stock: vial of Regular Insulin U 100/mL vial of NPH Iletin I Isophane Insulin Suspension U 100/mL

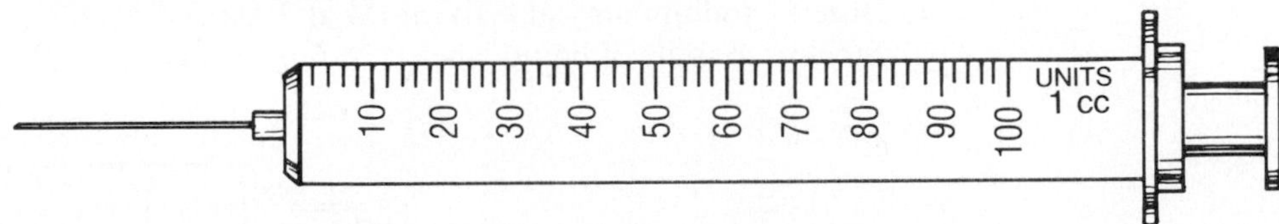

7. Order: Regular Insulin 3 Units SC stat
Stock: vial of Regular Insulin U 100/mL

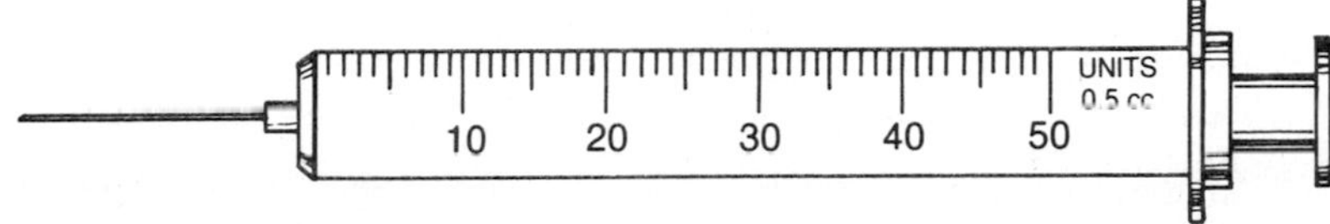

8. Order: Semilente Insulin Units 30 SC qd
Stock: vial of Semilente Insulin Prompt Insulin Zinc Suspension U 100/mL

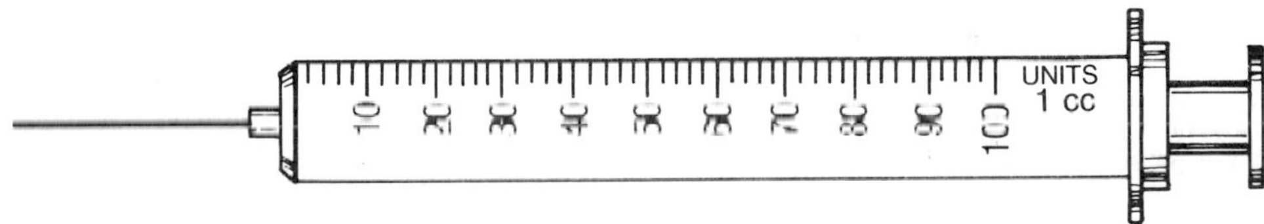

9. Order: Regular Insulin 10 Units with NPH Insulin 40 Units SC qd
Stock: vial of Regular Insulin U 100/mL vial of NPH Iletin I Isophane Insulin Suspension U 100/mL

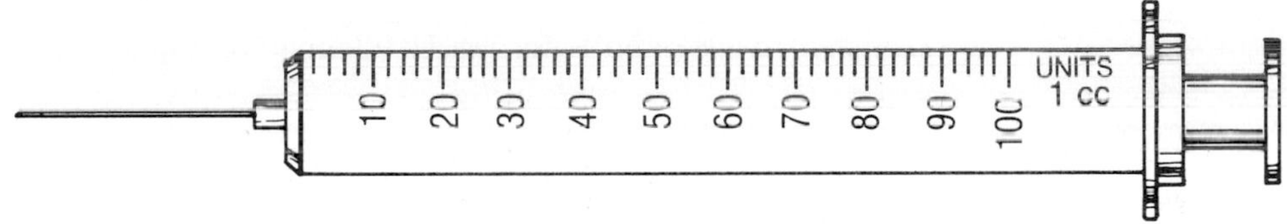

10. Order: Regular Humulin Insulin 13 Units SC stat
Stock: vial of Novolin R Regular Insulin U 100/mL

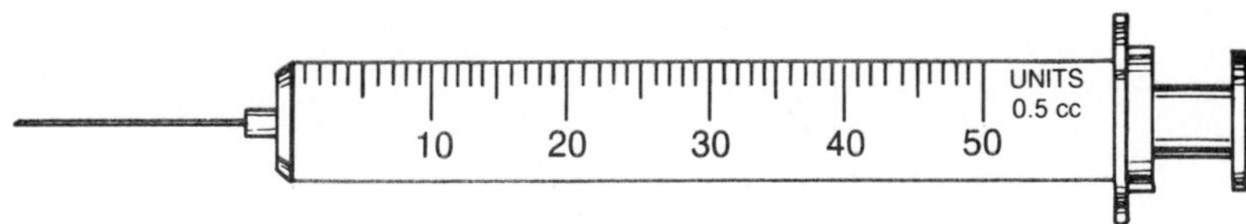

Proficiency Test 1

Solve these injection problems. Draw a line on the syringe indicating the amount you would prepare in milliliters (mL). Answers may be found at the end of the chapter. Aim for 100% accuracy!

1. Order: sodium amytal 0.1 Gm IM at 7 AM
Stock: ampule of liquid labeled 200 mg/3 mL

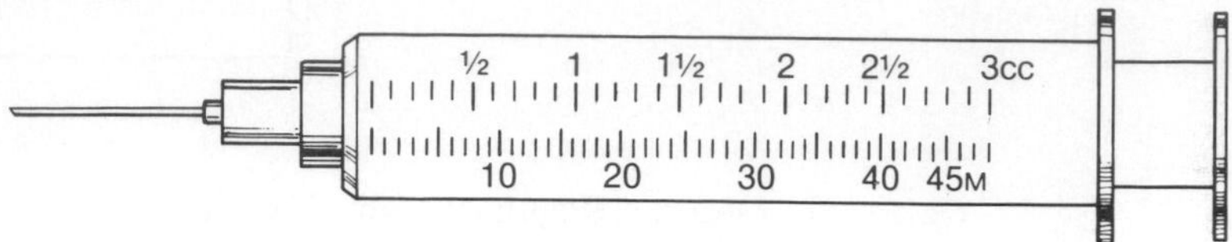

2. Order: morphine sulfate 5 mg SC stat
Stock: vial of liquid labeled 15 mg/mL

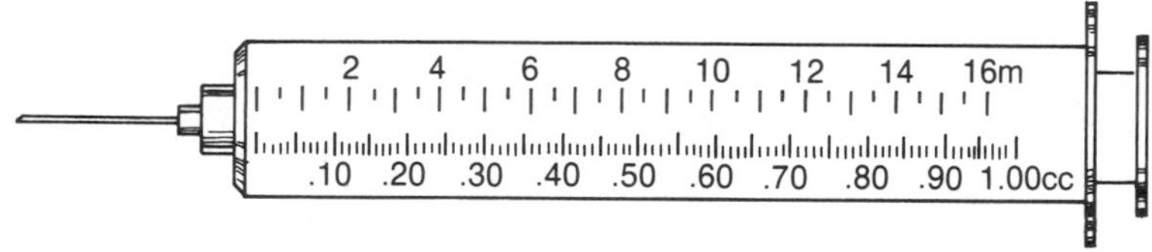

3. Order: Benadryl 25 mg IM q4h prn
Stock: ampule of liquid labeled 50 mg (2-cc size)

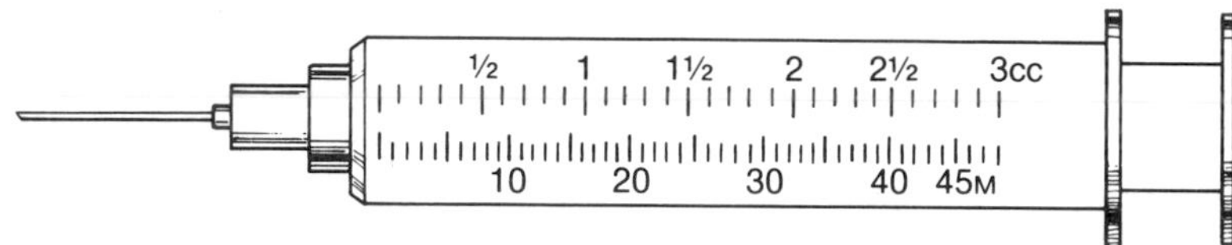

4. Order: NPH Insulin 15 units and Humulin Insulin 5 units SC qd 7 AM
Stock: vials of NPH Insulin U 100 and Humulin Insulin U 100

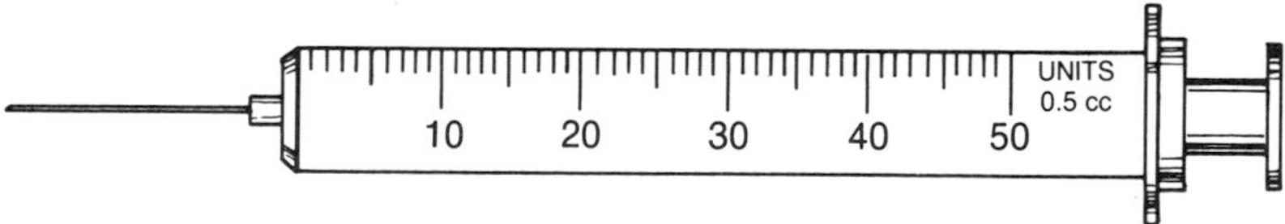

5. Order: add 20 mEq potassium chloride to IV stat
Stock: vial of liquid labeled 40 mEq (3 g) per 20 mL

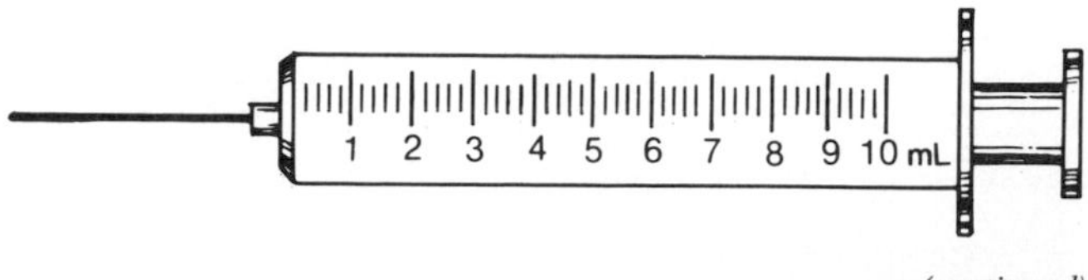

(continued)

Proficiency Test 1 (continued)

6. Order: scopolamine 0.6 mg SC stat
   Stock: vial labeled 0.4 mg/mL

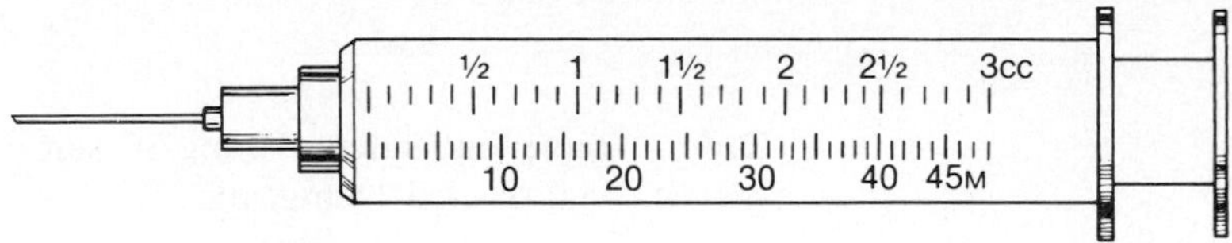

7. Order: atropine sulfate 0.8 mg IM at 7 AM
   Stock: vial labeled 0.4 mg/mL

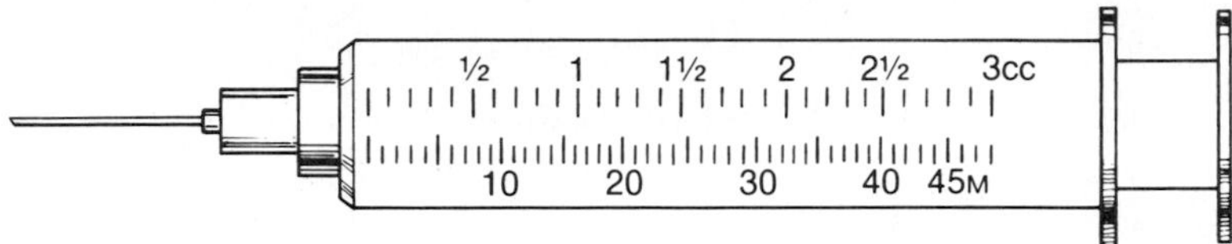

8. Order: add 0.5 Gm dextrose 25% to IV stat
   Stock: vial of liquid labeled Infant 25% Dextrose Injection 250 mg/mL

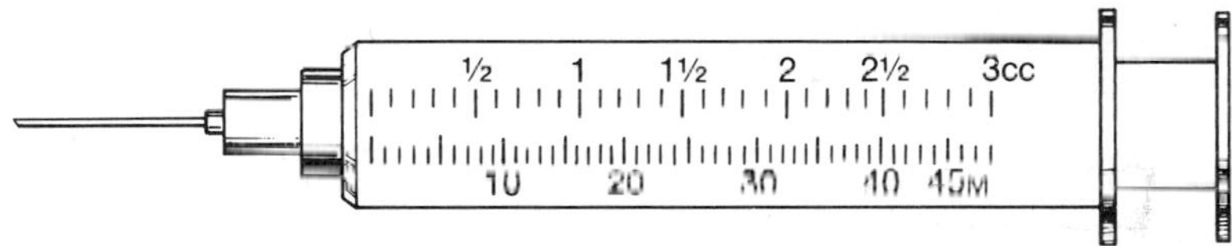

9. Order: ascorbic acid 200 mg IM bid
   Stock: ampule labeled 500 mg/2 mL

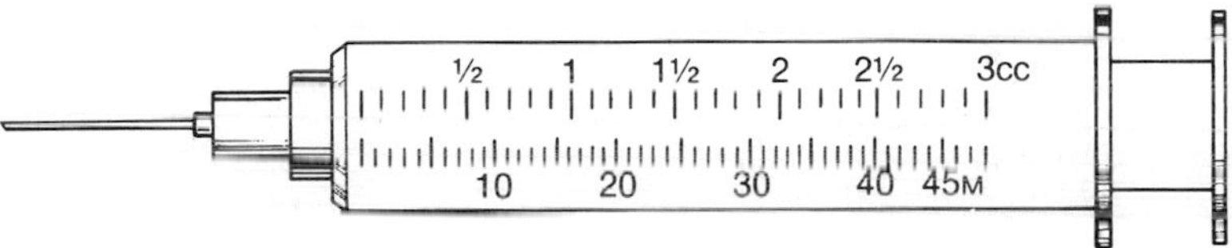

10. Order: epinephrine 7.5 mg SC stat
    Stock: ampule labeled 1:100

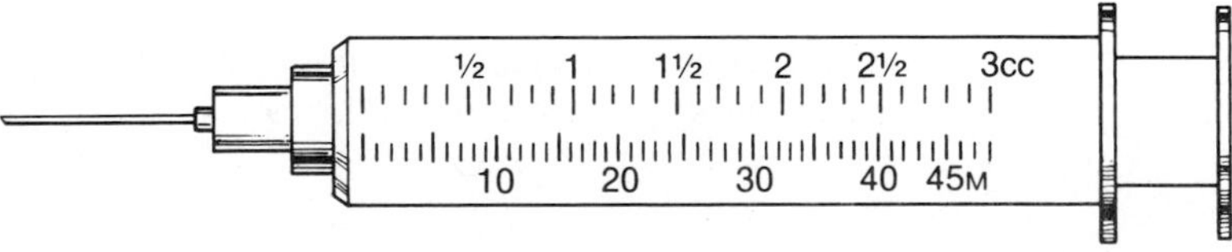

Proficiency Test 2

Solve these problems in injections from a liquid. Draw a line on the syringe indicating the amount you would prepare in milliliters (mL). Answers may be found at the end of the chapter. Aim for 100% accuracy!

1. Order: morphine sulfate 10 mg SC stat
   Stock: vial labeled 15 mg/mL

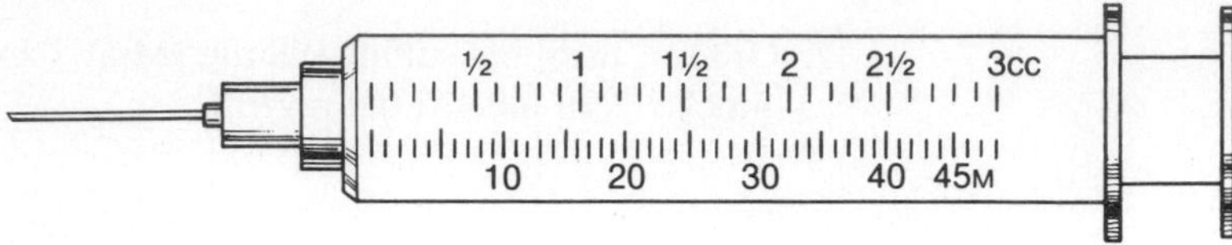

2. Order: Demerol 25 mg IM stat
   Stock: vial of liquid labeled 100 mg in 1 mL

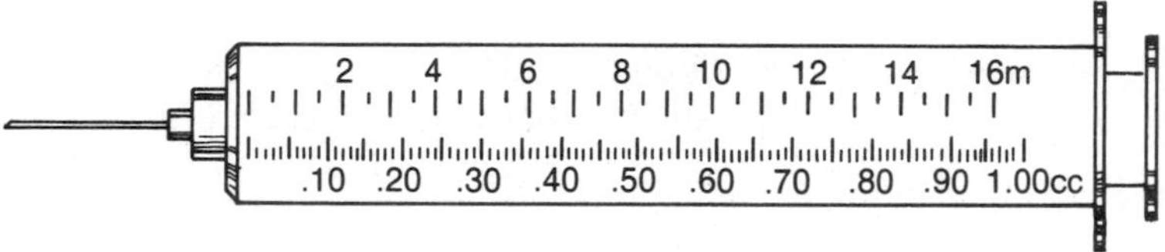

3. Order: phenobarbital 0.1 g IM q6h
   Stock: ampule of liquid labeled 200 mg/3 mL

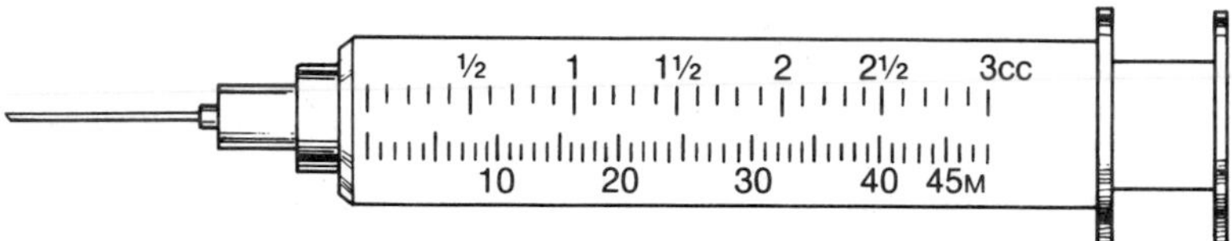

4. Order: vitamin B_{12} 1000 μg IM qd
   Stock: vial labeled 5000 μg/mL

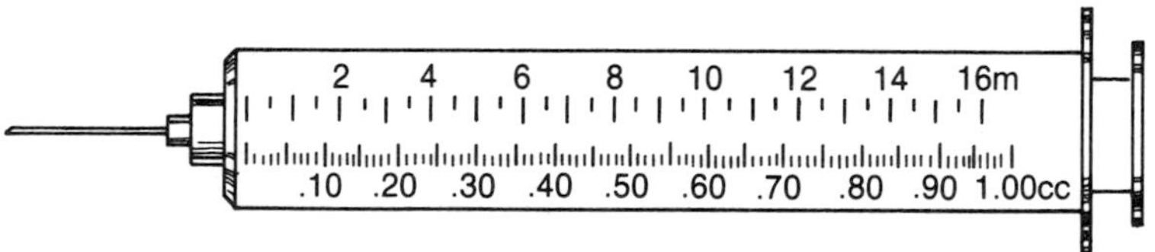

5. Order: prepare 25 mg lidocaine for physician to use
   Stock: vial of liquid labeled 1%

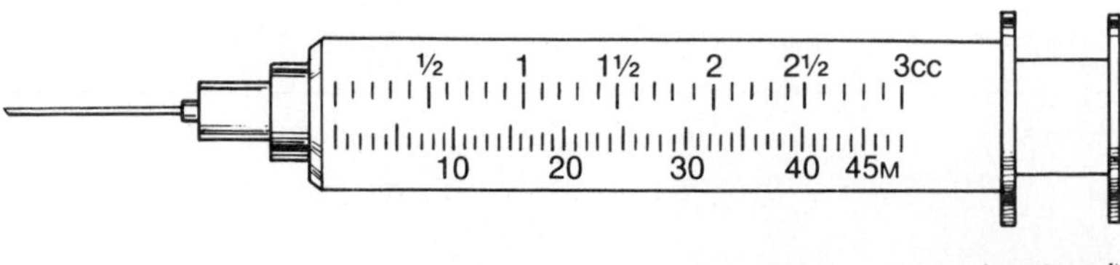

(continued)

Proficiency Test 2 (continued)

6. Order: scopolamine 0.5 mg SC stat
   Stock: vial labeled 0.4 mg/mL

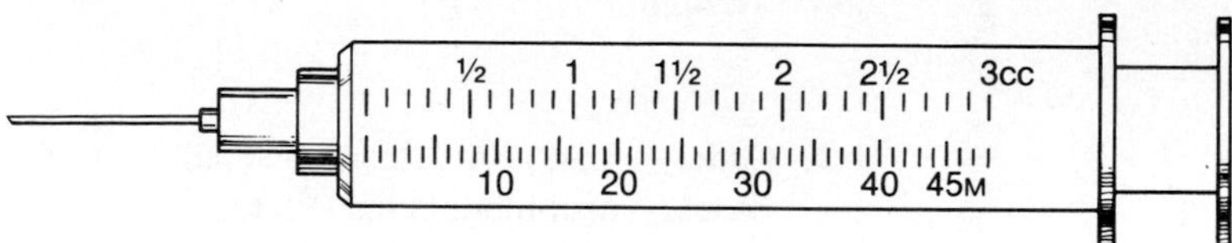

7. Order: NPH Insulin 10 units and Humulin Insulin 3 units SC qd 7 AM
   Stock: vials of NPH Insulin U 100 and Humulin Insulin U 100

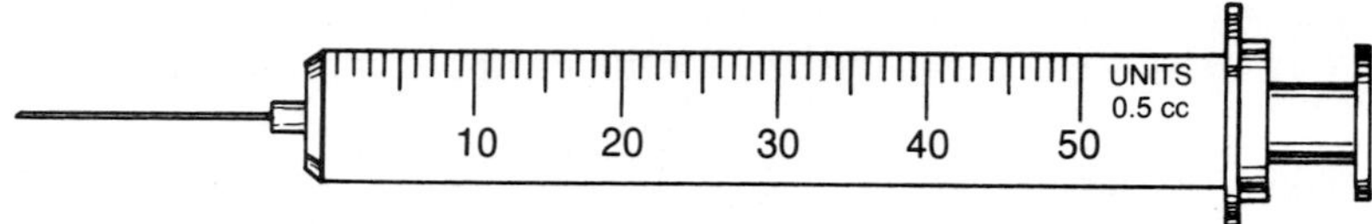

8. Order: add sodium bicarbonate 1.2 mEq to IV stat
   Stock: vial labeled Infant 4.2% Sodium Bicarbonate 5 mEq (0.5 mEq/mL)

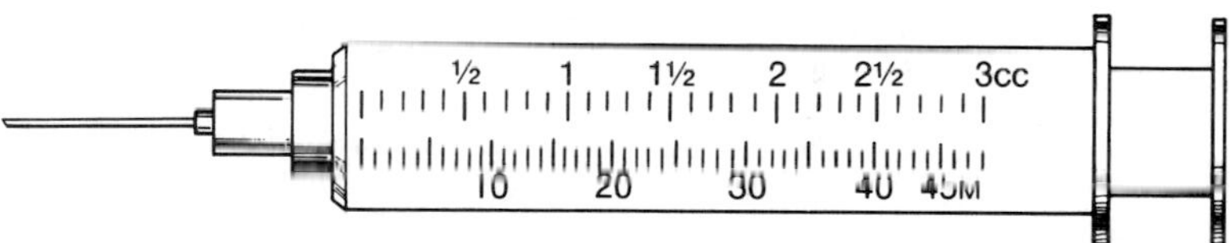

9. Order: dromostanolone proprionate 75 mg IM tiw
   Stock: vial labeled 50 mg/mL

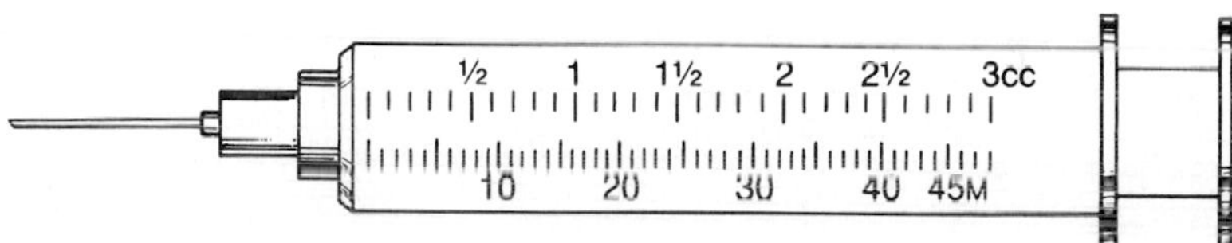

10. Order: adrenalin 500 μg SC stat
    Stock: ampule of liquid labeled 1:1000

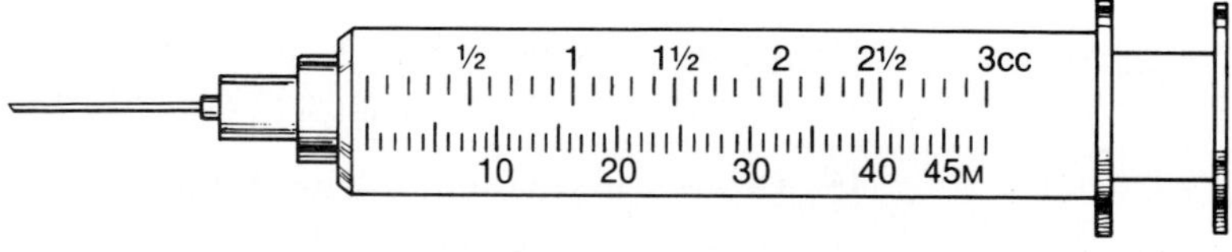

Proficiency Test 3

Aim for 90% or better on this test. There are 20 questions, each worth 5 points. If you have any difficulty, reread and study Chapter 7, which explains this information. Assume you have only a 3-cc syringe.

1. Order: Lanoxin 0.25 mg IM qd
Stock: ampule labeled 0.5 mg/2 mL

2. Order: diphenhydramine hydrochloride 40 mg IM stat
Stock: ampule labeled 50 mg (2-cc size)

3. Order: morphine sulfate 8 mg SC q4h prn
Stock: vial labeled 15 mg/mL

4. Order: Demerol Hydrochloride 25 mg IM q4h prn
Stock: vial labeled 100 mg/mL

5. Order: ascorbic acid 200 mg IM qd
Stock: ampule labeled 500 mg/2 mL

6. Order: vitamin B_{12} 1500 μg qd IM
Stock: vial labeled 5000 μg/mL

7. Order: atropine sulfate 0.6 mg SC at 7:30 AM
Stock: vial labeled 0.4 mg/mL

8. Order: Sodium Amytal 0.1 gm IM stat
Stock: ampule 200 mg/3 mL

9. Order: hydromorphone HCl 1.5 mg IM q4h prn
Stock: vial labeled 2 mg/mL

10. Order: penicillin G procaine 600,000 units IM q12h
Stock: vial labeled 500,000 USP units/mL

11. Order: add nitroglycerin 200 μg to IV stat
Stock: vial labeled 0.8 mg/mL

12. Order: neostigmine methylsulfate 500 mcg SC
Stock: ampule labeled 1:4000

13. Order: levorphanol tartrate 3 mg SC
Stock: vial labeled 2 mg/mL

14. Order: epinephrine 0.4 mg SC stat
Stock: ampule labeled 1:1000 (2-mL size)

15. Order: magnesium sulfate 500 mg IM
Stock: ampule labeled 50% (2-mL size)

16. Order: oxymorphone HCl 0.75 mg SC
Stock: vial labeled 1.5 mg/mL

(continued)

Proficiency Test 3 (continued)

17. Order: add lidocaine 100 mg to IV stat
Stock: ampule labeled 20%

18. Order: Lanoxin 0.125 mg IM 10 AM
Stock: ampule labeled 0.25 mg/2 mL

19. Order: nalbuphine HCl 12 mg IM
Stock: vial 10 mg/mL

20. Order: add 10 mEq KCl to IV
Stock: vial 40 mEq/20 mL

Exercise

Mental Drill in Liquids for Injection Problems

As you develop proficiency in solving problems, you will be able to calculate many answers without written work. This drill combines your knowledge of equivalents and dosages. Solve these problems mentally and write only the amount to give. Answers will be found at the end of the chapter. Keep the rule in mind as you solve each problem.

Order	*Stock*	*Give*
1. 0.5 g IM	250 mg/mL	______
2. 10 mEq IV	40 mEq/20 mL	______
3. 0.5 mg IM	0.25 mg/mL	______
4. 100 mg IM	0.2 Gm per 2 mL	______
5. 50 mg IM	100 mg = 1 mL	______
6. 0.25 mg IM	0.5 mg per 2 mL	______
7. 0.3 mg SC	0.4 mg/mL	______
8. 1 mg SC	1:1000 solution	______
9. 1 g IV	5% solution	______
10. 0.1 g IM	200 mg/5 mL	______
11. 400,000 units IM	500,000 U/mL	______
12. 0.5 mg IM	0.5 mg per 2 mL	______
13. 1 g IV	50% solution	______
14. 75 mg IM	100 mg per 2 mL	______
15. 15 mg IM	1:100 solution	______
16. 35 mg IM	100 mg/mL	______
17. 0.6 mg SC	0.4 mg per mL	______
18. 0.15 g IM	0.2 g/2 mL	______

ANSWERS

Self-Test 1

1. Equivalent 0.3 Gm = 300 mg

$$\frac{\overset{1}{\cancel{300\text{ mg}}}}{\underset{1}{\cancel{300\text{ mg}}}} \times 2\text{ mL} = 2\text{ mL}$$

Give 2 mL IM.

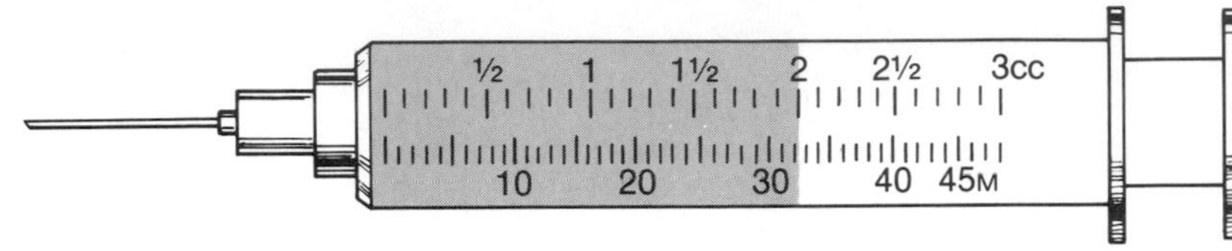

2. $$\frac{\overset{4}{\cancel{12}\text{ mg}}}{\underset{5}{\cancel{15}\text{ mg}}} \times 1\text{ mL} = \frac{4}{5}\ \ 5\overline{)4.0}^{\,.8}$$

Give 0.8 mL SC.

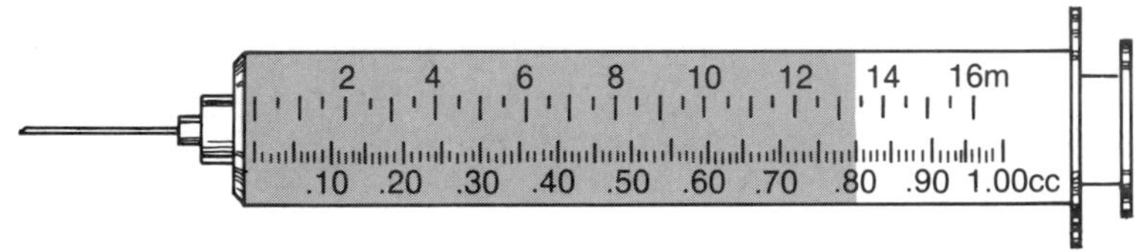

3. Equivalent 1 mg = 1000 μg

$$\frac{\overset{1}{\cancel{1000\ \mu\text{g}}}}{\underset{1}{\cancel{1000\ \mu\text{g}}}} \times 1\text{ mL} = 1\text{mL}$$

Give 1 mL IM.

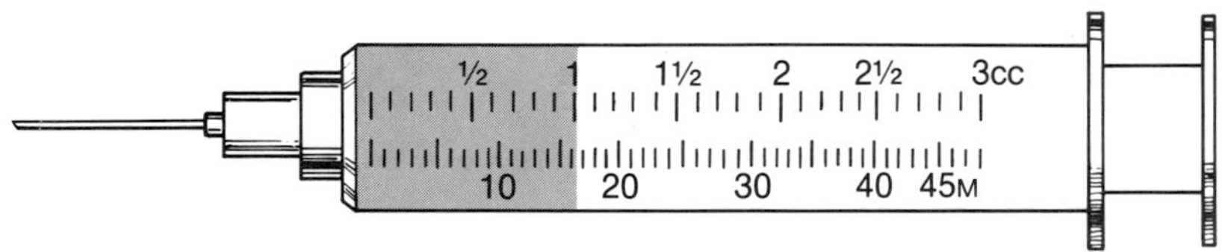

4. $$\frac{9\ \cancel{\text{mg}}}{20\ \cancel{\text{mg}}} \times 2\text{ mL} = \frac{18}{20}\ \ 20\overline{)18.0}^{\,.9}$$
$$\underline{18.0}$$

Give 0.9 mL IM. You are using a 1-mL precision syringe.

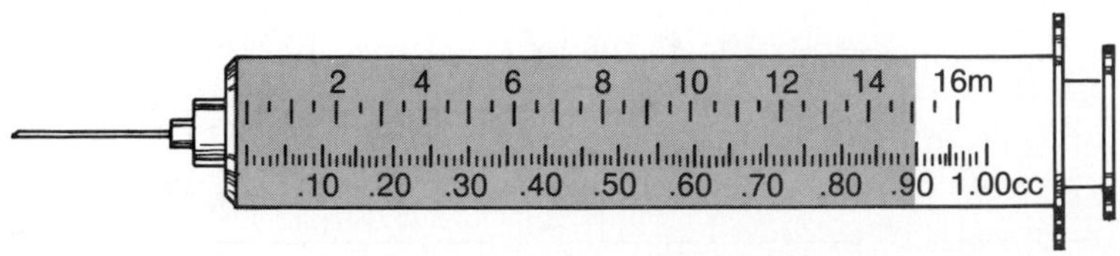

5. $\dfrac{\overset{2}{0.50\ \cancel{mg}}}{\underset{1}{0.25\ \cancel{mg}}} \times 1\ mL = 2\ mL$

Give 2 mL IM.

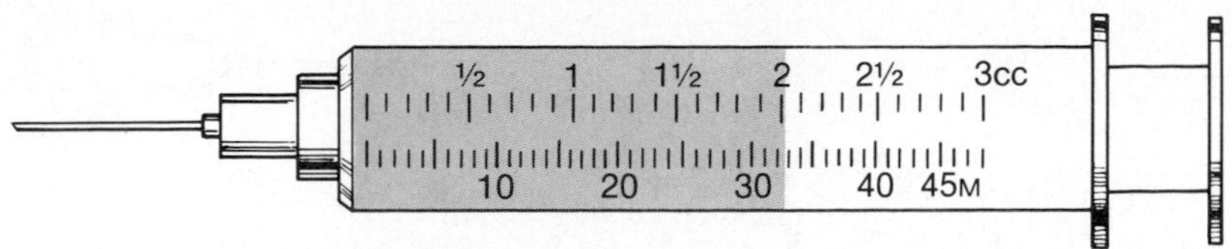

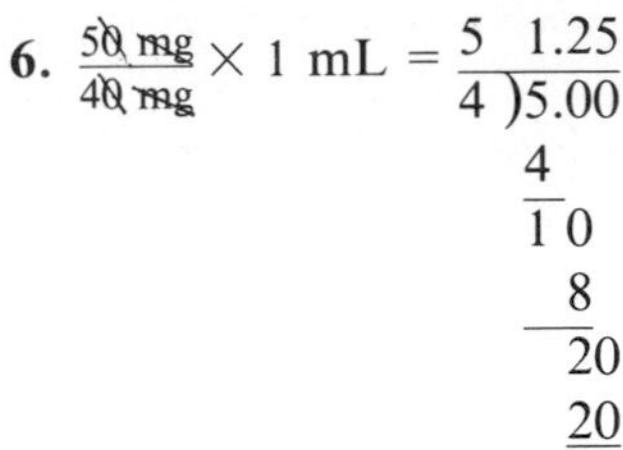

6. $\dfrac{5\cancel{0}\ \cancel{mg}}{4\cancel{0}\ \cancel{mg}} \times 1\ mL = \dfrac{5}{4}$

$$\begin{array}{r} 1.25 \\ 4\,\overline{)5.00} \\ \underline{4} \\ 10 \\ \underline{8} \\ 20 \\ \underline{20} \end{array}$$

Give 1.3 mL IM.

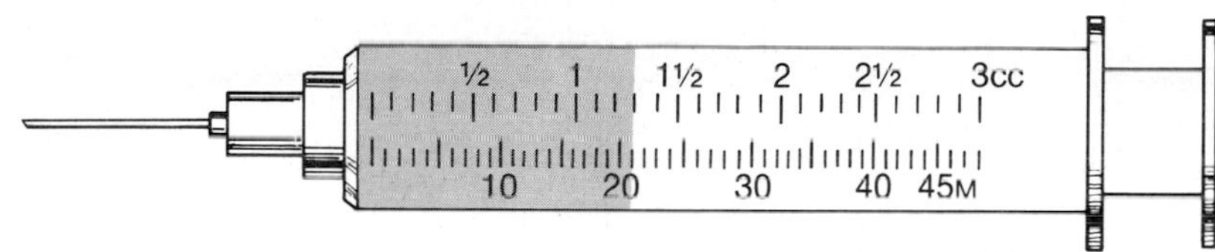

7. $\dfrac{10\cancel{0}\ \cancel{mg}}{13\cancel{0}\ \cancel{mg}} \times 1\ mL = \dfrac{10}{13}$

$$\begin{array}{r} .769 \\ 13\,\overline{)10.000} \\ \underline{91} \\ 90 \\ \underline{78} \\ 120 \\ \underline{117} \\ 3 \end{array}$$

Give 0.77 mL IM. You are using a 1-mL precision syringe, hence, milliliters to the nearest hundredth.

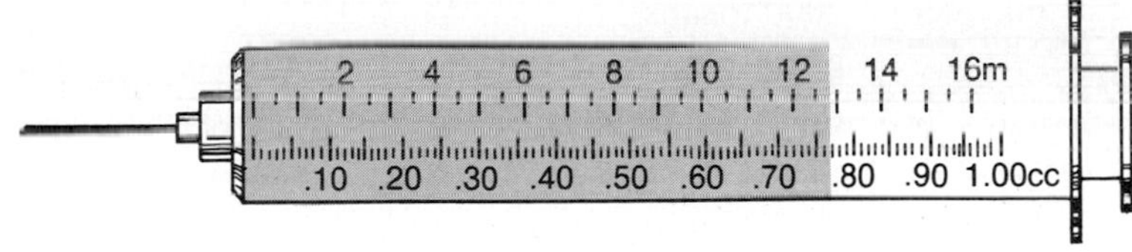

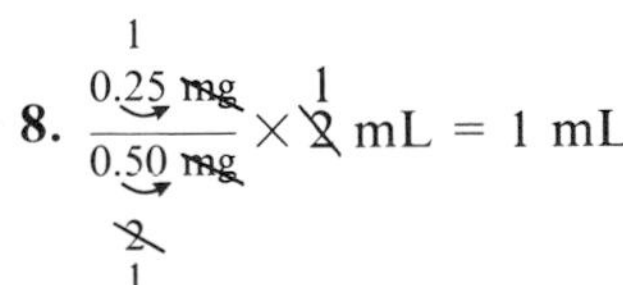

8. $\dfrac{\overset{1}{0.25\ \cancel{mg}}}{\underset{\underset{1}{\cancel{2}}}{0.50\ \cancel{mg}}} \times \overset{1}{\cancel{2}}\ mL = 1\ mL$

Give 1 mL IM.

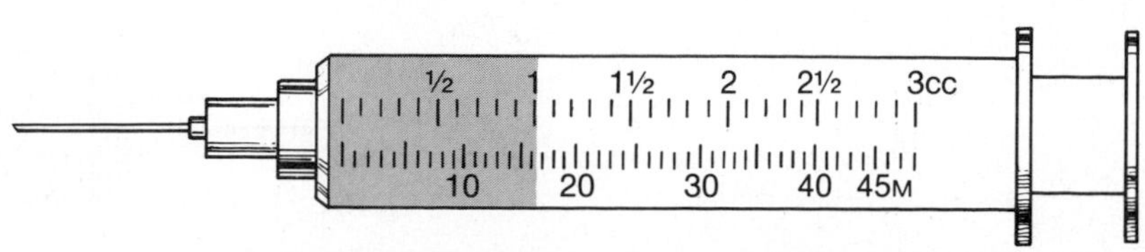

9. $\frac{6000 \text{ units}}{10000 \text{ units}} \times 1 \text{ cc} = \frac{6}{10} = 0.6$

Give 0.6 mL SC.

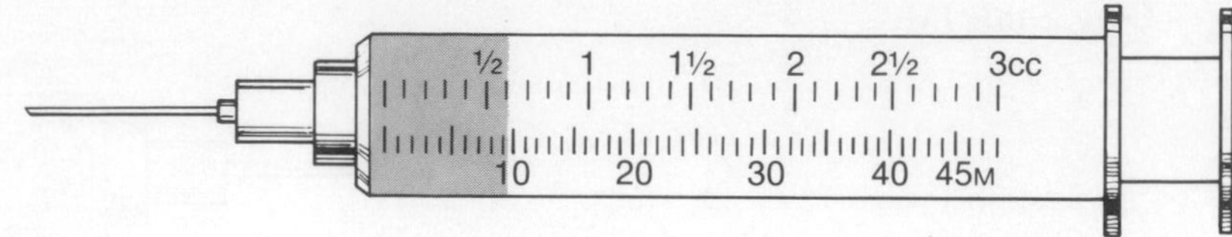

10. $\frac{70 \text{ mg}}{80 \text{ mg}} \times 2 \text{ mL} = \frac{7}{4} = 1.75$ (70 mg/80 mg reduced to 7/40, 2 mL reduced to 1)

$$\begin{array}{r} 1.75 \\ 4\overline{)7.00} \\ \underline{4} \\ 3\,0 \\ \underline{2\,8} \\ 20 \\ \underline{20} \end{array}$$

Give 1.8 mL IM.

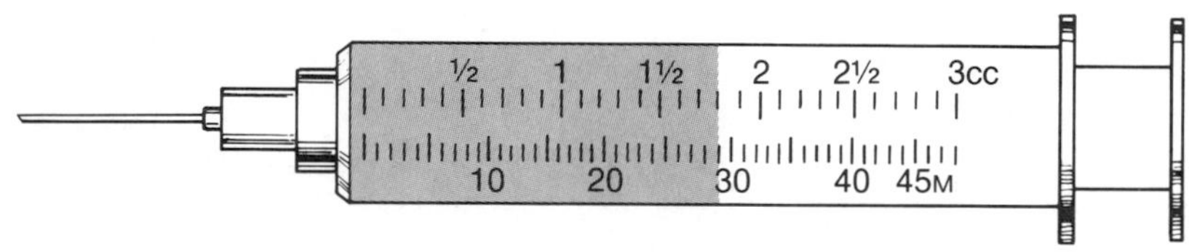

Exercise 1

1. 1 g per 20 mL; 1 g = 20 mL; 1 g/20 mL
2. 2 g per 15 mL; 2 g = 15 mL; 2 g/15 mL
3. 1 g per 500 mL; 1 g = 500 mL; 1 g/500 mL

Exercise 2

1. Equivalent 1:2000 means
   1 g in 2000 mL
   1 g = 1000 mg

   Hence, the solution is 1000 mg/2000 mL.

   $\frac{D}{H} \times S = A$

   $\frac{0.5 \text{ mg}}{1000 \text{ mg}} \times 2000 \text{ mL} = 0.5 \times 2 = 1.0$ (2000 reduced to 2)

   Give 1 mL SC.

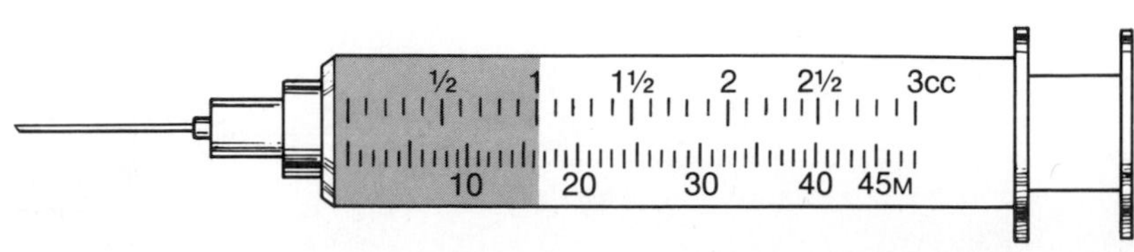

2. Equivalent 1:5000 means
   1 g in 5000 mL
   1 g = 1000 mg

   Hence, the solution is 1000 mg/5000 mL.

   $\frac{D}{H} \times S = A$

   $\frac{1\ \cancel{mg}}{\cancel{1000}\ \cancel{mg}} \times \overset{5}{\cancel{5000}}\ mL = 5\ mL$

   Add 5 mL to IV. (This is correct because route is IV, not IM.)

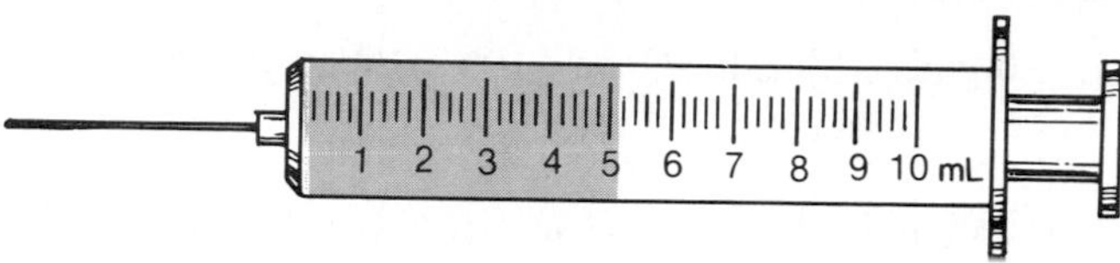

3. Equivalent 1:1000 means
   1 g in 1000 mL and 1 g = 1000 mg,

   hence the solution is 1000 mg/1000 mL or
   1 mg/mL

   $\frac{D}{H} \times S = A \qquad \frac{0.75\ \cancel{mg}}{1\ \cancel{mg}} \times 1\ mL = 0.75\ mL$

   You have a 1-cc syringe marked in hundredths.

   Draw up 0.75 mL. Do not round off.

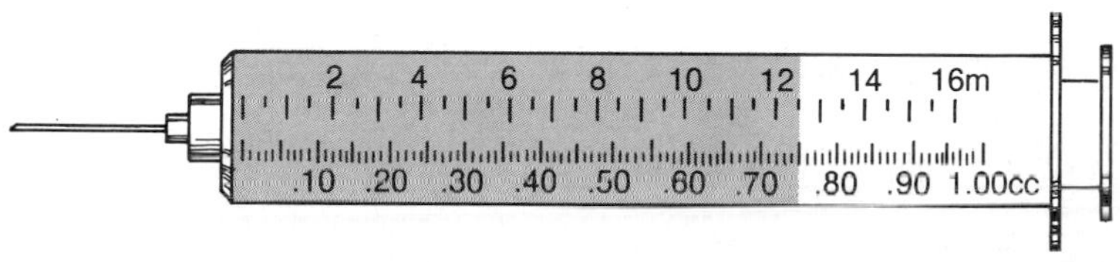

4. Equivalent 1:20 means
   1 g in 20 ml
   1 g = 1000 mg

   Hence, the solution is 1000 mg/20 mL.

   $\frac{\overset{1}{\cancel{50}}\ \cancel{mg}}{\underset{\underset{1}{20}}{\cancel{1000}}\ \cancel{mg}} \times \overset{1}{\cancel{20}}\ mL = 1\ mL$

   Give 1 mL IM.

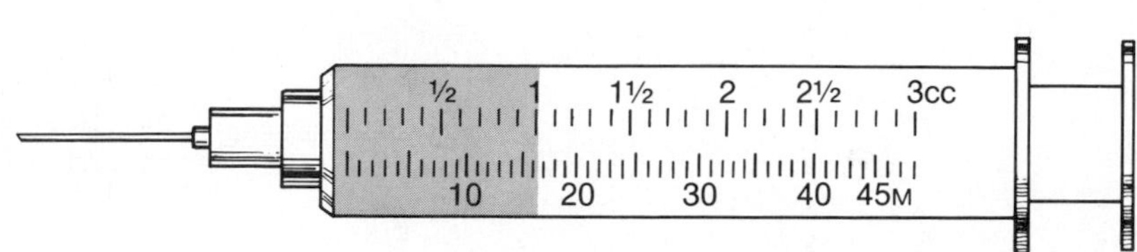

5. Equivalent 1:2000 = 1000 mg/2000 mL or
1 mg per 2 mL

$\frac{D}{H} \times S = A \qquad \frac{1.5 \text{ mg}}{1 \text{ mg}} \times 2 \text{ mL} = \begin{array}{r} 1.5 \\ \times 2 \\ \hline 3.0 \text{ mL} \end{array}$

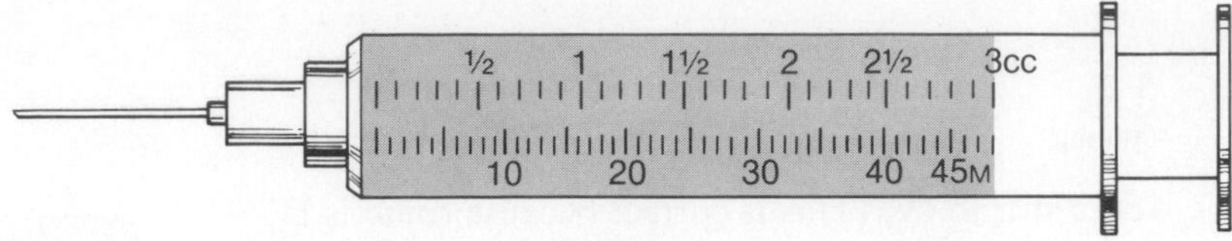

Exercise 3

1. 0.9 g per 100 mL; 0.9 g = 100 mL; 0.9 g/100 mL
2. 10 g per 100 mL; 10 g = 100 mL; 10 g/100 mL
3. 0.45 g per 100 mL; 0.45 g = 100 mL; 0.45 g/100 mL

Exercise 4

1. Equivalent 1% 1 g in 100 mL
1 g = 1000 mg

Hence, the solution is 1000 mg/100 mL.

$\frac{\overset{1}{\cancel{5}} \text{ mg}}{\underset{\underset{2}{\cancel{10}}}{\cancel{1000}} \text{ mg}} \times \overset{1}{\cancel{100}} \text{ mL} = \frac{1}{2} \text{ mL or } 0.5$

Give 0.5 mL SC.

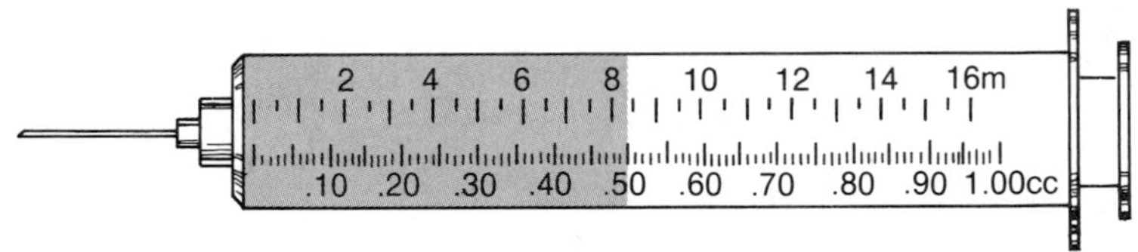

2. Equivalent 0.5% 0.5 g in 100 mL
0.5 g = 500 mg

Hence, the solution is 500 mg/100 mL.

$\frac{2.5 \text{ mg}}{\underset{5}{\cancel{500}} \text{ mg}} \times \overset{1}{\cancel{100}} \text{ mL} = \frac{2.5}{5} \quad 5\overline{)2.5}^{\,0.5}$

Give 0.5 mL IM.

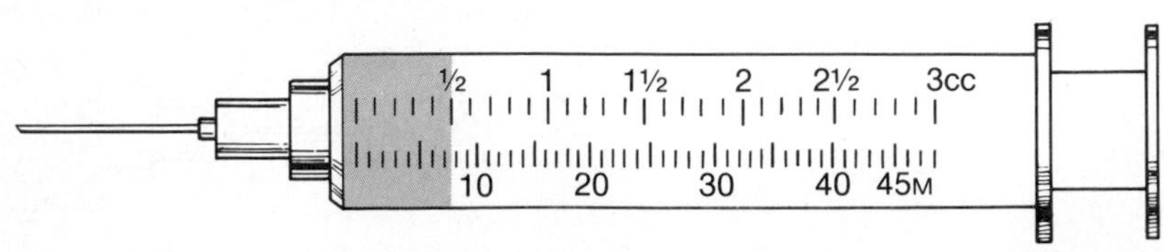

3. Equivalent 1% 1 g in 100 mL
1 g = 1000 mg

Hence, the solution is 1000 mg per 100 mL.

$$\frac{3 \text{ mg}}{\underset{10}{1000} \text{ mg}} \times \overset{1}{100} \text{ mL} = \frac{3}{10} = 0.3 \text{ mL}$$

Give 0.3 mL SC.

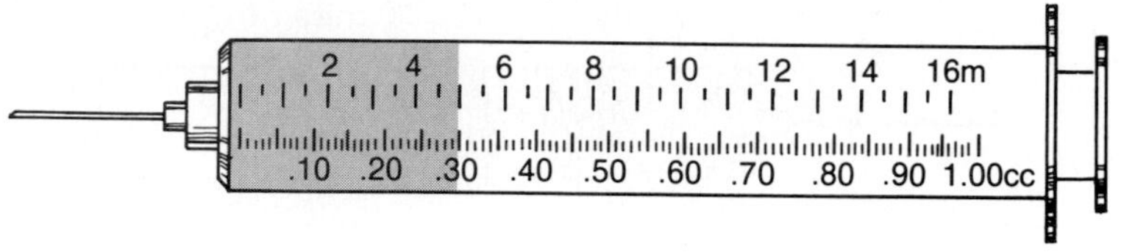

4. Equivalent 10% means 10 g in 100 mL or
1 g in 10 mL

$$\frac{D}{H} \times S = A \qquad \frac{0.3 \text{ g}}{1 \text{ g}} \times 10 \text{ mL} \qquad \begin{array}{r} 10 \\ \times\, 0.3 \\ \hline 3.0 \text{ mL} \end{array}$$

Prepare the syringe with 3 mL for IV use.

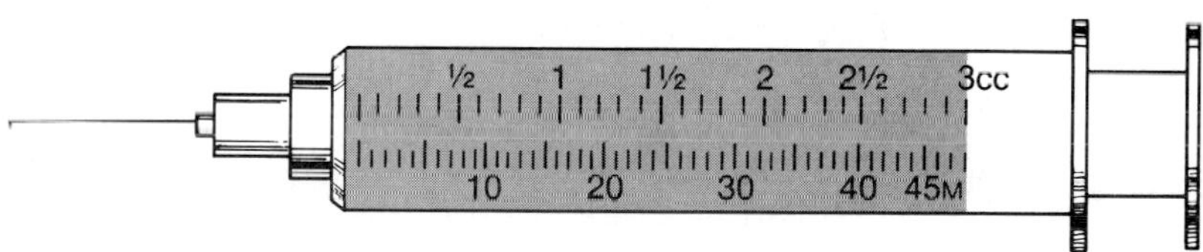

5. Equivalent 3% means 3 g in 100 mL or
3000 mg in 100 mL. This
can be reduced $\frac{3000 \text{ mg}}{100 \text{ mL}} = 30 \text{ mg/mL}$

Equivalent 0.015 g = 15 mg

$$\frac{D}{H} \times S = A \qquad \frac{\overset{1}{15} \text{ mg}}{\underset{2}{30} \text{ mg}} \times 1 \text{ mL} = \frac{1}{2} \text{ mL}$$

Prepare 0.5 mL ($\frac{1}{2}$ mL) for IV use.

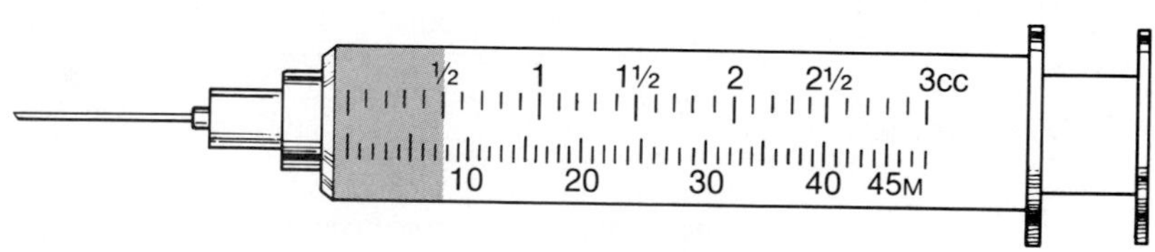

Exercise 5

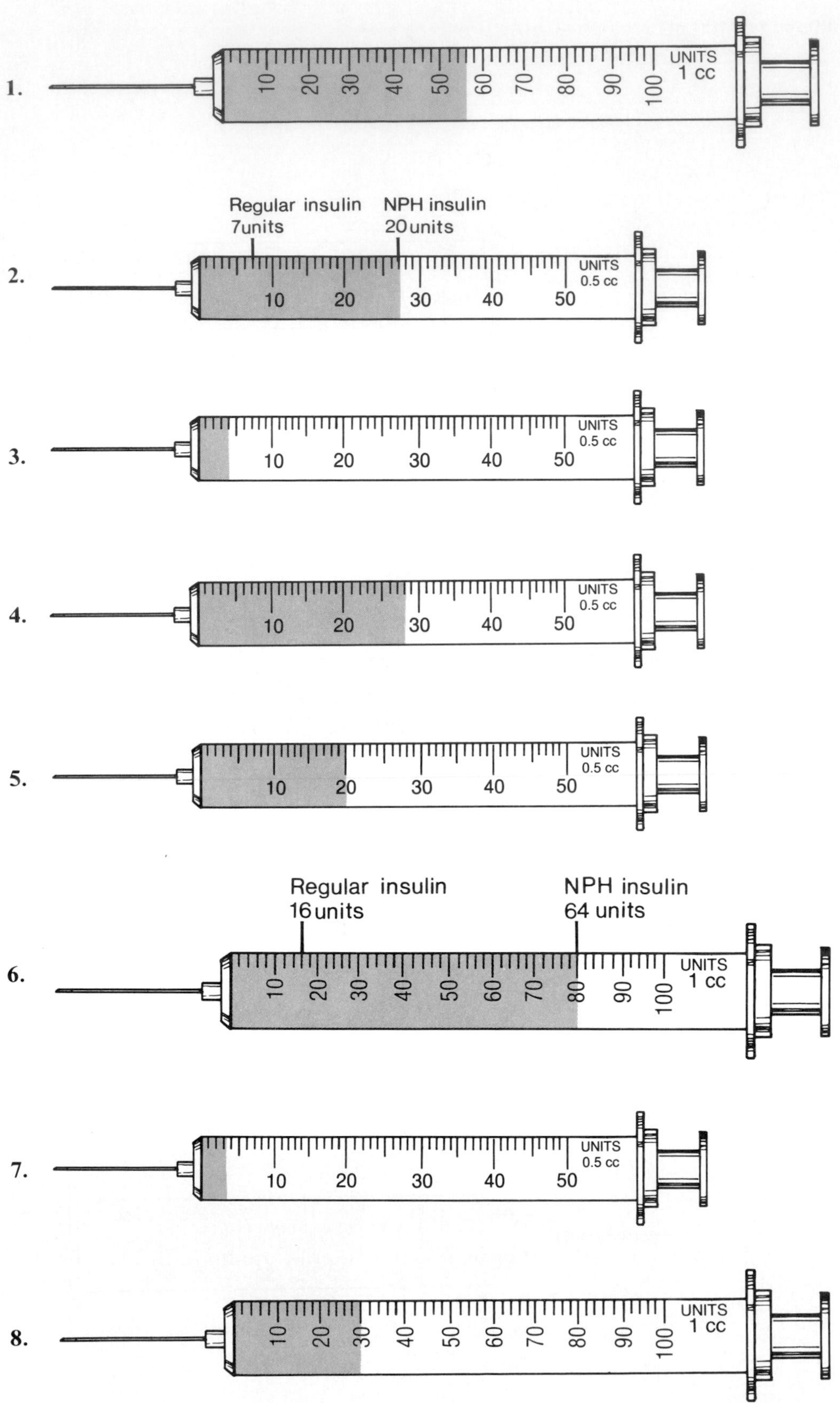
1.
UNITS
1 cc
10 20 30 40 50 60 70 80 90 100
2.
Regular insulin
7units
NPH insulin
20units
UNITS
0.5 cc
10 20 30 40 50
3.
UNITS
0.5 cc
10 20 30 40 50
4.
UNITS
0.5 cc
10 20 30 40 50
5.
UNITS
0.5 cc
10 20 30 40 50
6.
Regular insulin
16units
NPH insulin
64 units
UNITS
1 cc
10 20 30 40 50 60 70 80 90 100
7.
UNITS
0.5 cc
10 20 30 40 50
8.
UNITS
1 cc
10 20 30 40 50 60 70 80 90 100

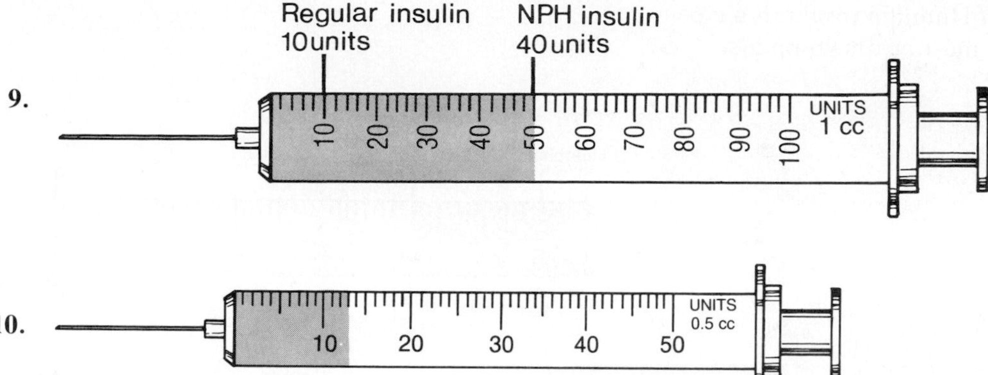

Proficiency Test 1

1. Equivalent 0.1 Gm = 100 mg

$$\frac{\overset{1}{\cancel{100\text{ mg}}}}{\underset{2}{\cancel{200\text{ mg}}}} \times 3\text{ mL} = \frac{3}{2} \quad 2\overline{)3.0}\ \ 1.5$$

Give 1.5 mL IM.

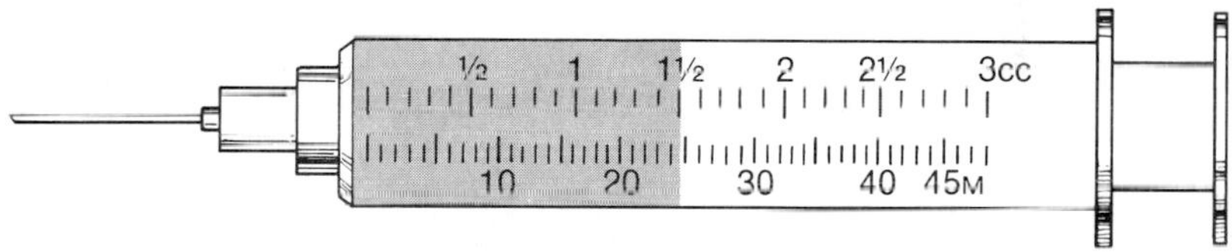

2. $$\frac{\overset{1}{\cancel{5\text{ mg}}}}{\underset{3}{\cancel{15\text{ mg}}}} \times 1\text{ mL} = \frac{1}{3} \quad 3\overline{)1.000}\ \ .333$$

Give 0.33 mL SC.

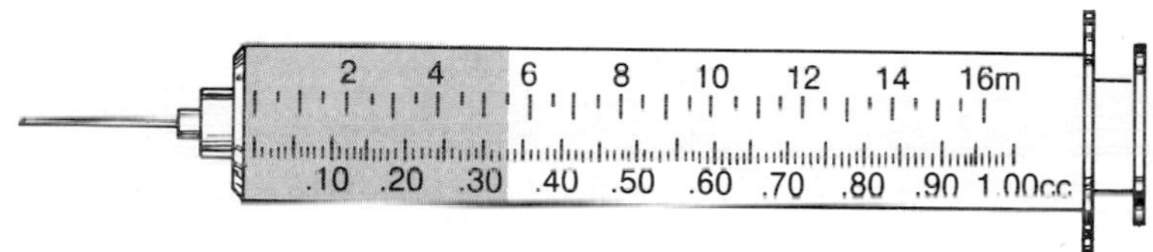

3. $$\frac{\overset{1}{\cancel{25\text{ mg}}}}{\underset{\underset{1}{\cancel{2}}}{\cancel{50\text{ mg}}}} \times \overset{1}{\cancel{2}}\text{ cc} = 1\text{ cc}$$

Give 1 cc IM.

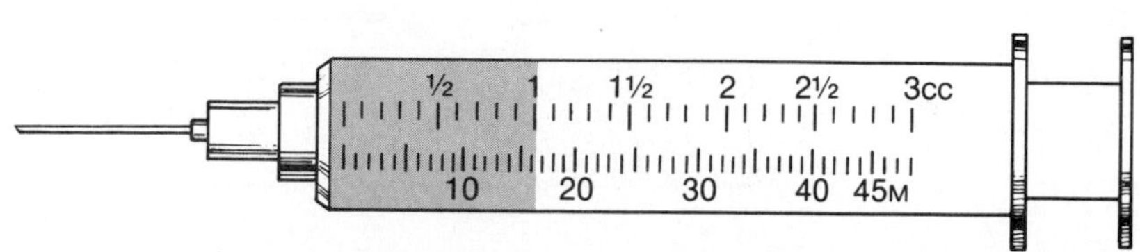

4. 20 units. Remember that Humulin insulin is a type of regular insulin and so must be drawn up first into the syringe!

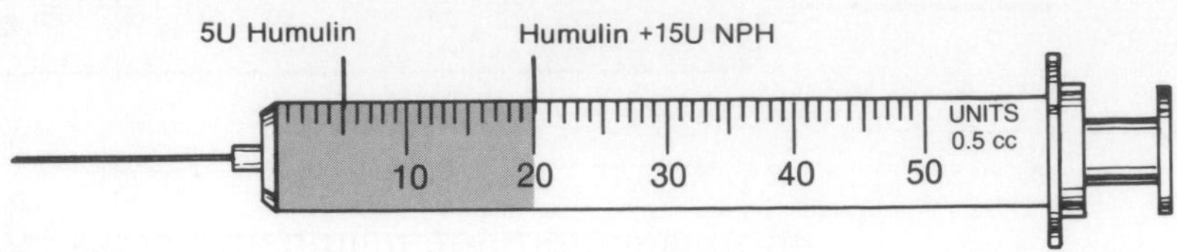

5. 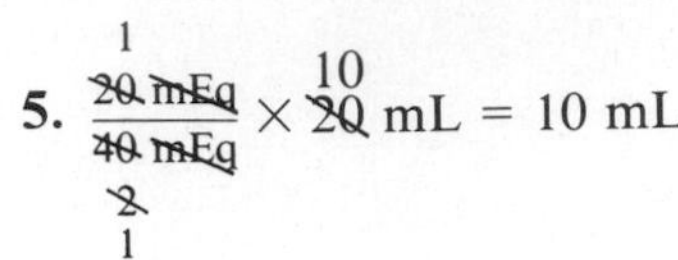

$$\frac{\overset{1}{\cancel{20}}\ \cancel{\text{mEq}}}{\underset{\underset{1}{\cancel{2}}}{\cancel{40}}\ \cancel{\text{mEq}}} \times \overset{10}{\cancel{20}}\ \text{mL} = 10\ \text{mL}$$

Add 10 mL to IV.

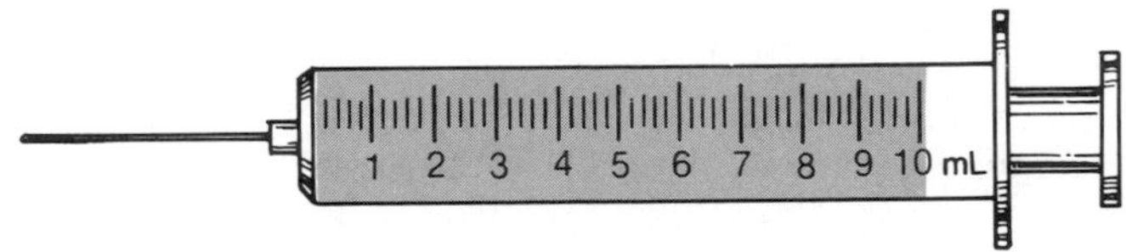

6. $$\frac{\overset{3}{0.\cancel{6}}\ \cancel{\text{mg}}}{\underset{2}{0.\cancel{4}}\ \cancel{\text{mg}}} \times 1\ \text{mL} = \frac{3}{2} \quad 2\overline{)3.0}^{\ 1.5}$$

Give 1.5 mL SC.

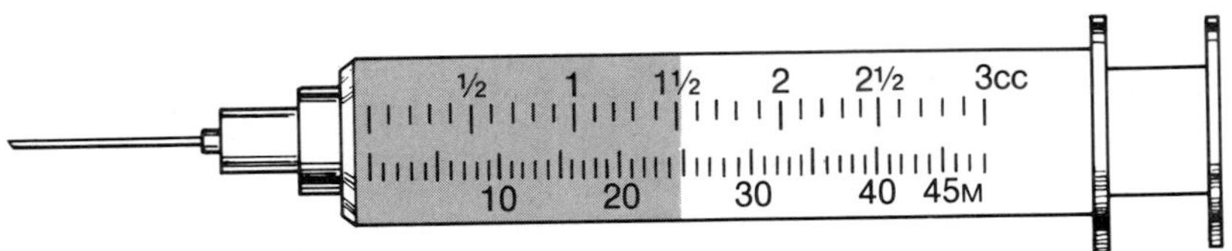

7. $$\frac{\overset{2}{0.\cancel{8}}\ \cancel{\text{mg}}}{\underset{1}{0.\cancel{4}}\ \cancel{\text{mg}}} \times 1\ \text{mL} = 2\ \text{mL}$$

Give 2 mL IM.

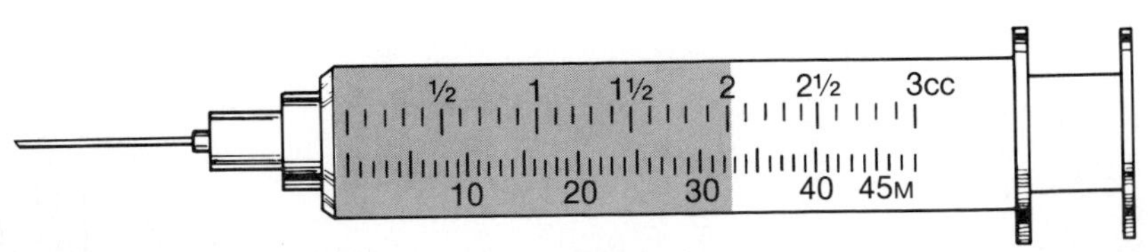

8. Equivalent 0.5 Gm = 500 mg

$$\frac{\overset{2}{\cancel{500}\ \cancel{\text{mg}}}}{\underset{1}{\cancel{250}\ \cancel{\text{mg}}}} \times 1\ \text{mL} = 2\ \text{mL}$$

Add 2 mL to IV. Were you confused by the 25%?
No reason to use it to solve this problem!

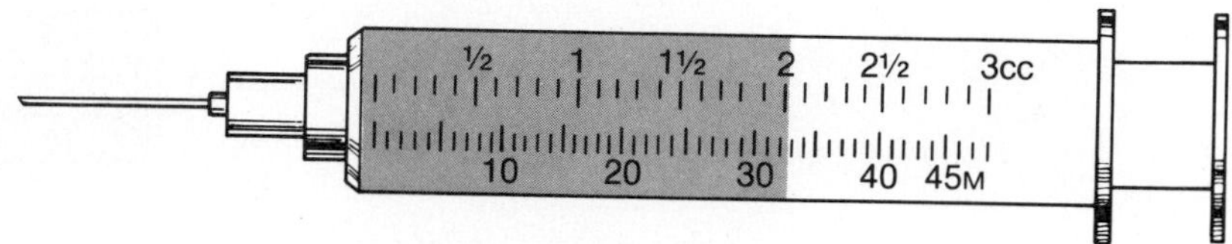

9. $\frac{\cancel{200}\ \cancel{\text{mg}}}{\cancel{500}\ \cancel{\text{mg}}} \times 2\ \text{mL} = \frac{4}{5} \quad 5\overline{)4.0}$ = .8

Give 0.8 mL IM.

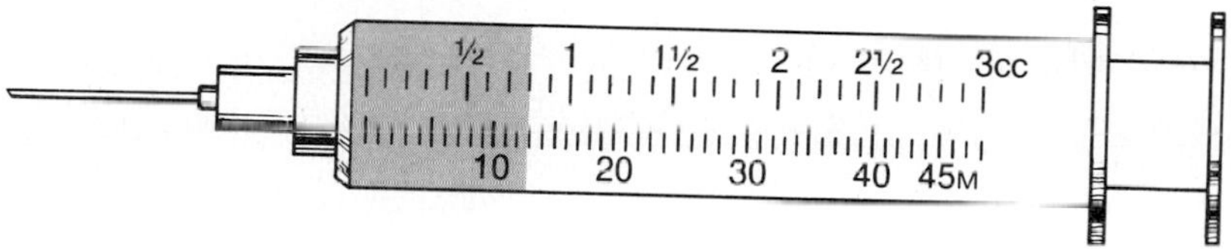

10. Equivalent 1:100 means 1 g in 100 mL
1 g = 1000 mg

Hence, the solution is 1000 mg/100 mL.

$$\frac{7.5\ \cancel{\text{mg}}}{10\cancel{00}\ \cancel{\text{mg}}} \times 1\cancel{00}\ \text{mL} = \frac{7.5}{10} \quad 10\overline{)7.50} = .75$$

$$\begin{array}{r} 7\,0 \\ \hline 50 \\ \underline{50} \end{array}$$

Give 0.8 mL SC.

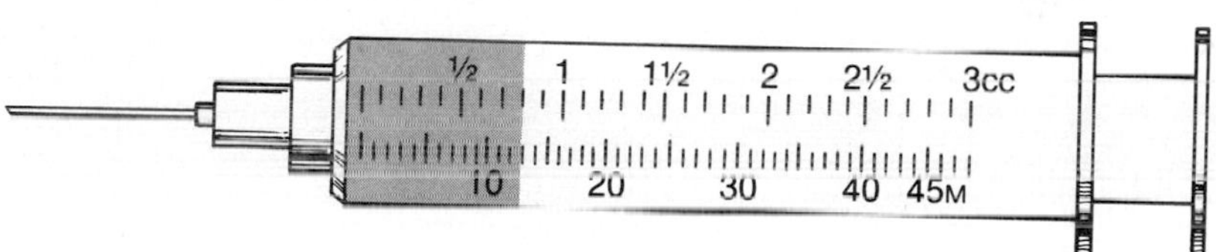

Proficiency Test 2

1. $\frac{\overset{2}{\cancel{10}\ \cancel{\text{mg}}}}{\underset{3}{\cancel{15}\ \cancel{\text{mg}}}} \times 1\ \text{mL} = \frac{2}{3} \quad 3\overline{)2.00}$ = .66

Give 0.7 mL SC.

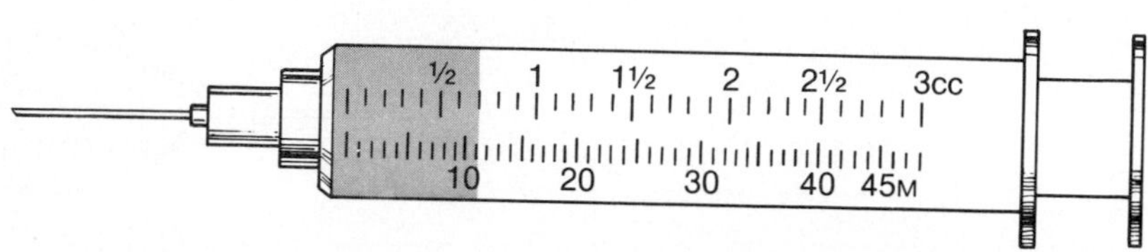

2. $$\frac{\overset{1}{\cancel{25}\text{ mg}}}{\underset{4}{\cancel{100}\text{ mg}}} \times 1\text{ mL} = \frac{1}{4} \quad \begin{array}{r} .25 \\ 4\,\overline{)1.00} \end{array}$$

Give 0.25 mL. You are using a 1-mL precision syringe; therefore, the answer is the nearest hundredth.

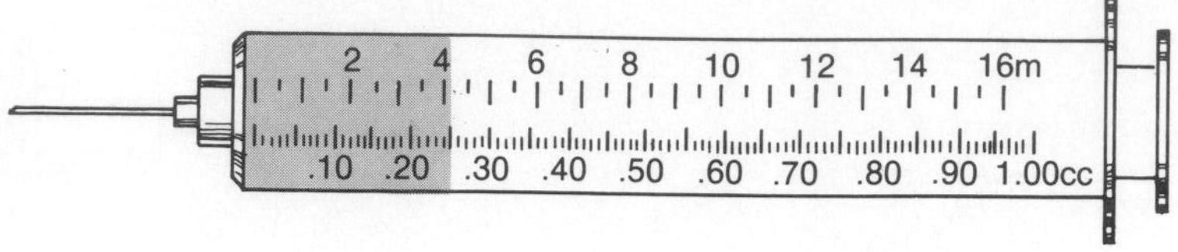

3. Equivalent 0.1 g = 100 mg

$$\frac{\overset{1}{\cancel{100}\text{ mg}}}{\underset{2}{\cancel{200}\text{ mg}}} \times 3\text{ mL} = \frac{3}{2} \quad \begin{array}{r} 1.5 \\ 2\,\overline{)3.0} \end{array}$$

Give 1.5 mL IM.

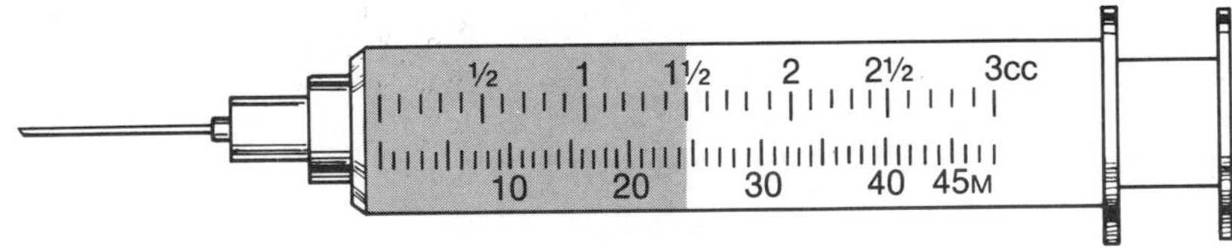

4. $$\frac{\overset{1}{\cancel{1000}\ \cancel{\mu\text{g}}}}{\underset{5}{\cancel{5000}\ \cancel{\mu\text{g}}}} \times 1\text{ mL} = \frac{1}{5} \quad \begin{array}{r} .2 \\ 5\,\overline{)1.0} \end{array}$$

Give 0.2 mL IM.

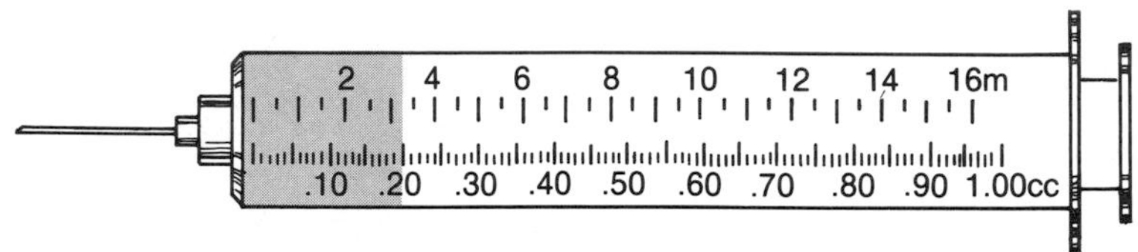

5. Equivalent 1% means 1 g in 100 mL
1 g = 1000 mg

Hence, the solution is 1000 mg in 100 mL.

$$\frac{\overset{5}{\cancel{25}\text{ mg}}}{\underset{\underset{2}{\cancel{10}}}{\cancel{1000}\text{ mg}}} \times \overset{1}{\cancel{100}}\text{ mL} = \frac{5}{2} \quad \begin{array}{r} 2.5 \\ 2\,\overline{)5.0} \end{array}$$

Prepare 2.5 mL for the physician.

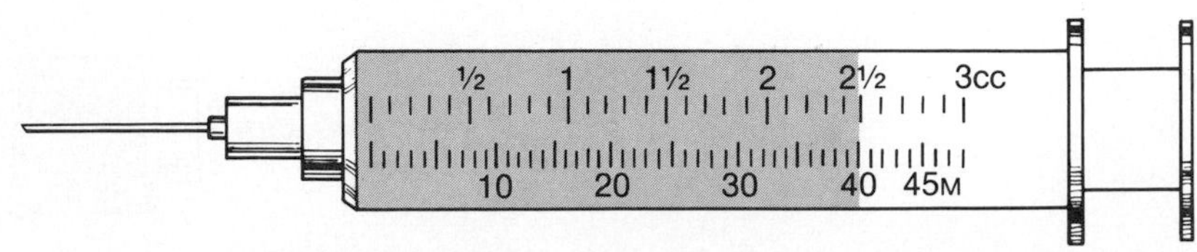

6. $\dfrac{0.5\ \cancel{\text{mg}}}{0.4\ \cancel{\text{mg}}} \times 1\ \text{mL} = \dfrac{5}{4}\ \begin{array}{r}1.25\\ \overline{)5.00}\end{array}$

Give 1.3 mL SC.

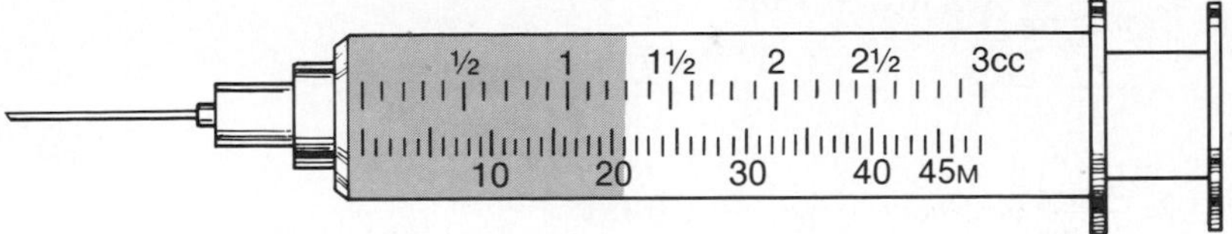

7. 13 units. Remember that Humulin insulin is a type of regular insulin and so must be drawn up first into the syringe!

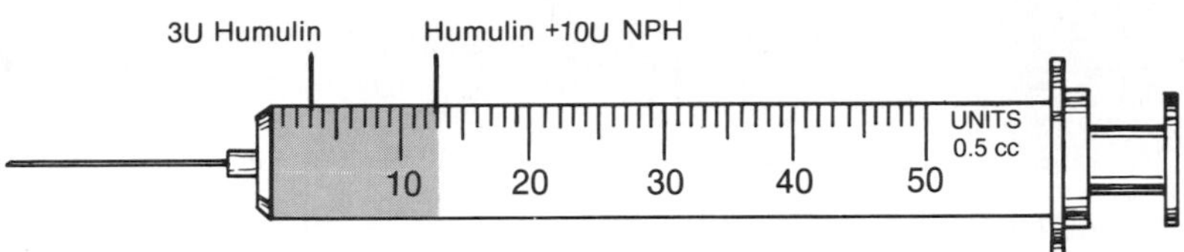

8. $\dfrac{1.2\ \cancel{\text{mEq}}}{0.5\ \cancel{\text{mEq}}} \times 1\ \text{mL} = \dfrac{1.2}{0.5}\ \begin{array}{r}2.4\\ 0.5\overline{)1.20}\end{array}$

Add 2.4 mL to the IV stat.

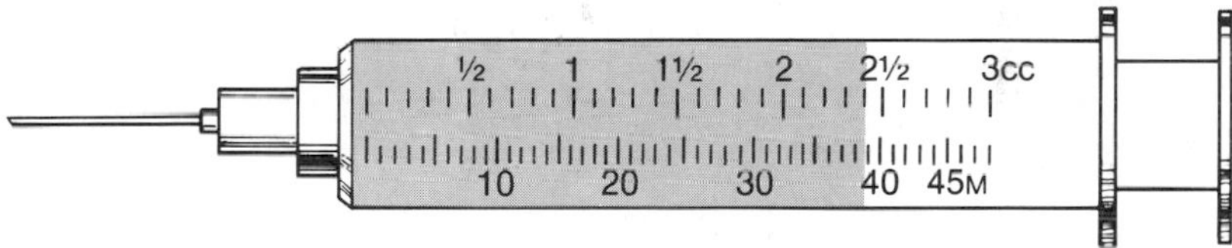

9. $\dfrac{\overset{3}{\cancel{75}}\ \cancel{\text{mg}}}{\underset{2}{\cancel{50}}\ \cancel{\text{mg}}} \times 1\ \text{mL} = \dfrac{3}{2}\ \begin{array}{r}1.5\\ \overline{)3.0}\end{array}$

Give 1.5 mL IM.

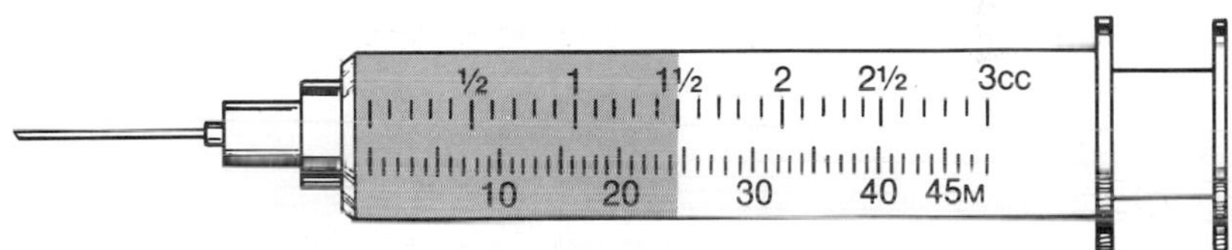

10. Equivalent 1:1000 means 1 g in 1000 mL
1 g = 1000 mg

Hence, the solution is 1000 mg in 1000 mL.

500 μg = 0.5 mg

$\dfrac{0.5\ \cancel{\text{mg}}}{\underset{1}{\cancel{1000}}\ \cancel{\text{mg}}} \times \cancel{1000}\ \text{mL} = 0.5\ \text{mL}$

Give 0.5 mL SC stat.

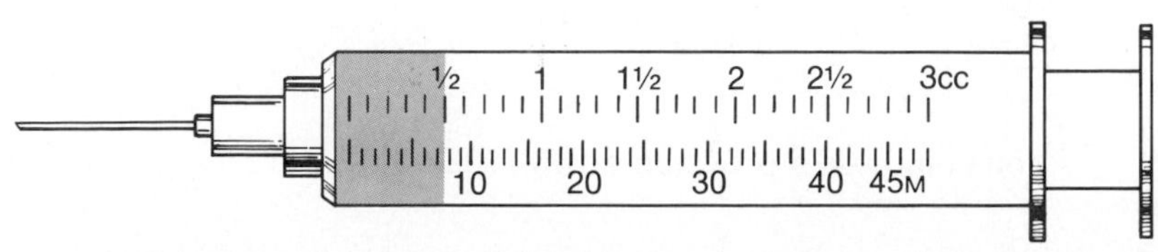

Proficiency Test 3

1. $\frac{0.25 \text{ mg}}{0.50 \text{ mg}} \times 2 \text{ mL} = 1 \text{ mL}$

2. $\frac{40 \text{ mg}}{50 \text{ mg}} \times 2 \text{ cc} = 5\overline{)8.0}^{\,1.6} = 1.6 \text{ mL}$

3. $\frac{8 \text{ mg}}{15 \text{ mg}} \times 1 \text{ mL} = 15\overline{)8.00}^{\,.53} = 0.5 \text{ mL}$

$$\begin{array}{r} 15\overline{)8.00} \\ 7\,5 \\ \hline 50 \\ \underline{45} \end{array}$$

4. $\frac{25 \text{ mg}}{100 \text{ mg}} \times 1 \text{ mL} = 4\overline{)1.00}^{\,.25} = 0.3 \text{ mL}$

You could use the 1-mL precision syringe (0.25 mL).

5. $\frac{200 \text{ mg}}{500 \text{ mg}} \times 2 \text{ mL} \; 5\overline{)4.0}^{\,.8} = 0.8 \text{ mL}$

6. $\frac{1500 \; \mu g}{5000 \; \mu g} \times 1 \text{ mL} = 10\overline{)3.0}^{\,.3} = 0.3 \text{ mL}$

7. $\frac{0.6 \text{ mg}}{0.4 \text{ mg}} \times 1 \text{ mL} = 2\overline{)3.0}^{\,1.5} = 1.5 \text{ mL}$

8. 0.1 gm = 100 mg

$\frac{100 \text{ mg}}{200 \text{ mg}} \times 3 \text{ mL} = 2\overline{)3.0}^{\,1.5} = 1.5 \text{ mL}$

9. $\frac{1.5 \text{ mg}}{2.0 \text{ mg}} \times 1 \text{ mL} = 4\overline{)3.00}^{\,.75} = 0.8 \text{ mL}$

You could use a 1-mL precision syringe (0.75 mL).

10. $\frac{600{,}000 \text{ units}}{500{,}000 \text{ units}} \times 1 \text{ mL} = 5\overline{)6.0}^{\,1.2} = 1.2 \text{ mL}$

11. 200 μg = 0.2 mg

$\frac{0.2 \text{ mg}}{0.8 \text{ mg}} \times 1 \text{ mL} = 4\overline{)1.00}^{\,.25} = 0.3 \text{ mL}$

You could use a precision syringe (0.25 mL).

12. 1:4000 means 1 g in 4000 mL

1 g = 1000 mg

500 mcg = 0.5 mg

$\frac{0.5 \text{ mg}}{1000 \text{ mg}} \times 4000 \text{ mL} = \begin{array}{r} 0.5 \\ \times 4 \\ \hline 2.0 \end{array} \text{ mL}$

13. $\frac{3 \text{ mg}}{2 \text{ mg}} \times 1 \text{ mL} = 2\overline{)3.0}^{\,1.5} = 1.5 \text{ mL}$

14. 1:1000 means 1 g = 1000 mL

1 g = 1000 mg

$\frac{0.4 \text{ mg}}{1000 \text{ mg}} \times 1000 \text{ mL} = 0.4 \text{ mL}$

15. 50% means 50 g in 100 mL

500 mg = 0.5 g

$\frac{0.5 \text{ g}}{50 \text{ g}} \times 100 \text{ mL} = 1.0 \text{ mL}$

16. $\frac{0.75 \text{ mg}}{1.50 \text{ mg}} \times 1 \text{ mL} = \frac{1}{2} \text{ mL or } 0.5 \text{ mL}$

17. 20% means 20 g in 100 mL

100 mg = 0.1 g

$\frac{0.1 \text{ g}}{20 \text{ g}} \times 100 \text{ mL} = 0.5 \text{ mL}$

18. $\frac{0.125 \text{ mg}}{0.250 \text{ mg}} \times 2 \text{ mL} = 1 \text{ mL}$

19. $\frac{12 \text{ mg}}{10 \text{ mg}} \times 1 \text{ mL} = 5\overline{)6.0}^{\,1.2} = 1.2 \text{ mL}$

20. $\frac{10 \text{ mEq}}{40 \text{ mEq}} \times 20 \text{ mL} = 5 \text{ mL}$

This is correct because the route is IV.

Mental Drill in Liquids for Injection Problems

1. 2 mL IM
2. 5 mL IV
3. 2 mL IM
4. 1 mL IM
5. 0.5 mL IM
6. 1 mL IM
7. 0.75 mL or 0.8 mL SC
8. 1 cc SC
9. 20 mL IV
10. 2.5 mL IM
11. 0.8 mL IM
12. 2 mL IM
13. 2 mL IV
14. 1.5 mL IM
15. 1.5 mL IM
16. 0.35 mL or 0.4 mL IM
17. 1.5 mL SC
18. 1.5 mL IM

8 Injections From Powders

CONTENT TO MASTER

Principles for reconstituting drugs from powder form

Reading and understanding drug manufacturer's label and package insert directions when:

- dissolving powders accurately;
- storing reconstituted drugs safely;
- labelling reconstituted drugs

Acceptable fluids for diluting powders for injection

Terms used when reconstituting powders:

displacement, dilution, sterile technique, concentration, new stock, diluting fluids

Some medications are prepared in a dry form, powder or crystal. As liquids they are unstable and lose potency over time. The drug must be reconstituted according to the manufacturer's directions, which will give the type and amount of diluent to use.

▼ INJECTIONS FROM POWDERS

The rule used to solve injection from powder problems is the same as that for oral medications and for injection from a liquid, because the powdered drug *becomes a liquid* once the powder is dissolved.

Application of the Rule for Injections From Powders

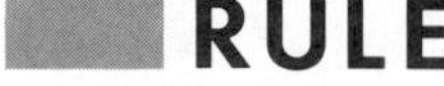

RULE $\frac{\text{Desire}}{\text{Have}} \times \text{Stock} = \text{Amount}$

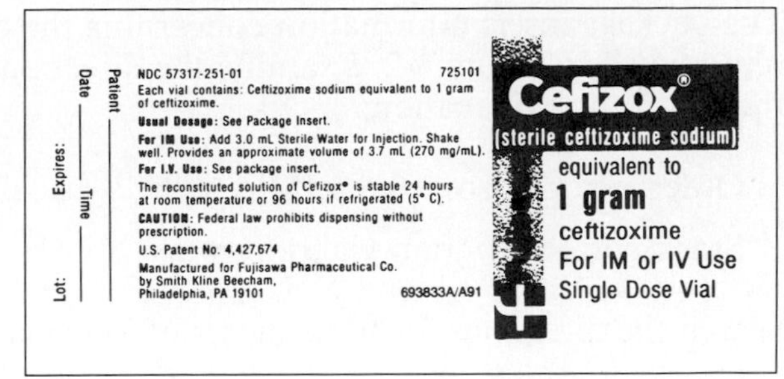

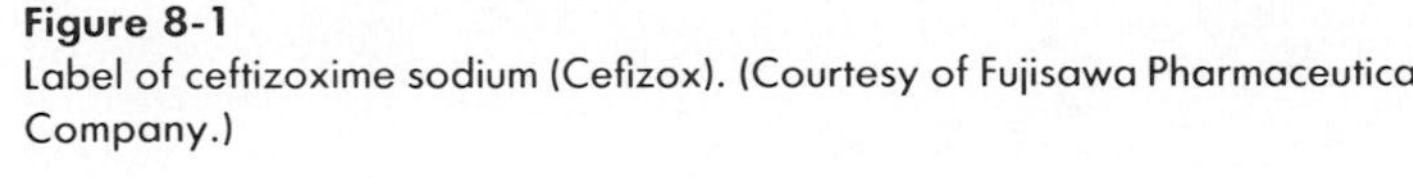

Figure 8-1
Label of ceftizoxime sodium (Cefizox). (Courtesy of Fujisawa Pharmaceutical Company.)

EXAMPLE Order: ceftizoxime sodium 270 mg IM q6h

Label (Fig. 8-1):

Label directions: Add 3.0 mL of sterile water for injection. Shake well. Provides a volume of 3.7 mL (270 mg/mL). Stable for 24 hours at room temperature or 96 hours if refrigerated.

Desire: The order in the example is 270 mg IM.

Have: The strength of the drug supplied. In the example it is 1 g as a dry powder; when it is reconstituted, it is 270 mg/mL. Remember that the manufacturer gives the solution strength; the nurse does not have to determine it.

Stock: The fluid portion of the solution made: in this example it is *1 mL* = 270 mg.

Answer: How much liquid to give (stated as mL, cc). In the example given, the nurse has a solution of 270 mg/mL and an order for 270 mg IM. The answer is obvious: give 1 mL IM. The remaining solution is stored in the refrigerator. The vial is labeled with the date, the solution made, and the nurse's initials.

▼ DISTINCTIVE FEATURES OF INJECTIONS FROM POWDERS

Sterile technique is used to prepare and administer the medication, which is given parenterally (usually IM, IV, or IVPB). The dry drug is supplied in vials of powder or crystals and may come in different strengths. Because powders deteriorate in solution, choose the strength closest to the amount ordered.

The powder is usually diluted with one of the following:

Sterile water for injection

Bacteriostatic water for injection that has a preservative added

Normal saline for injection (0.9% sodium chloride)

Directions will state which fluids may be used. Read this information carefully because some fluids may be incompatible (i.e., unsuitable) as diluents. When the powder goes into solution, *displacement* occurs. This means that the *volume* added to the vial is *increased* by the powder as it is dissolved. There is no uniformity in the way powders go into solution.

Refer to the label in Figure 8-1 again. The manufacturer tells the nurse to add 3.0 mL of sterile water to provide an approximate volume of 3.7 mL. In this example 0.7 mL is the displacement volume. *Injections from powder problems are solved by using the solution made, not the displacement volume.* The manufacturer will give the solution.

The package insert information concerning the dilution of cefoperazone sodium (Cefobid) injection is reproduced in Figure 8-2. Examine the directions with the intention of solving the following problem, then read the explanation:

Order: cefoperazone 0.5 g IM q 12 h

Stock powder: 1 gram vial of powder

Search the directions for three pieces of information to dissolve your stock, which is 1 gram:

- The type of fluid needed to dissolve the powder
- The amount of fluid to add
- The solution made

Explanation

1. Figure 8-2 gives *Solutions for Initial Reconstitution:* sterile water for injection, bacteriostatic water for injection, and 0.9% sodium chloride injection. Choose one.

RECONSTITUTION

The following solutions may be used for the initial reconstitution of CEFOBID sterile powder:

Table 1. Solutions for Initial Reconstitution

5% Dextrose Injection (USP)	0.9% Sodium Chloride Injection (USP)
5% Dextrose and 0.9% Sodium Chloride Injection (USP)	Normosol* M and Dextrose Injection
5% Dextrose and 0.2% Sodium Chloride Injection (USP)	Normosol* R
10% Dextrose Injection (USP)	Sterile Water for Injection*
Bacteriostatic Water for Injection [Benzyl Alcohol or Parabens] (USP)*†	

*Not to be used as a vehicle for intravenous infusion

†Preparations containing Benzyl Alcohol should not be used in neonates.

Preparation for Intramuscular Injection

Any suitable solution listed above may be used to prepare CEFOBID sterile powder for intramuscular injection. When concentrations of 250 mg/ml or more are to be administered, a lidocaine solution should be used. These solutions should be prepared using a combination of Sterile Water for Injection and 2% Lidocaine Hydrochloride Injection (USP) that approximates a 0.5% Lidocaine Hydrochloride Solution. A two-step dilution process as follows is recommended: First, add the required amount of Sterile Water for Injection and agitate until CEFOBID powder is completely dissolved. Second, add the required amount of 2% lidocaine and mix.

	Final Cefoperazone Concentration	Step 1 Volume of Sterile Water	Step 2 Volume of 2% Lidocaine	Withdrawable Volume*†
1 g vial	333 mg/ml	2.0 ml	0.6 ml	3 ml
	250 mg/ml	2.8 ml	1.0 ml	4 ml
2 g vial	333 mg/ml	3.8 ml	1.2 ml	6 ml
	250 mg/ml	5.4 ml	1.8 ml	8 ml

When a diluent other than Lidocaine HCI Injection (USP) is used reconstitute as follows:

	Cefoperazone Concentration	Volume of Diluent to be Added	Withdrawable Volume*
1 g vial	333 mg/ml	2.6 ml	3 ml
	250 mg/ml	3.8 ml	4 ml
2 g vial	333 mg/ml	5.0 ml	6 ml
	250 mg/ml	7.2 ml	8 ml

*There is sufficient excess present to allow for withdrawal of the stated volume.

†Final lidocaine concentration will approximate that obtained if a 0.5% Lidocaine Hydrochloride Solution is used as diluent

STORAGE AND STABILITY

CEFOBID sterile powder is to be stored at or below 25°C (77°F) and protected from light prior to reconstitution. After reconstitution, protection from light is not necessary.

The following parenteral diluents and approximate concentrations of CEFOBID provide stable solutions under the following conditions for the indicated time periods. (After the indicated time periods, unused portions of solutions should be discarded.)

Controlled Room Temperature (15°–25°C/59°–77°F)

24 Hours	Approximate
Bacteriostatic Water for Injection [Benzyl Alcohol or Parabens] (USP)	300 mg/ml
5% Dextrose Injection (USP)	2 mg to 50 mg/ml
5% Dextrose and Lactated Ringer's Injection	2 mg to 50 mg/ml
5% Dextrose and 0.9% Sodium Chloride Injection (USP)	2 mg to 50 mg/ml
5% Dextrose and 0.2% Sodium Chloride Injection (USP)	2 mg to 50 mg/ml
10% Dextrose Injection (USP)	2 mg to 50 mg/ml
Lactated Ringer's Injection (USP)	2 mg/ml
0.5% Lidocaine Hydrochloride Injection (USP)	300 mg/ml
0.9% Sodium Chloride Injection (USP)	2 mg to 300 mg/ml
Normosol* M and 5% Dextrose Injection	2 mg to 50 mg/ml
Normosol* R	2 mg to 50 mg/ml
Sterile Water for Injection	300 mg/ml

Reconstituted CEFOBID solutions may be stored in glass or plastic syringes, or in glass or flexible plastic parenteral solution containers.

Refrigerator Temperature (2°–8°C/36°–46°F)

5 Days	Approximate Concentrations
Bacteriostatic Water for Injection [Benzyl Alcohol or Parabens] (USP)	300 mg/ml
5% Dextrose Injection (USP)	2 mg to 50 mg/ml
5% Dextrose and 0.9% Sodium Chloride Injection (USP)	2 mg to 50 mg/ml
5% Dextrose and 0.2% Sodium Chloride Injection (USP)	2 mg to 50 mg/ml
Lactated Ringer's Injection (USP)	2 mg/ml
0.5% Lidocaine Hydrochloride Injection (USP)	300 mg/ml
0.9% Sodium Chloride Injection (USP)	2 mg to 300 mg/ml
Normosol* M and 5% Dextrose Injection	2 mg to 50 mg/ml
Normosol* R	2 mg to 50 mg/ml
Sterile Water for Injection	300 mg/ml

Reconstituted CEFOBID solutions may be stored in glass or plastic syringes, or in glass or flexible plastic parenteral solution containers.

Figure 8-2

Reconstitution directions for cefoperazone sodium (Cefobid). (Courtesy of Roerig-Pfizer Laboratories.)

2. The heading *Preparation for Intramuscular Injection* states that when a concentration of 250 mg or more is to be administered, a 2% lidocaine solution should be used together with sterile water for injection in a two-step dilution.
3. Two tables are given. The upper table has the two-step dilution, the lower one does not. Because the order requires two steps, use the directions in the top table.
4. Two strengths of powder are listed in the upper table. Look at the extreme left. They are 1-g vial and 2-g vial. Our supply is a 1-g vial. Follow directions for 1 g.
5. The next heading is *Final Cefoperazone Concentration.* Two possibilities are given for the dilution: 333 mg/mL and 250 mg/mL. Because the order calls for 0.5 g, choose 250 mg/mL. This concentration makes the arithmetic easy. Do you see that the answer will be 2 mL?
6. To make the solution of 250 mg/mL, the following are added: 2.8 mL of sterile water and 1.0 mL of 2% lidocaine.
7. The last column to the right is headed *Withdrawable Volume* and lists 4 mL. Ignore this column; it does not affect the answer: When you add 2.8 mL and 1.0 mL, you expect to have 3.8 mL. The package insert states you will end up with 4 mL. The manufacturer is giving the displacement.
8. You now have all the information needed to prepare the dose ordered. Your solution is 250 mg/mL. Equivalent 0.5 g = 500 mg.

   $$\frac{D}{H} \times S = A$$

   $$\frac{\overset{2}{\cancel{500}\ \cancel{mg}}}{\underset{1}{\cancel{250}\ \cancel{mg}}} \times 1\ mL = 2\ mL$$

   Give 2 mL IM.
9. Write on the label the solution you made, the date, and your initials.
10. Note the storage directions and stability expiration.

Steps for Reconstituting Powders With Directions

1. Read the order
2. Identify the stock
3. Dilute the fluid
4. Identify the solution and new stock
5. Apply the rule and arithmetic
6. Obtain the amount to give
7. Write on label
8. Store according to directions

EXAMPLE Order: cefoperazone 0.5 g IM = 500 mg (Refer to Fig. 8-2.)

Stock powder: 1 g

Diluting fluid and number of milliliters

Step 1. Add 2.8 mL sterile water

Step 2. Add 1 mL 2% lidocaine

Solution and new stock: 250 mg/mL

Rule and arithmetic: $\frac{D}{H} \times S = A$

$$\frac{\overset{2}{\cancel{500 \text{ mg}}}}{\underset{1}{\cancel{250 \text{ mg}}}} \times 1 \text{ mL} = 2 \text{ mL}$$

Amount to give: 2 mL IM

Write on label: 250 mg/mL; date; initials

Store: Refrigerate. Stable for 5 days

▼ WHERE TO FIND INFORMATION ABOUT RECONSTITUTION OF POWDERS

Information about reconstitution of powders may be found from

- The label on the vial of powder
- The package insert that comes with the vial of powder
- Nursing drug handbooks
- Other references such as the *Physician's Desk Reference (PDR)*

EXAMPLE

Example 1:

Order: cefazolin sodium 0.3 g IM (Fig. 8-3)

Stock powder: 500 mg

Diluting fluid: 2.0 mL sterile water for injection

Solution and new stock: 225 mg/mL

RECONSTITUTION

Preparation of Parenteral Solution

Parenteral drug products should be SHAKEN WELL when reconstituted, and inspected visually for particulate matter prior to administration. If particulate matter is evident in reconstituted fluids, the drug solutions should be discarded. When reconstituted or diluted according to the instructions below, Ancef (sterile cefazolin sodium, SK&F) is stable for 24 hours at room temperature or for 96 hours if stored under refrigeration. Reconstituted solutions may range in color from pale yellow to yellow without a change in potency.

Single-Dose Vials

For I.M. injection, I.V. direct (bolus) injection, or I.V. infusion, reconstitute with Sterile Water for Injection according to the following table. SHAKE WELL.

Vial Size	Amount of Diluent	Approximate Concentration	Approximate Available Volume
250 mg.	2.0 ml.	125 mg./ml.	2.0 ml.
500 mg.	2.0 ml.	225 mg./ml.	2.2 ml.
1 gram	2.5 ml.	330 mg./ml.	3.0 ml.

Figure 8-3
Reconstitution directions for cefazolin sodium (Ancef). (Courtesy of Smith Kline Beecham Pharmaceuticals.)

Rule and arithmetic: $\frac{D}{H} \times S = A$

Equivalent 0.3 g = 300 mg

$$\frac{\overset{\overset{4}{\cancel{12}}}{\cancel{300}\ \text{mg}}}{\underset{\underset{3}{\cancel{9}}}{\cancel{225}\ \text{mg}}} \times 1\ \text{mL} = \frac{4}{3} \quad 3\,\overline{)4.00}^{\,1.33}$$

Give 1.3 mL IM.

Write on label: 225 mg/mL, date, initials

Storage: Refrigerate. Stable for 96 hours.

Example 2:

Order: penicillin G potassium 1 million units IM q6h (Fig. 8-4)

Stock powder: 5 million unit vial

Diluting fluid and number of milliliters: Use sterile water for injection. The reconstitution directions are difficult to read. The word "respectively" at the end of the sentence means "in order." Write out the directions for the 5 million unit vial (stock).

23 mL will provide 200,000 U/mL
18 mL will provide 250,000 U/mL
8 mL will provide 500,000 U/mL
3 mL will provide 1 million U/mL

Choose 3 mL to dilute the powder.

Solution and new stock: 1 million units/mL

Rule: not needed because

$$\frac{D}{H} \times S = A$$

$$\frac{1\ \text{million units}}{1\ \text{million units}} \times 1\ \text{mL} = 1\ \text{mL}$$

Preparation of Solutions

Solutions of penicillin should be prepared as follows: Loosen powder. Hold vial horizontally and rotate it while *slowly* directing the stream of diluent against the wall of the vial. Shake vial vigorously after all the diluent has been added. Depending on the route of administration, use Sterile Water for Injection USP, isotonic Sodium Chloride Injection USP, or Dextrose Injection USP. NOTE: Penicillins are rapidly inactivated in the presence of carbohydrate solutions at alkaline pH.

RECONSTITUTION: 1,000,000 u vial—add 9.6 ml, 4.6 ml, or 3.6 ml diluent to provide 100,000 u, 200,000 u, or 250,000 u per ml, respectively: 5,000,000 u vial—add 23 ml, 18 ml, 8 ml, or 3 ml diluent to provide 200,000 u, 250,000 u, 500,000 u, or 1,000,000 u per ml, respectively. *For IV infusion only:* 10,000,000 u vial—add 15.5 ml or 5.4 ml diluent to provide 500,000 u or 1,000,000 u per ml, respectively: 20,000,000 u vial—add 31.6 ml diluent to provide 500,000 u per ml.

HOW SUPPLIED

Penicillin G Potassium for Injection USP is available in vials providing 1, 5, 10 and 20 million u of crystalline penicillin G potassium.

Storage

The dry powder is relatively stable and may be stored at room temperature without significant loss of potency. Sterile solutions may be kept in the refrigerator one week without significant loss of potency. Solutions prepared for intravenous infusion are stable at room temperature for at least 24 hours.

Figure 8-4
Preparation of solution for the 1-million-unit and the 5-million-unit vial of penicillin G potassium. (Package insert used by permission of E. R. Squibb & Sons, Inc., copyright owner.)

Give 1 mL IM.

Write on label: 1 million units/mL; date; initials

Storage: Refrigerate. Stable for 1 week

Note: This solution (1 million units/mL) may be so concentrated that it is painful when injected. The nurse could decide to dilute the powder with 8 mL to make 500,000 U/mL and give 2 mL to the patient. This more dilute solution may be less painful.

Here are a few tips before you begin Practice Exercise 1.

- When you read the directions for reconstitution, look first at the solutions you can make. Think the problem through mentally and choose one dilution. This provides a focus as you read.
- If your answer is more than 3 mL for an IM injection, consider using two syringes and injecting in two different sites.
- Experience in administering injections will guide you in choosing the concentration of the solution. Stronger concentrations, although smaller in volume, may be more painful; a more dilute solution may be more suitable despite its larger volume.
- Each powder problem is unique. Read the directions carefully!
- Choose one diluting fluid—generally sterile water or 0.9% sodium chloride for injection. Do not list all of them in your answer.
- For the following practice problems and self-tests, assume that the doses ordered and the order are correct. Chapter 12 discusses the nurse's responsibilities in drug knowledge. Dosages for infants and children are discussed in Chapter 10.

Practice Exercise 1

Solve the following problems in injections from powders and write your answers using the steps. Answers are found at the end of the chapter.

1. Order: carbenicillin disodium 1 g IM q6h (for an adult) (Fig. 8-5)
Stock: vial of powder labeled 2 g

a. Diluting fluid and number of milliliters:
b. Solution and new stock:
c. Rule and arithmetic:
d. Answer:
e. Write on label:
f. Storage:

For Intramuscular Use: The 2 g vial should be reconstituted with 4.0 ml of Sterile Water for Injection, 0.5% Lidocaine Hydrochloride (without epinephrine), or Bacteriostatic Water containing 0.9% benzyl alcohol. (Preparations containing benzyl alcohol should not be used in neonates.) In order to facilitate reconstitution up to 7.2 ml of diluent can be used.

Amount of Diluent to be Added to the 2 g Vial	Volume to be Withdrawn for a 1 g Dose
4.0 ml	2.5 ml
5.0 ml	3.0 ml
7.2 ml	4.0 ml

The 5 g vial should be reconstituted with 7.0 ml of Sterile Water for Injection, 0.5% Lidocaine Hydrochloride (without epinephrine), or Bacteriostatic Water containing 0.9% benzyl alcohol. (Preparations containing benzyl alcohol should not be used in neonates.) In order to facilitate reconstitution, up to 17 ml of diluent can be used.

Amount of Diluent to be Added to the 5 g Vial	Volume to be Withdrawn for a 1 g Dose
7.0 ml	2.0 ml
9.5 ml	2.5 ml
12.0 ml	3.0 ml
17.0 ml	4.0 ml

After reconstitution, no significant loss of potency occurs for up to 24 hours at room temperature, and for 72 hours if refrigerated. Any of these unused solutions should be discarded.

Figure 8-5
Preparation of solution of carbenicillin sodium (Geopen). (Courtesy of Roerig-Pfizer Laboratories.)

(continued)

Practice Exercise 1 (continued)

2. Order: ceftazidime 1 g IM q6h (Fig. 8-6)
   Stock: 1 g powder
   a. Diluting fluid and number of milliliters:
   b. Solution and new stock:
   c. Rule and arithmetic:
   d. Answer:
   e. Write on label:
   f. Storage:

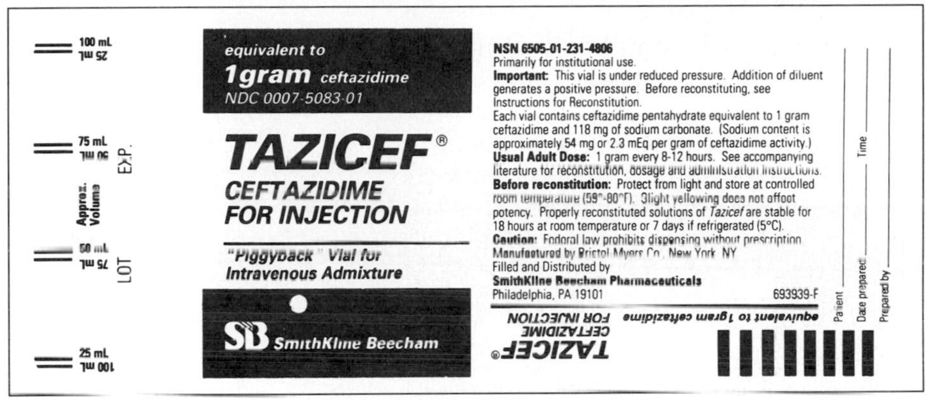

RECONSTITUTION
Single Dose Vials:
For I.M. injection, I.V. direct (bolus) injection, or I.V. infusion, reconstitute with Sterile Water for Injection according to the following table. The vacuum may assist entry of the diluent. SHAKE WELL.

Table 5

Vial Size	Diluent to Be Added	Approx. Avail. Volume	Approx. Avg. Concentration
Intramuscular or Intravenous Direct (bolus) Injection			
1 gram	3.0 mL	3.6 mL	280 mg/ml
Intravenous Infusion			
1 gram	10 mL	10.6 mL	95 mg/mL
2 gram	10 mL	11.2 mL	180 mg/ml

Withdraw the total volume of solution into the syringe (the pressure in the vial may aid withdrawal). The withdrawn solution may contain some bubbles of carbon dioxide.

NOTE: **As with the administration of all parenteral products, accumulated gases should be expressed from the syringe immediately before injection of *Tazicef*.**

These solutions of *Tazicef* are stable for 18 hours at room temperature or seven days if refrigerated (5°C). Slight yellowing does not affect potency.

Figure 8-6
Label and reconstitution directions for ceftazidime (Tazicef) 1 g. (Courtesy of Smith Kline Beecham Laboratories.)

(continued)

Practice Exercise 1 (continued)

3. Order: Omnipen 250 mg IM q6h (Fig. 8-7)
   Stock: 500-mg vial of powder
   a. Diluting fluid and number of milliliters:
   b. Solution and new stock:
   c. Rule and arithmetic:
   d. Answer:
   e. Write on label:
   f. Storage:

For dilution of 500-mg, 1-gram, and 2-gram vials, dissolve contents of a vial with the amount of Sterile water for Injection, USP, or Bacteriostatic Water for Injection, USP, listed in the table below:

Label Claim	Recommended Amount of Diluent	With-draw-able Volume	Concen-tration in mg/ml
500 mg	1.8 ml	2.0 ml	250 mg
1.0 gram	3.4 ml	4.0 ml	250 mg
2.0 gram	6.8 ml	8.0 ml	250 mg

While the 1-gram and 2-gram vials are primarily for intravenous use, they may be administered intramuscularly when the 250-mg or 500-mg vials are unavailable. In such instances, dissolve in 3.4 or 6.8 ml Sterile Water for Injection, USP, or Bacteriostatic Water for Injection, USP, to give a final concentration of 250 mg/ml
The above solutions must be used within one hour after reconstitution.

Figure 8-7
Reconstitution directions for ampicillin sodium (Omnipen-N) for IM or IV injection. (Courtesy of Wyeth-Ayerst Laboratories, Philadelphia, PA.)

Practice Exercise 2

Solve the following problems in injections from powders using the steps. Answers can be found at the end of the chapter.

1. Order: Ancef 225 mg IM q6h (Fig. 8-8)
   Stock: On the shelf there are three vial sizes of powder: 250 mg, 500 mg, 1 g
   a. Stock chosen:
   b. Diluting fluid and number of milliliters:
   c. Solution and new stock:
   d. Rule and arithmetic:
   e. Answer:
   f. Write on label:
   g. Storage:

RECONSTITUTION

Preparation of Parenteral Solution

Parenteral drug products should be SHAKEN WELL when reconstituted, and inspected visually for particulate matter prior to administration. If particulate matter is evident in reconstituted fluids, the drug solutions should be discarded. When reconstituted or diluted according to the instructions below, Ancef (sterile cefazolin sodium, SK&F) is stable for 24 hours at room temperature or for 96 hours if stored under refrigeration. Reconstituted solutions may range in color from pale yellow to yellow without a change in potency.

Single-Dose Vials

For I.M. injection, I.V. direct (bolus) injection, or I.V. infusion, reconstitute with Sterile Water for Injection according to the following table. SHAKE WELL.

Vial Size	Amount of Diluent	Approximate Concentration	Approximate Available Volume
250 mg.	2.0 ml.	125 mg./ml.	2.0 ml.
500 mg.	2.0 ml.	225 mg./ml.	2.2 ml.
1 gram	2.5 ml.	330 mg./ml.	3.0 ml.

Figure 8-8
Reconstitution directions for cefazolin sodium (Ancef). (Courtesy of Smith Kline Beecham Laboratories.)

(continued)

Practice Exercise 2 (continued)

2. Order: cefazolin sodium 0.5 g IM q8h (refer to Fig. 8-8)
   Stock: vial of powder labeled 1 Gm

   a. Diluting fluid and number of milliliters:
   b. Solution made and new stock:
   c. Rule and arithmetic:
   d. Answer:
   e. Write on label:
   f. Storage:

3. Order: Fortaz 500 mg IM q 6 h (Fig. 8-9)
   Stock: 1 g powder

   a. Diluting fluid and number of milliliters:
   b. Solution and new stock:
   c. Rule and arithmetic:
   d. Answer:
   e. Write on label:
   f. Storage:

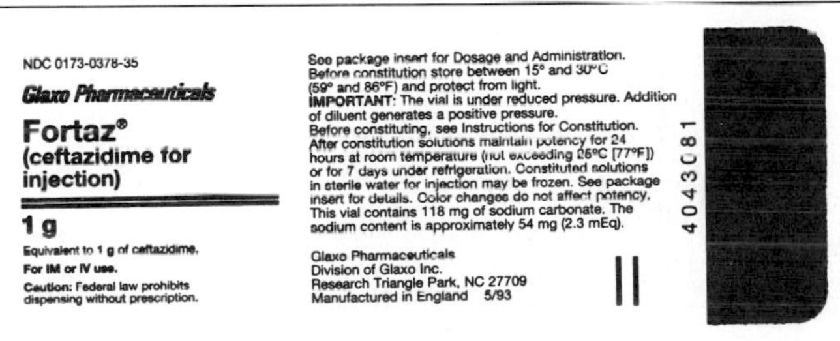

Table 5: Preparation of Fortaz Solutions

Size	Amount of Diluent to Be Added (mL)	Approximate Available Volume (mL)	Approximate Ceftazidime Concentration (mg/mL)
Intramuscular			
500-mg vial	1.5	1.8	280
1-gram vial	3.0	3.6	280
Intravenous			
500-mg vial	5.0	5.3	100
1-gram vial	10.0	10.6	100
2-gram vial	10.0	11.5	170
Infusion pack			
1-gram vial	100*	100	10
2-gram vial	100*	100	20
Pharmacy bulk package			
6-gram vial	26	30	200

***Note:** Addition should be in two stages (see Instructions for Constitution).

COMPATIBILITY AND STABILITY:
Intramuscular: Fortaz®, when constituted as directed with sterile water for injection, bacteriostatic water for injection, or 0.5% or 1% lidocaine hydrochloride injection, maintains satisfactory potency for 24 hours at room temperature or for 7 days under refrigeration. Solutions in sterile water for injection that are frozen immediately after constitution in the original container are stable for 3 months when stored at -20°C. Once thawed, solutions should not be refrozen. Thawed solutions may be stored for up to 8 hours at room temperature or for 4 days in a refrigerator.

Figure 8-9
Preparation of Fortaz solutions. (Courtesy of Glaxo Pharmaceuticals.)

Self-Test 1

Solve these problems. Check your answers at the end of the chapter.

1. Order: cefoxitin sodium 200 mg IM q4h (Fig. 8-10)
   Stock: vial of powder labeled 1 g

Table 3 — Preparation of Solution

Strength	Amount of Diluent to be Added (mL)+ +	Approximate Withdrawable Volume (mL)	Approximate Average Concentration (mg/mL)
1 gram Vial	2 (Intramuscular)	2.5	400
2 gram Vial	4 (Intramuscular)	5	400
1 gram Vial	10 (IV)	10.5	95
2 gram Vial	10 or 20 (IV)	11.1 or 21.0	180 or 95
1 gram Infusion Bottle	50 or 100 (IV)	50 or 100	20 or 10
2 gram Infusion Bottle	50 or 100 (IV)	50 or 100	40 or 20
10 gram Bulk	43 or 93 (IV)	49 or 98.5	200 or 100

+ +Shake to dissolve and let stand until clear.

Intramuscular
MEFOXIN, as constituted with Sterile Water for Injection, Bacteriostatic Water for Injection, or 0.5 percent or 1 percent lidocaine hydrochloride solution (without epinephrine), maintains satisfactory potency for 24 hours at room temperature, for one week under refrigeration (below 5°C), and for at least 30 weeks in the frozen state.

Figure 8-10
Directions to reconstitute cefoxitin sodium (Mefoxin). (Courtesy of Merck Sharp & Dohme.)

   a. Diluting fluid and number of milliliters:
   b. Solution made and new stock:
   c. Rule and arithmetic:
   d. Answer:
   e. Write on label:
   f. Storage:

2. Order: Mefoxitin 0.6 g IM q6h (refer to Fig. 8-10)
   Stock powder: 1 gram

   a. Diluting fluid and number of milliliters:
   b. Solution made and new stock:
   c. Rule and arithmetic:
   d. Amount to give:
   e. Write on label:
   f. Storage:

(continued)

Self-Test 1 (continued)

3. Order: Claforan 800 mg IM q12h (Fig. 8-11)
   Stock: vials of powder 1 g, and 2 g

PREPARATION OF CLAFORAN STERILE

Claforan for IM or IV administration should be reconstituted as follows:

Strength	Diluent (mL)	Withdrawable Volume (mL)	Approximate Concentration (mg/mL)
1g vial (IM)*	3	3.4	300
2g vial (IM)*	5	6.0	330
1g vial (IV)*	10	10.4	95
2g vial (IV)*	10	11.0	180
1g infusion	50-100	50-100	20-10
2g infusion	50-100	50-100	40-20
10g bottle	47	52.0	200
10g bottle	97	102.0	100

(*) in conventional vials

Shake to dissolve; inspect for particulate matter and discoloration prior to use. Solutions of Claforan range from very pale yellow to light amber, depending on concentration, diluent used, and length and condition of storage.

For intramuscular use: Reconstitute VIALS with Sterile Water for Injection or Bacteriostatic Water for Injection as described above.

COMPATIBILITY AND STABILITY

Solutions of Claforan Sterile reconstituted as described above **(Preparation of Claforan Sterile)** maintain satisfactory potency for 24 hours at room temperature (at or below 22°C), 10 days under refrigeration (at or below 5°C), and for at least 13 weeks frozen.

Figure 8-11
Preparation of solution of cefotaxime sodium (Claforan). (Courtesy of Hoechst–Roussel Pharmaceuticals.)

a. Stock chosen:
b. Diluting fluid and number of milliliters:
c. Solution made and new stock:
d. Rule and arithmetic:
e. Amount to give:
f. Write on label:
g. Storage:

4. Order: amytal sodium 250 mg IM stat
   Stock: ampule of crystals labeled 0.5 g
   Directions: To derive a 20% solution add 2.5 mL of sterile water for injection.
   Note: You may wish to review Chapter 7, "When Stock Is a Percent."

a. Diluting fluid and number of milliliters:
b. Solution made and new stock:
c. Rule and arithmetic:
d. Amount to give:
e. Write on label:
f. Storage:

Self-Test 2 *Solve these problems. Write the steps. Answers can be found at the end of the chapter.*

1. Order: Pentacef 0.25 g IM q 12 h (Fig. 8-12)
   Stock powder: 1 gram

RECONSTITUTION

Single Dose Vials:
For I.M. injection, I.V. direct (bolus) injection, or I.V. infusion, reconstitute with Sterile Water for Injection according to the following table. SHAKE WELL.

Table 5

Vial Size	Diluent to Be Added	Approx. Avail. Volume	Approx. Avg. Concentration
Intramuscular or Intravenous Direct (bolus) Injection			
1 gram	3.0 mL	3.6 mL	280 mg/mL

COMPATIBILITY AND STABILITY
Intramuscular: *Pentacef*, when reconstituted as directed with Sterile Water for Injection, maintains satisfactory potency for 24 hours at room temperature or for seven days under refrigeration (5°C). Solutions in Sterile Water for Injection that are frozen immediately after reconstitution in the original container are stable for three months when stored at -20°C. Components of the solution may precipitate in the frozen state and will dissolve upon reaching room temperature with little or no agitation. Potency is not affected. Frozen solutions should only be thawed at room temperature. Do not force thaw by immersion in water baths or by microwave irradiation. Once thawed, solutions should not be refrozen. Thawed solutions may be stored for up to eight hours at room temperature or for four days in a refrigerator (5°C).

Figure 8-12
Reconstitution directions for ceftazidime (Pentacef). (Courtesy of Smith Kline Beecham and Bristol Meyers Squibb Company—joint manufacturers.)

2. Order: penicillin G potassium 300,000 units IM (refer to Figure 8-4 for directions)
   Stock powder: 1 million unit vial

3. Order: Velosef 350 mg IM q8h (Fig. 8-13)
   Stock: vial of powder labeled 1 g for injection

VELOSEF FOR INJECTION
(Cephradine for Injection USP)

IM DILUTION TABLE

Vial Size	Volume of Diluent	Approximate Available Volume	Approximate Available Concentration
250 mg	1.2 mL	1.2 mL	208 mg/mL
500 mg	2.0 mL	2.2 mL	227 mg/mL
1 g	4.0 mL	4.5 mL	222 mg/mL

For I.M. Use.—Aseptically add Sterile Water for Injection or Bacteriostatic Water for Injection (containing 0.9% [w/v] benzyl alcohol, or 0.12% methylparaben and 0.014% propylparaben) according to the following table [i.e., the table entitled "IM Dilution Table" below].

Intramuscular solutions should be used within two hours at room temperature; if stored in the refrigerator at 5° C., solutions retain full potency for 24 hours. Constituted solutions may vary in color from light straw to yellow; however, this does not affect the potency.

Figure 8-13
Directions to reconstitute cephradine (Velosef) for IM injection. (Package insert used by permission of E. R. Squibb & Sons, Inc., copyright owner.)

4. Order: ceftazidime 0.5 g IM q12h (refer to Fig. 8-6 for directions)
   Stock powder: 1 gram

Exercise

Mental Drill in Injection From Powder Problems

As you develop proficiency in solving these problems, you will be able to calculate many answers without written work. Here are two drills to sharpen your skill. The first drill ***should be easy*** *because the specific directions needed are given to you. In the second exercise you must choose the direction you need. Aim for 100%! We will not indicate storage directions. Answers will be shown as follows at the end of the chapter:*

a. Diluting fluid and number of milliliters:
b. Solution made and new stock:
c. Answer:
d. Label:

Set A

1. Order: penicillin G 300,000 units IM
Stock: powder labeled 1 million units
Directions: dissolve with 4.6 mL sterile water for injection to make 200,000 units/mL.

2. Order: acetazolamide sodium 200 mg IM
Stock: vial of powder labeled 500 mg
Directions: dissolve powder with 5 cc sterile water for injection. Each cc = 100 mg.

3. Order: hydrocortisone sodium succinate 100 mg IM
Stock: vial of powder labeled 100 mg and an ampule of 2 mL diluent
Directions: add diluent to powder. Each 2 mL = 100 mg.

4. Order: penicillin G 400,000 units IM
Stock: vial of powder labeled 1 million units
Directions: dissolve powder with 4.6 mL sterile water for injection to make 200,000 U/mL.

5. Order: acetazolamide 150 mg IM
Stock: vial of powder labeled 500 mg
Directions: reconstitute powder with 5 mL sterile water for injection. Solution will be 100 mg/mL.

(continued)

Exercise (continued)

6. Order: Amytal sodium 200 mg IM
   Stock: ampule of crystals labeled 250 mg
   Dirctions: add 5 mL sterile water for injection to make a solution of 50 mg/mL, or add 2.5 mL sterile water for injection to make a solution of 100 mg/mL.

7. Order: colycillin 250 mg IM
   Stock: vial of powder labeled 1 g.
   Directions: add 1.5 mL sterile water for injection to prepare a solution of 500 mg/cc.

8. Order: phenytoin sodium 100 mg IM
   Stock: vial of powder labeled 250 mg
   Directions: add 3.5 mL sterile water for injection. Solution will be 75 mg/mL.

9. Order: ampicillin 400 mg IM
   Stock: vial of powder labeled 500 mg
   Directions: add 1.8 mL sterile water for injection to make a solution of 250 mg/mL.

10. Order: cefazolin sodium 150 mg IM
    Stock: vial of powder labeled 250 mg
    Directions: Add 2 mL sterile water for injection to make a solution of 125 mg/mL.

Set B

Directions for these problems are located throughout Chapter 8. Choose the directions you need to give the ordered dose. Aim for 100%.

1. Order: ceftizoxime sodium 90 mg IM q12h
   Stock: vial of powder labeled Cefizox 1 gram (refer to Fig. 8-1)

2. Order: carbenicillin disodium 0.5 Gm q8h
   Stock: vial of powder labeled Geopen 2 grams (refer to Fig. 8-5)

(continued)

Exercise (continued)

3. Order: penicillin G potassium 40,000 units q4h IM
Stock: vial of powder labeled Pfizerpen 1,000,000 U (refer to Fig. 8-14)

Pfizerpen

Approx. Desired Concentration (units/ml)	Approx. Volume (ml) 1,000,000 units	Solvent for Vial of 5,000,000 units	Infusion Only 20,000,000 units
50,000	20.0	. . .	. . .
100,000	10.0	. . .	. . .
250,000	4.0	18.2	75.0
500,000	1.8	8.2	33.0
750,000	. . .	4.8	. . .
1,000,000	. . .	3.2	11.5

(1) Intramuscular Injection: Keep total volume of injection small. The intramuscular route is the preferred route of administration. Solutions containing up to 100,000 units of penicillin per ml of diluent may be used with a minimum of discomfort. Greater concentration of penicillin G per ml is physically possible and may be employed where therapy demands. When large dosages are required, it may be advisable to administer solutions of penicillin by means of continuous intravenous drip.

Buffered Pfizerpen (penicillin G potassium) for Injection is highly water soluble. It may be dissolved in small amounts of Water for Injection, or Sterile Isotonic Sodium Chloride Solution for Parenteral Use. All solutions should be stored in a refrigerator. When refrigerated, penicillin solutions may be stored for seven days without significant loss of potency. Buffered Pfizerpen (penicillin G potassium) for Injection may be given intramuscularly or by continuous intravenous drip for dosages of 500,000, 1,000,000, or 5,000,000 units.

Figure 8-14
Preparation of solution of penicillin G potassium (Pfizerpen). (Courtesy of Roerig-Pfizer Laboratories.)

4. Order: cefazolin sodium 0.45 g IM q12h
Stock: vial of powder labeled cefazolin sodium 500 mg (refer to Fig. 8-3)

5. Order: ampicillin sodium 400 mg IM q 6 h (refer to Fig. 8-7)
Stock powder: 500 mg

6. Order: cefotaxime sodium 1 g IM 1 hr before surgery
Stock: vial of powder labeled Claforan 1 gram (refer to Fig. 8-11)

7. Order: ceftazidime 0.5 g IM q 6 h (refer to Fig. 8-6)
Stock powder: 1 gram

8. Order: cefoxitin sodium 0.5 gm IM q12h
Stock: vial of powder labeled Mefoxin 1 gram (refer to Fig. 8-10)

9. Order: cefazolin sodium 150 mg IM q8h
Stock: vial of powder labeled 250 mg (refer to Fig. 8-3)

10. Order: penicillin G potassium 250,000 U IM q8h
Stock: vial of powder labeled 5 million units (refer to Fig. 8-4)

Proficiency Test

There are 10 questions, each worth 10 points. Aim for 90% or better on this test. If you have any difficulty doing the problems, review and study Chapter 8. Answers may be found at the end of the chapter in milliliters to the nearest tenth.

1. Order: penicillin G potassium 600,000 units IM q8h
Stock: vial of powder labeled 1 million units (refer to Fig. 8-14)

a. Diluting fluid and number of milliliters:
b. Solution and new stock:
c. Rule and arithmetic:
d. Amount to give:
e. Write on label:
f. Storage:

2. Order: ticarcillin disodium 1 g IM
Stock: vial of powder labeled Ticar 1 gram (Fig. 8-15)

a. Diluting fluid and number of milliliters:
b. Solution and new stock:
c. Rule and arithmetic:
d. Amount to give:
e. Write on label:
f. Storage:

DIRECTIONS FOR USE

—1 Gm, 3 Gm and 6 Gm Standard Vials—

INTRAMUSCULAR USE: (Concentration of approximately 385 mg/ml).
For initial reconstitution use Sterile Water for Injection, USP, Sodium Chloride Injection, USP or 1% Lidocaine Hydrochloride solution* (without epinephrine).
Each gram of Ticarcillin should be reconstituted with 2 ml of Sterile Water for Injection, U.S.P., Sodium Chloride Injection, U.S.P. or 1% Lidocaine Hydrochloride solution* (without epinephrine) and **used promptly.** Each 2.6 ml of the resulting solution will then contain 1 Gm of Ticarcillin.
*[For full product information, refer to manufacturer's package insert for Lidocaine Hydrochloride.]
As with all intramuscular preparations, TICAR (Ticarcillin Disodium) should be injected well within the body of a relatively large muscle, using usual techniques and precautions.

Figure 8-15
Directions for use of ticarcillin disodium (Ticar). (Courtesy of Beecham Laboratories.)

3. Order: ceftazidime 200 mg IM q8h
Stock: vial of powder labeled 500 mg (Fig. 8-16)

a. Diluting fluid and number of milliliters:
b. Solution and new stock:
c. Rule and arithmetic:
d. Amount to give:
e. Write on label:
f. Storage:

Preparation of Solutions of Tazidime

	Amount of Diluent to Be Added (mL)	Approximate Available Volume (mL)	Approximate Ceftazidime Concentration (mg/mL)
Intramuscular			
500 mg, Vial No. 7230	1.5	1.8	280
1 g, Vial No. 7231	3.0	3.6	280
Intravenous			
500 mg, Vial No. 7230	5	5.3	100
1 g, Vial No. 7231	5 or 10	5.6 or 10.6	180 or 100
2 g, Vial No. 7234	10	11.2	180
Piggyback (100 mL)			
1 g, Vial No. 7238	50* or 100*	50 or 100	20 or 10
2 g, Vial No. 7239	50* or 100*	50 or 100	40 or 20

COMPATIBILITY AND STABILITY

Intramuscular: Vials of Tazidime, when reconstituted as directed with Sterile Water for Injection, Bacteriostatic Water for Injection, or 0.5% or 1% Lidocaine Hydrochloride Injection, maintain satisfactory potency for 24 hours at room temperature or for 10 days under refrigeration. Solutions in Sterile Water for Injection that are frozen immediately after reconstitution in the original container are stable for 3 months when stored at −20°C. Once thawed, solutions should not be refrozen. Thawed solutions may be stored for up to 24 hours at room temperature or for 4 days in a refrigerator.

Figure 8-16
Preparation of solution of ceftazidime (Tazidime). (Courtesy of Eli Lilly and Co.)

(continued)

Proficiency Test (continued)

4. Order: carbenicillin disodium 1 g IM q6h
   Stock: vial of powder 5 grams (Fig. 8-17)
   a. Diluting fluid and number of milliliters:
   b. Solution and new stock:
   c. Rule and arithmetic:
   d. Amount to give:
   e. Write on label:
   f. Storage:

For Intramuscular Use: The 2 g vial should be reconstituted with 4.0 ml of Sterile Water for Injection, 0.5% Lidocaine Hydrochloride (without epinephrine), or Bacteriostatic Water containing 0.9% benzyl alcohol. (Preparations containing benzyl alcohol should not be used in neonates.) In order to facilitate reconstitution up to 7.2 ml of diluent can be used.

Amount of Diluent to be Added to the 2 g Vial	Volume to be Withdrawn for a 1 g Dose
4.0 ml	2.5 ml
5.0 ml	3.0 ml
7.2 ml	4.0 ml

The 5 g vial should be reconstituted with 7.0 ml of Sterile Water for Injection, 0.5% Lidocaine Hydrochloride (without epinephrine), or Bacteriostatic Water containing 0.9% benzyl alcohol. (Preparations containing benzyl alcohol should not be used in neonates.) In order to facilitate reconstitution, up to 17 ml of diluent can be used.

Amount of Diluent to be Added to the 5 g Vial	Volume to be Withdrawn for a 1 g Dose
7.0 ml	2.0 ml
9.5 ml	2.5 ml
12.0 ml	3.0 ml
17.0 ml	4.0 ml

After reconstitution, no significant loss of potency occurs for up to 24 hours at room temperature, and for 72 hours if refrigerated. Any of these unused solutions should be discarded.

Figure 8-17
Preparation of solution of carbenicillin disodium. (Courtesy of Roerig-Pfizer Laboratories.)

5. Order: ampicillin sodium 300 mg IM q8h
   Stock: vial of 500 mg powder (refer to Fig. 8-18)
   a. Diluting fluid and number of milliliters:
   b. Solution and new stock:
   c. Rule and arithmetic:
   d. Amount to give:
   e. Write on label:
   f. Storage:

Intramuscular Use: 125 mg vial: Add 1 ml Sterile Water for Injection, USP, or Bacteriostatic Water for Injection, USP (TUBEX® Sterile Cartridge-Needle Unit) to give a final concentration of 125 mg per ml. For fractional doses, withdraw the ampicillin sodium solution as follows:

Dose	Withdraw
25 mg	0.2 ml
50 mg	0.4 ml
75 mg	0.6 ml
100 mg	0.8 ml
125 mg	1 ml

250 mg vial: Add 0.9 ml Sterile Water for Injection, USP, or Bacteriostatic Water for Injection, USP (TUBEX) to give a final concentration of 250 mg/ml. For fractional doses, withdraw the ampicillin sodium solution as follows:

Dose	Withdraw
125 mg	0.5 ml
150 mg	0.6 ml
175 mg	0.7 ml
200 mg	0.8 ml
225 mg	0.9 ml
250 mg	1 ml

For dilution of 500-mg, 1-gram, and 2-gram vials, dissolve contents of a vial with the amount of Sterile water for Injection, USP, or Bacteriostatic Water for Injection, USP, listed in the table below:

Label Claim	Recommended Amount of Diluent	With-draw-able Volume	Concen-tration in mg/ml
500 mg	1.8 ml	2.0 ml	250 mg
1.0 gram	3.4 ml	4.0 ml	250 mg
2.0 gram	6.8 ml	8.0 ml	250 mg

While the 1-gram and 2 gram vials are primarily for intravenous use, they may be administered intramuscularly when the 250-mg or 500-mg vials are unavailable. In such instances, dissolve in 3.4 or 6.8 ml Sterile Water for Injection, USP, or Bacteriostatic Water for Injection, USP, to give a final concentration of 250 mg/ml
The above solutions must be used within one hour after reconstitution.

Figure 8-18
Reconstitutions directions for ampicillin sodium. (Omnipen®-N) for IM or IV injection. (Courtesy of Wyeth-Ayerst Laboratories, Philadelphia, PA)

(continued)

Proficiency Test (continued)

6. Order: ampicillin sodium 200 mg IM q8h
   Stock: vial of powder labeled 250 mg (Fig. 8-18)

   a. Diluting fluid and number of milliliters:
   b. Solution and new stock:
   c. Rule and arithmetic:
   d. Amount to give:
   e. Write on label:
   f. Storage:

7. Order: Mefoxitin 300 mg IM q4h
   Stock: vial of powder 1 gram (Fig. 8-19)

   a. Diluting fluid and number of milliliters:
   b. Solution and new stock:
   c. Rule and arithmetic:
   d. Amount to give:
   e. Write on label:
   f. Storage:

— Preparation of Solution

Strength	Amount of Diluent to be Added (mL)+ +	Approximate Withdrawable Volume (mL)	Approximate Average Concentration (mg/mL)
1 gram Vial	2 (Intramuscular)	2.5	400
2 gram Vial	4 (Intramuscular)	5	400
1 gram Vial	10 (IV)	10.5	95
2 gram Vial	10 or 20 (IV)	11.1 or 21.0	180 or 95
1 gram Infusion Bottle	50 or 100 (IV)	50 or 100	20 or 10
2 gram Infusion Bottle	50 or 100 (IV)	50 or 100	40 or 20
10 gram Bulk	43 or 93 (IV)	49 or 98.5	200 or 100

+ +Shake to dissolve and let stand until clear.

Intramuscular
MEFOXIN, as constituted with Sterile Water for Injection, Bacteriostatic Water for Injection, or 0.5 percent or 1 percent lidocaine hydrochloride solution (without epinephrine), maintains satisfactory potency for 24 hours at room temperature, for one week under refrigeration (below 5°C), and for at least 30 weeks in the frozen state.

Figure 8-19
Directions to reconstitute Mefoxitin (cefoxitin sodium). (Courtesy of Merck & Co. Inc.)

(continued)

Proficiency Test (continued)

8. Order: Claforan 200 mg IM q6h
Stock: vial of powder labeled 1 gram (Fig. 8-20)

a. Diluting fluid and number of milliliters:
b. Solution and new stock:
c. Rule and arithmetic:
d. Amount to give:
e. Write on label:
f. Storage:

PREPARATION OF CLAFORAN STERILE

Claforan for IM or IV administration should be reconstituted as follows:

Strength	Diluent (mL)	Withdrawable Volume (mL)	Approximate Concentration (mg/mL)
1g vial (IM)*	3	3.4	300
2g vial (IM)*	5	6.0	330
1g vial (IV)*	10	10.4	95
2g vial (IV)*	10	11.0	180
1g infusion	50-100	50-100	20-10
2g infusion	50-100	50-100	40-20
10g bottle	47	52.0	200
10g bottle	97	102.0	100

(*) in conventional vials

Shake to dissolve; inspect for particulate matter and discoloration prior to use. Solutions of Claforan range from very pale yellow to light amber, depending on concentration, diluent used, and length and condition of storage.

For Intramuscular use: Reconstitute VIALS with Sterile Water for Injection or Bacteriostatic Water for Injection as described above.

COMPATIBILITY AND STABILITY

Solutions of Claforan Sterile reconstituted as described above **(Preparation of Claforan Sterile)** maintain satisfactory potency for 24 hours at room temperature (at or below 22°C), 10 days under refrigeration (at or below 5°C), and for at least 13 weeks frozen.

Figure 8-20
Preparation of cefotaxime sodium (Claforan) solution. (Courtesy of Hoechst–Roussel Pharmaceuticals, Inc.)

(continued)

Proficiency Test (continued)

9. Order: cephradine 108 mg IM q8h
   Stock: vial of 250 mg of powder (Fig. 8-21)

   a. Diluting fluid and number of milliliters:
   b. Solution and new stock:
   c. Rule and arithmetic:
   d. Amount to give:
   e. Write on label:
   f. Storage:

VELOSEF FOR INJECTION
(Cephradine for Injection USP)

IM DILUTION TABLE

Vial Size	Volume of Diluent	Approximate Available Volume	Approximate Available Concentration
250 mg	1.2 mL	1.2 mL	208 mg/mL
500 mg	2.0 mL	2.2 mL	227 mg/mL
1 g	4.0 mL	4.5 mL	222 mg/mL

For I.M. Use.—Aseptically add Sterile Water for Injection or Bacteriostatic Water for Injection (containing 0.9% [w/v] benzyl alcohol, or 0.12% methylparaben and 0.014% propylparaben) according to the following table [i.e., the table entitled "IM Dilution Table" below].

Intramuscular solutions should be used within two hours at room temperature; if stored in the refrigerator at 5° C., solutions retain full potency for 24 hours. Constituted solutions may vary in color from light straw to yellow; however, this does not affect the potency.

Figure 8-21
IM dilution table for Velosef (cephradine for injection). (Package insert used by permission of E. R. Squibb & Sons, Inc., copyright owner.)

10. Order: cefazolin sodium 0.33 g IM q8h
    Stock: vial of powder labeled 1 gram (Fig. 8-22)

    a. Diluting fluid and number of milliliters:
    b. Solution and new stock:
    c. Rule and arithmetic:
    d. Amount to give:
    e. Write on label:
    f. Storage:

Vial Size	Diluent to Be Added	Approximate Available Volume	Approximate Average Concentration
250 mg	2 ml	2 ml	125 mg/ml
500 mg	2 ml	2.2 ml	225 mg/ml
1 g*	2.5 ml	3 ml	330 mg/ml

* The 1-g vial should be reconstituted only with Sterile Water for Injection or Bacteriostatic Water for Injection.

STABILITY
Reconstituted Kefzol (cefazolin sodium, Lilly) and dilutions of Kefzol in the recommended intravenous fluids are stable for 24 hours at room temperature and for 96 hours stored under refrigeration (5°C).

Figure 8-22
Dilution table for cefazolin sodium (Kefzol). (Courtesy of Eli Lilly & Company.)

ANSWERS

Practice Exercise 1

1. There are two ways to prepare carbenicillin. We could make a solution of

   1 g = 2.5 mL

   or

   1 g = 3.0 mL

   Either one is correct. Both are shown. The last dilution 1 g = 4.0 mL is too much. It would require two syringes.

   a. 4 mL sterile water
   b. 1 g = 2.5 mL
   c. Not necessary
   d. Give 2.5 mL
   e. 1 g = 2.5 mL, date, initials
   f. Refrigerate. Stable for 72 hours

   a. 5 mL sterile water
   b. 1 g = 3 mL
   c. Not necessary
   d. Give 3 mL
   e. 1 g = 3 mL, date, initials
   f. Refrigerate. Stable for 72 hours

2. You want 1 g. The stock is 1 g. When you dilute the powder, you will give the whole amount of fluid, *whatever the amount is.* The manufacturer states it will be 3.6 mL/1 g. If you solve the arithmetic you have:

   $\frac{D}{H} \times S = A$

   $\frac{100\not{0}\text{ }\not{mg}}{28\not{0}\text{ }\not{mg}} \times 1 \text{ mL} = \frac{100}{28} = 3.57 = 3.6 \text{ mL}$

   $$\begin{array}{r} 3.57 \\ 28\overline{)100.00} \\ \underline{84} \\ 160 \\ \underline{140} \\ 200 \\ \underline{196} \end{array}$$

   a. 3 mL sterile water for injection
   b. 1 g in 3.6 mL, 280 mg/mL
   c. Not necessary
   d. Give 3.6 mL in two syringes
   e. Discard the vial; it is empty.
   f. Discard the vial in appropriate receptacle.

3. **a.** 1.8 mL sterile water for injection
   b. 250 mg/mL
   c. $\frac{D}{H} \times S = A \qquad \frac{25\not{0}\text{ }\not{mg}}{25\not{0}\text{ }\not{mg}} \times 1 \text{ mL} = 1 \text{ mL}$
   d. Give 1 mL IM
   e. Nothing! Read the last line: "The above solutions must be used within 1 hour after reconstitution." You must discard the remaining fluid!
   f. None

Practice Exercise 2

1. **a.** Choose 500 mg powder (Can you see why?)
   b. Add 2 mL sterile water for injection
   c. 225 mg/mL
   d. Not necessary: you want 225 mg; you made 225 mg/mL
   e. Give 1 mL IM
   f. 225 mg/mL, date, initials
   g. Refrigerate. Stable for 96 hours

2. **a.** 2.5 mL sterile water for injection
   b. 330 mg/mL
   c. 0.5 g = 500 mg

   $\frac{D}{H} \times S = A \qquad \frac{50\not{0}\text{ }\not{mg}}{33\not{0}\text{ }\not{mg}} \times 1 \text{ mL} = \frac{50}{33}$

   $$\begin{array}{r} 1.51 \\ 33\overline{)50.00} \\ \underline{33} \\ 170 \\ \underline{165} \\ 50 \\ \underline{33} \\ 17 \end{array}$$

   d. Give 1.5 mL IM
   e. 330 mg/mL, date, initials
   f. Refrigerate. Stable for 96 hours

3. a. 3.0 mL sterile water for injection
   b. 280 mg/mL
   c. $\frac{D}{H} \times S = A \quad \frac{500 \text{ mg}}{280 \text{ mg}} \times 1 \text{ mL} = \frac{50}{28} = 1.8 \text{ mL}$

$$\begin{array}{r} 1.78 \\ 28\overline{)50.00} \\ \underline{28} \\ 220 \\ \underline{196} \\ 240 \\ \underline{224} \\ 16 \end{array}$$

   d. Give 1.8 mL IM
   e. 280 mg/mL, date, initials
   f. Refrigerate. Stable for 7 days

Self-Test 1

1. a. Add 2 mL of sterile water for injection
   b. 400 mg/mL
   c. $\frac{D}{H} \times S = A \quad \frac{\overset{1}{200 \text{ mg}}}{\underset{4}{400 \text{ mg}}} \times 1 \text{ mL} = \frac{1}{2} \text{ mL or } 0.5 \text{ mL}$
   d. Give $\frac{1}{2}$ mL (0.5 mL)
   e. 400 mg/mL, date, initials
   f. Refrigerate. Stable for 1 week

2. a. Add 2 mL sterile water for injection
   b. 400 mg/mL
   c. $\frac{D}{H} \times S = A \quad 0.6 \text{ g} = 600 \text{ mg}$

$$\frac{\overset{3}{600 \text{ mg}}}{\underset{2}{400 \text{ mg}}} \times 1 \text{ mL} = \frac{3}{2} \quad \begin{array}{r} 1.5 \\ 2\overline{)3.0} \end{array}$$

   d. Give 1.5 mL IM
   e. 400 mg/mL, date, initials
   f. Refrigerate. Stable for 1 week

3. a. Choose 1 g. It is closest to the order.
   b. Add 3 mL of sterile water for injection
   c. 300 mg/mL
   d. $\frac{D}{H} \times S = A \quad \frac{800 \text{ mg}}{300 \text{ mg}} \times 1 \text{ mL} = \frac{8}{3} \quad \begin{array}{r} 2.66 \\ 3\overline{)8.00} \end{array}$
   e. Give 2.7 mL IM
   f. 300 mg/mL, date, initials
   g. Refrigerate. Stable for 10 days

4. a. Diluting fluid and number of milliliters: Add 2.5 mL sterile water for injection
   b. Solution made and new stock: 20% solution means

   20 g in 100 mL or reducing that $\frac{\overset{1}{20 \text{ g}}}{\underset{5}{100 \text{ mL}}} = \frac{1 \text{ g}}{5 \text{ mL}}$

   New stock: 1 g = 5 mL; 1 g = 1000 mg; therefore, 1000 mg = 5 mL
   c. Rule and arithmetic:

$$\frac{D}{H} \times S = A \quad \frac{\overset{1}{250 \text{ mg}}}{\underset{4}{1000 \text{ mg}}} \times 5 \text{ mL} = \frac{5}{4} \quad \begin{array}{r} 1.25 \\ 4\overline{)5.0} \end{array}$$

   d. Amount to give 1.3 mL IM
   e. Write on label: Nothing. An ampule must be discarded.
   f. Storage: No. Discard in a suitable receptacle.

Self-Test 2

1. a. Diluting fluid and number of milliliters: Add 3 mL sterile water for injection
   b. Solution made and new stock: 280 mg/mL
   c. Rule and arithmetic: 0.25 g = 250 mg

$$\frac{D}{H} \times S = A \quad \frac{250 \text{ mg}}{280 \text{ mg}} \times 1 \text{ mL} = \frac{25}{28} = 0.9 \text{ mL}$$

$$\begin{array}{r} .89 \\ 28\overline{)25.00} \\ \underline{22\ 4} \\ 2\ 60 \\ \underline{2\ 52} \\ 8 \end{array}$$

   d. Give 0.9 mL IM
   e. 280 mg/mL, date, initials
   f. Refrigerate. Stable for 7 days.

2. Actually all three ways to dilute the powder are possible! (A) If you made 100,000 U/mL—give 3 mL. (B) If you made 200,000 U/mL—give 1.5 mL. (C) If you made 250,000 U/mL—give 1.2 mL. The steps for all three ways are shown.

	A	B	C
Diluting fluid and no. mL	9.6 ml sterile water	4.6 ml sterile water	3.6 ml sterile water
Solution made	100,000 U/mL	200,000 U/mL	250,000 U/mL
Rule (and arithmetic)			
$\frac{D}{H} \times S = A$	$\frac{\cancel{300,000\ U}}{\cancel{100,000\ U}} \times 1\ mL = 3\ mL$	$\frac{\cancel{300,000\ U}}{\cancel{200,000\ U}} \times 1\ mL =$	$\frac{\overset{6}{\cancel{300,000\ U}}}{\underset{5}{\cancel{250,000\ U}}} \times 1\ mL =$
		$\frac{3}{2} \quad \begin{array}{r} 1.5 \\ 2\overline{)3.0} \end{array}$	$\frac{6}{5} \quad \begin{array}{r} 1.2 \\ 5\overline{)6.0} \end{array}$
Answer	Give 3 mL IM	Give 1.5 mL IM	Give 1.2 mL IM
Write on label	100,000 U/mL, date, initials	200,000 U/mL, date, initials	250,000 U/mL, date, initials
Storage	Refrigerate. Stable for 1 week	Refrigerate. Stable for 1 week	Refrigerate. Stable for 1 week

3. a. Diluting fluid and number of milliliters: Add 4 mL sterile water for injection
   b. Solution made and new stock: 222 mg/mL
   c. Rule and arithmetic:

$$\frac{D}{H} \times S = A \qquad \frac{350\ \cancel{mg}}{222\ \cancel{mg}} \times 1\ mL = \frac{350}{222} \quad \begin{array}{r} 1.57 \\ 222\overline{)350.00} \\ \underline{222} \\ 128\ 0 \\ \underline{111\ 0} \\ 17\ 00 \\ \underline{15\ 54} \\ 1\ 46 \end{array}$$

   d. Amount to give: 1.6 mL IM
   e. Write on label: 222 mg/mL, date, initials
   f. Storage: Refrigerate. Stable for 24 hours

4. a. Diluting fluid and number of milliliters: Add 3 mL sterile water for injection
   b. Solution and new stock: 280 mg/mL
   c. Rule and arithmetic:

$$\frac{D}{H} \times S = A \qquad \frac{\overset{25}{\cancel{500\ mg}}}{\underset{14}{\cancel{280\ mg}}} \times 1\ mL = \frac{25}{14} \quad \begin{array}{r} 1.78 \\ 14\overline{)25.00} \\ \underline{14} \\ 110 \\ \underline{98} \\ 120 \\ \underline{112} \\ 8 \end{array} = 1.8$$

   d. Amount to give: 1.8 mL IM
   e. 280 mg/mL, date, initials
   f. Refrigerate. Stable for 7 days.

Mental Drill in Injection From Powder Problems

Set A

1. a. 4.6 mL sterile water for injection
   b. 200,000 units/mL
   c. Give 1.5 mL IM
   d. 200,000 U/mL, date, initials

2. a. 5 cc sterile water for injection
   b. 100 mg/cc
   c. Give 2 cc IM
   d. 100 mg/cc, date, initials

3. a. 2 mL diluent with the vial
   b. 100 mg = 2 mL
   c. Give entire amount (give 2 mL) IM
   d. None. Discard empty vial.

4. a. 4.6 cc sterile water for injection
   b. 200,000 U/mL
   c. give 2 mL IM
   d. 200,000 U/mL, date, initials

5. a. 5 mL sterile water for injection
   b. 100 mg/mL
   c. $1\frac{1}{2}$ mL or 1.5 mL IM
   d. 100 mg/mL, date, initials

6. **a.** 2.5 mL sterile water for injection. *Note:* Should not be diluted with 5 mL. The answer would be to give 4 mL—this is too much fluid.
   b. 100 mg/mL
   c. Give 2 mL IM
   d. None; stock was an ampule. Discard in a suitable receptacle.

7. **a.** 1.5 mL sterile water for injection
   b. 500 mg/cc
   c. Give $\frac{1}{2}$ cc or 0.5 cc IM
   d. 500 mg/cc, date, initials

8. **a.** 3.5 mL sterile water for injection
   b. 75 mg/mL
   c. Give 1.3 mL IM
   d. 75 mg/mL, date, initials

9. **a.** 1.8 mL of sterile water for injection
   b. 250 mg/mL
   c. Give 1.6 mL IM
   d. 250 mg/mL, date, initials

10. **a.** 2 mL sterile water for injection
    b. 125 mg/mL
    c. Give 1.2 mL
    d. 125 mg/mL, date, initials

Set B

1. **a.** 3.0 mL sterile water for injection
   b. 270 mg/mL
   c. Give 0.3 mL IM (3-mL syringe) or 0.33 mL (1-mL precision syringe)
   d. 270 mg/mL, date, initials

2. Two ways are possible: use either one.

A	B
a. 4 mL sterile water for injection	5 mL sterile water for injection
b. 1 g/2.5 mL	1 g/3 mL
c. Give 1.3 mL	Give 1.5 mL
d. 1 g/2.5 mL, date, initials	1 g/3 mL, date, initials

3. Two ways are possible: the nurse must assess the patient to determine which is better. The other solutions would yield too small a dose.

A	B
a. 20 mL sterile water for injection	10 mL sterile water for injection
b. 50,000 U/mL	100,000 U/mL
c. Give 0.8 mL IM	Give 0.4 mL IM
d. 50,000 U/mL, date, initials	100,000 U/mL, date, initials

4. **a.** 2 mL sterile water for injection
   b. 225 mg/mL
   c. 2 mL IM
   d. 225 mg/mL, date, initials

5. **a.** 1.8 mL sterile water for injection
   b. 250 mg/mL
   c. 1.6 mL
   d. 250 mg/mL, date, initials

6. **a.** 3 mL sterile water for injection
   b. 300 mg/mL
   c. Entire amount. Under the heading *Withdrawable Volume* the manufacturer says 3.4 mL. Consider two injection sites. Split the dose into two injections of 1.7 mL.
   d. Nothing! Entire amount has been used. Discard vial in an appropriate receptacle.

7. **a.** 3 mL sterile water for injection
   b. 280 mg/mL
   c. 1.8 mL
   d. 280 mg/mL, date, initials

8. **a.** 2 mL sterile water for injection
   b. 400 mg/mL
   c. 1.3 mL IM
   d. 400 mg/mL, date, initials

9. **a.** 2 mL sterile water for injection
   b. 125 mg/mL
   c. 1.2 mL IM
   d. 125 mg/mL, date, initials

10. Three ways are possible:

A	B	C
a. 23 mL	18 mL	8 mL
b. 200,000 U/mL	250,000 U/mL	500,000 U/mL
c. 1.3 mL IM	1 mL IM	0.5 mL IM
d. 200,000 U/mL, date, initials	250,000 U/mL, date, initials	500,000 U/mL, date, initials

Proficiency Test

1. a. 1.8 mL sterile water for injection
   b. 500,000 units/mL
   c. $\frac{D}{H} \times S = A$ $\frac{600{,}000\ U}{500{,}000\ U} \times 1\ mL = 5\overline{)6.0}$ 1.2
   d. 1.2 mL IM
   e. 500,000 units/mL; date; initials
   f. Refrigerate. Stable for 7 days

2. a. 2 mL sterile water for injection
   b. 1 g/2.6 mL
   c. $\frac{D}{H} \times S = A$ $\frac{1\ g}{1\ g} \times 2.6\ mL = 2.6$
   d. 2.6 mL
   e. Nothing is left in the vial.
   f. *Discard the vial in a proper receptacle.*

3. a. 1.5 mL sterile water for injection
   b. 280 mg/mL
   c. $\frac{D}{H} \times S = A$ $\frac{200\ mg}{280\ mg} \times 1\ mL = 7\overline{)5.00}$ .71; 4 9; 10; 7
   d. 0.7 mL IM
   e. 280 mg/mL; date; initials
   f. Refrigerate. Stable for 10 days

4. a. 7 mL sterile water for injection
   b. 1 g/2.0 mL
   c. Not necessary. Order is 1 g
   d. 2 mL IM
   e. 1 g/mL; date; initials
   f. Refrigerate. Stable for 72 hours

5. a. 1.8 mL sterile water for injection
   b. 250 mg/mL
   c. $\frac{D}{H} \times S = A$ $\frac{300\ mg}{250\ mg} \times 1\ mL = 5\overline{)6.0}$ 1.2
   d. 1.2 mL IM
   e. Nothing! Discard the vial. Directions say solution must be used within 1 hour.
   f. No. *Discard the vial in an appropriate receptacle.*

6. a. 0.9 mL sterile water for injection
   b. 250 mg/mL
   c. Not necessary. Directions state to give 0.8 mL
   d. 0.8 mL
   e. Discard the vial. Directions say that the solution must be used within 1 hour.
   f. No. *Discard the vial in a proper receptacle.*

7. a. 2 mL sterile water for injection
   b. 400 mg/mL
   c. $\frac{D}{H} \times S = A$ $\frac{300\ mg}{400\ mg} \times 1\ mL = 4\overline{)3.00}$ .75; 2 8; 20; 20
   d. 0.8 mL IM
   e. 400 mg/mL; date; initials
   f. Refrigerate. Stable for 1 week

8. a. 3 mL sterile water for injection
   b. 300 mg/mL
   c. $\frac{D}{H} \times S = A$ $\frac{200\ mg}{300\ mg} \times 1\ mL = 3\overline{)2.00}$ .66; 1 8; 20; 18
   d. 0.7 mL IM
   e. 300 mg/mL; date; initials
   f. Refrigerate. Stable for 10 days

9. a. 1.2 mL sterile water for injection
   b. 208 mg/mL
   c. $\frac{D}{H} \times S = A$ $\frac{108\ mg}{208\ mg} \times 1\ mL = 208\overline{)108.00}$ .51; 104 0; 4 00; 2 08
   d. 0.5 mL IM
   e. 208 mg/mL; date; initials
   f. Refrigerate. Stable for 24 hours

10. a. 2.5 mL sterile water for injection
    b. 330 mg/mL
    c. $\frac{D}{H} \times S = A$ Not necessary. 0.33 g is 330 mg
    d. 1 mL IM
    e. 330 mg/mL; date; initials
    f. Refrigerate. Stable for 96 hours

Intravenous Drip Rates and Intravenous Piggyback Intermittent Infusions

CONTENT TO MASTER

- Types of intravenous fluids
- Kinds of intravenous drip factors
- Infusion pumps
- Labeling IVs
- Calculating IV orders
  - Continuous vs intermittent IVPB
  - mL over a number of hours
  - mL/hr
  - units/hr
  - mcg/min
  - mcg/kg/min
- Calculating intravenous drip rate
- Choosing the infusion set
- Adding medications
  - Continuous IVs
  - IV piggyback
- Calculating and recording parenteral intake

▼ OVERVIEW

Some medications are given intravenously (IV), with the use of sterile technique, to achieve an immediate effect and a high blood level. These drugs, in a powder or liquid form, are diluted and then administered continuously through the primary IV tubing, or through a secondary line attached to the primary IV. The secondary IV is termed an intravenous piggyback infusion or an IVPB (Fig. 9-1).

To learn how to prepare these medications and set the drip rate, nurses must first learn about types of IV fluids, IV drip factors, how orders can be written for IVs and IVPBs, and how the nurse calculates the drip rate.

▼ TYPES OF INTRAVENOUS FLUIDS

A partial listing of IV fluids available at one hospital is shown in Figure 9-2. These fluids are packaged in sterile plastic bags or glass bottles and distributed to the patient care units. The nurse selects the IV fluid needed and prepares the solution. An error in choosing fluid may result in serious fluid and electrolyte

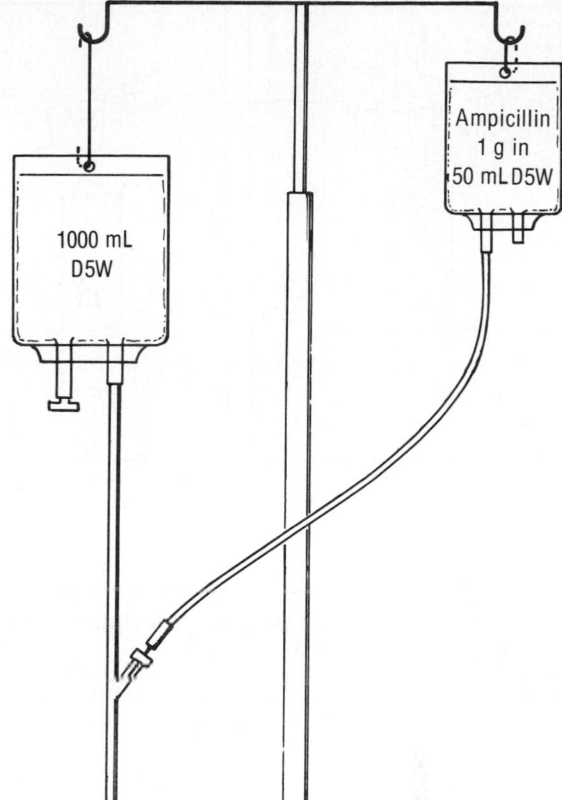

Figure 9-1
Drawing of a main IV line and an IVPB line. Fluid flows continuously through the main line **(left)** into the patient's vein. At timed intervals medication **(right)** placed in an intravenous piggyback bag (IVPB) is attached by needle and tubing to the main IV for delivery to the patient.

QUANTITY REQUESTED	UNIT MEASURE	DESCRIPTION	
		SOLUTIONS	
		DEXTROSE IN WATER	
	EACH	1000cc D2.5% W GLASS	2A0014
	EACH	50cc D5% W (Pk of 4)	2B0081
	EACH	100cc D5% W (Pk of 4)	2B0082
	EACH	250cc D5% W	2B0062
	EACH	500cc D5% W	2B0063
	EACH	1000cc D5% W	2B0064
	EACH	250cc D5% W GLASS	2A0062
	EACH	500cc D10% W	2B0163
		DEXTROSE AND SODIUM CHLORIDE	
	EACH	500cc D5% W .9 NS	2B1063
	EACH	1000cc D5% W .9 NS	2B1064
	EACH	500cc D5% W .2 NS	2B1093
	EACH	250cc D5% W .33 NS	2B1082
	EACH	500cc D5% W .33 NS	2B1083
	EACH	1000cc D5% W .33 NS	2B1084
	EACH	500cc D5% W .45 NS	2B1073
	EACH	1000cc D5% W .45 NS	2B1074
	EACH	500cc D2.5% W .45 NS	2B1023
	EACH	1000cc D2.5% W .45 NS	2B1024
	EACH	1000cc D10% W .9 NS	2B1164
		ISOTONIC SODIUM CHLORIDE NS	
	EACH	50cc .9% (Pk of 4)	2B1301
	EACH	100cc .9% (Pk of 4)	2B1302
	EACH	250cc .9%	2B1322
	EACH	500cc .9%	2B1323
	EACH	1000cc .9%	2B1324

Figure 9-2
Partial list of IV fluids available at one hospital. (Courtesy of Central Distribution, St. Vincent Hospital and Medical Center, New York City)

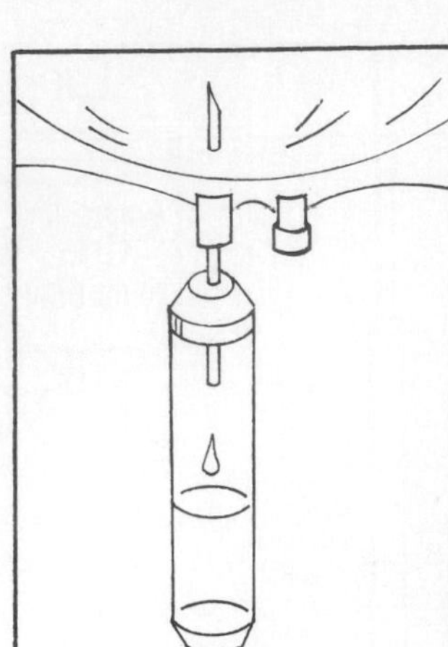

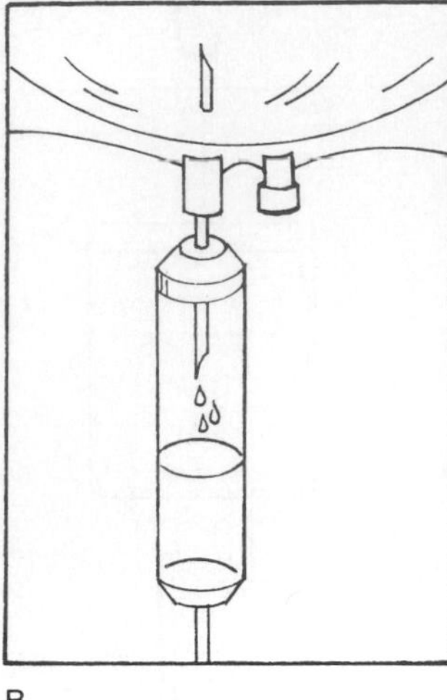

Figure 9-3
Infusion set chambers. **(A)** Macrodrip chamber has no needle. **(B)** Microdrip chamber with a needle delivers 1 mL in 60 separate gtt.

imbalance. The stock label may be printed in a different way than the written order. The nurse should *always seek assistance* when in doubt about which solution to use.

EXAMPLES

Stock Label	Written Order
1000 cc D5%W	1000 mL D5W
500 cc D5%.9NS	500 mL D5NS
250 cc D5W.45NS	250 mL D5$\frac{1}{2}$NS
500 cc D5.33NS	500 mL D5$\frac{1}{3}$NS

▼ KINDS OF INTRAVENOUS DRIP FACTORS

Intravenous fluids are administered through infusion sets that consist of plastic tubing attached at one end to the IV bag and at the other end to a needle or catheter inserted into a blood vessel. The top of the infusion set contains a chamber (Fig. 9-3). Sets that contain a needle in the chamber are called *microdrip* because the drops are small. To deliver 1 mL of fluid to the patient, 60 drops (gtt) must fall (60 gtt = 1 mL). *All microdrip sets deliver 60 gtt/mL.*

Infusion sets that do not have a needle in the chamber are called *macrodrip.* These sets are not standard. Different manufacturers have a different number of drops per milliliter. Table 9-1 lists examples of macrodrip infusion sets. The package label will state the drops per milliliter (gtt/mL). You need to know this information to calculate the IV drip rates.

The tubing for these sets will include a clamp that the nurse can open or close to regulate the drip rate while using a second-hand on a watch or clock to count the drops per minute.

TABLE 9-1
Examples of Different Macrodrip Factors

Manufacturer	Drops per Milliliter (gtt/mL)
Travenol	10
Abbott	15
McGaw	15
Cutter	20

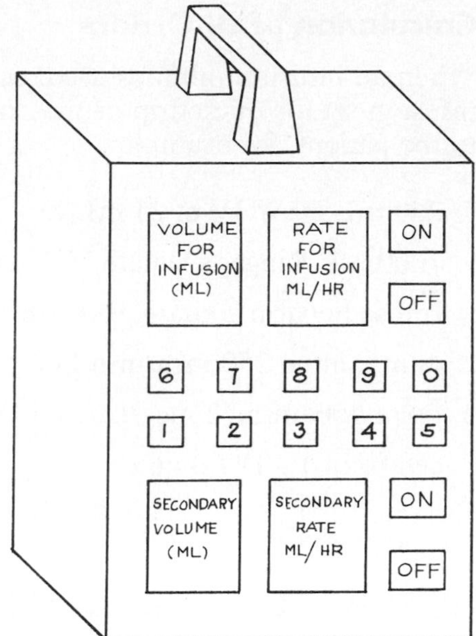

Figure 9-4
Schematic diagram of the face of an infusion pump that delivers mL/hr.

Infusion Pumps

Many health care institutions use electrical infusion pumps to deliver IV fluid. These are excellent timesaving devices. Some are simple to operate, others are more elaborate. The most basic ones require the nurse to enter two pieces of information: the total number of milliliters to be infused and the number of milliliters per hour. Figure 9-4 shows a schematic diagram of the face of an infusion pump. IV tubing would be connected to the pump. If an order read: "500 mL D5W. Run 50 mL/hr," the nurse would press *Volume for Infusion,* 500; *Rate for Infusion,* 50; On. The pump would automatically deliver 50 mL/hr over a 10-hour period. Note that the pump delivers milliliters per hour (mL/hr). The lower buttons in Figure 9-4 are used to add an IVPB. If an order read: "Ampicillin 2 g IVPB in 100 mL NS over 1 hour," the nurse would press *Secondary Volume,* 100; *Secondary Rate,* 100; On. The pump would interrupt the main IV to administer the IVPB over one hour, then resume the primary flow.

Labeling IVs

IV fluids are labeled with the following information:

Patient name, room, and bed number

Date

Physician's order as written

Time for infusion

Rate of flow of the IV

Initials of the nurse who prepared the IV

Patient	Fred Jones	Room	1503–4
Date	6/28	Rate	50 mL/hr.
Order	500 mL D5W ½NS. Run 50 mL/hr.		
Time	10a – 8p	Initials	JS

Calculation of IV Orders

When an infusion pump is used, calculations are in mL/hr. Other IVs require the nurse to choose an infusion set for microdrip or macrodrip rate. Orders may be written in different ways to deliver IV fluid to the patient, for example:

250 mL D5W IV at 25 mL/hr

1000 mL Ringer's lactate IV 8 AM–8 PM

Infuse heparin sodium 1000 units/hr

dobutamine 250 mcg/min IV

renal dopamine 2 mcg/kg/min IV

cefazolin 1 g IVPB q6h

RULE

CALCULATING INTRAVENOUS DRIP RATE

Problems in IV calculations are solved in two steps. Step 1 is used to solve problems requiring an infusion pump and to simplify the arithmetic needed for microdrip and macrodrip. Step 2 will solve micro- and macrodrip problems.

Step 1. $\frac{\text{Total number of milliliters ordered}}{\text{number of hours to run}} = \text{number of mL/hr}$

Step 2. $\frac{\text{Number of milliliters per hour} \times \text{tubing drip factor}}{\text{number of minutes}} = \text{drops per minute}$

◀ ***Learning Aid***

Step 1. $\frac{\text{\# mL}}{\text{\# hr}} = \text{mL/hr}$

Step 2. $\frac{\text{mL/hr} \times \text{TF}}{\text{\# min}} = \text{gtt/min}$

Explanation

Step 1. $\frac{\text{\# mL}}{\text{\# hr}} = \text{mL/hr}$

mL: The physician will indicate the number of milliliters to be infused in the order.

hr: The number of hours to run depends on the way the order is written. For example, if the order is written:

q8h = 8 hours at a time

10 AM–4 PM = 6 hours

25 mL/hr = the answer to Step 1. No calculation is required.

Step 2. $\frac{\text{mL/hr} \times \text{TF}}{\text{\# min}} = \text{gtt/min}$

mL/hr: mL/hr is the answer to Step 1.

TF: TF (tubing drip factor) is either microdrip (60 gtt = 1 mL) or macrodrip.

Depending on the manufacturer, macrodrip could be 10 gtt = 1 mL; 15 gtt = 1 mL; or 20 gtt = 1 mL.

min: Number of minutes is always 60 for this problem. In Step 1 you found mL/hr, but you need gtt/min; because there are 60 minutes in an hour, divide by 60.

gtt/min: gtt/min is the drip factor calculated to deliver an even flow of fluid over a specified time. The nurse regulates the drip rate using a second hand on a watch or a clock. If the drip rate was calculated to be 80 gtt/min, the nurse would open the clamp and regulate the drip until there were 20 gtts in 15 seconds. This would provide 80 gtt/minute.

In the problems requiring calculation in this text, the drip factor will be given to you. In the clinical area, you must read the package label to identify the gtt/mL.

Application of the Rule

EXAMPLE

Example 1:

Order: 1000 mL Ringer's lactate IV 8 AM–8 PM

Available: An infusion pump

Logic: 8 AM–8 PM is 12 hours for the IV to run. The infusion pump regulates the rate in milliliters per hour. Only Step 1 is necessary.

$$\frac{\text{\# mL}}{\text{\# hr}} = \text{mL/hr}$$

> ◀ ***Learning Aid***
> *Carry out arithmetic one decimal place and round off the answer to the nearest whole number.*

$$\frac{1000 \text{ mL}}{12 \text{ hr}} = \frac{\cancel{1000}}{12} \quad 12\overline{)1000.0} = 83.3$$

```
      83.3
12 )1000.0
     96
      40
      36
       40
       36
```

Label the IV

Set the pump as follows:

Total # mL: 1000

mL/hr: 83

Example 2:

Order: 500 mL D5NS IV 12 N–4 PM

Available: microdrip at 60 gtt/mL; macrodrip at 20 gtt/mL

Logic: The IV will run 4 hours. Since no pump is available, the nurse must choose the drip factor; two steps are necessary. Solve for both drip factors and choose one.

Step 1. $\frac{\text{\# mL}}{\text{\# hr}} = \text{mL/hr}$

$$\frac{\cancel{500}}{4} \quad 4\overline{)500.} = 125. = 125 \text{ mL/hr}$$

> ◀ ***Learning Aid***
> *Note that the answer to Step 1 is 125 mL/hr.*
> *The answer to Step 2 is 125 gtt/min for microdrip.*

Step 2. $\frac{\text{mL/hr} \times \text{TF}}{\text{\# min}} = \text{gtt/min}$

Macrodrip

$$\frac{125 \times \overset{1}{\cancel{20}}}{\underset{3}{\cancel{60}}} = \frac{\cancel{125}}{3} \quad 3\overline{)125.0} = 41.6$$

```
     41.6
3 )125.0
   12
     5
     3
     20
```

Macrodrip at 42 gtt/min.

Microdrip

$$\frac{125 \times \overset{1}{\cancel{60}}}{\underset{1}{\cancel{60}}} = 125 \text{ gtt/min}$$

Microdrip at 125 gtt/min.

◀ ***Learning Aid***
Important:
mL/hr = gtt/min microdrip. Why? The TF is always 60 and the # minutes is always 60. These cancel each other.

Logic: Answers are macrodrip at 42 gtt/min and microdrip at 125 gtt/min. Choose one. (See explanation for choosing the infusion set, following this discussion.)

Label the IV

Set drip rate

Example 3:

Order: 500 mL D5 $\frac{1}{3}$ NS IVKVO for 24°

Available: microdrip at 60 gtt/mL; macrodrip 10 gtt/mL

Logic: Because no pump is available, choose the IV set. This is a two-step problem. The IV will run 24 hr.

Step 1. $\frac{\text{\# mL}}{\text{\# hr}} = \text{mL/hr}$

$$\frac{\cancel{500}}{24} \quad 24\overline{)500.0}^{\,20.8} = 21 \text{ mL/hr}$$

```
     20.8
 24 )500.0
     48
     20 0
     19 2
```

◀ ***Learning Aid***
1. *Note that the order reads 24°. This abbreviation is used by some physicians to denote hours.*
2. *Carry out arithmetic one decimal place. Round off the milliliter answer to the nearest whole number.*

Step 2. $\frac{\text{mL/hr} \times \text{TF}}{\text{\# min}} = \text{gtt/min}$

Logic: The answer to Step 1 is 21 mL/hr. The number of minutes is 60. Work out the problem for micro- and macrodrip and make a nursing judgment about which tube to use.

Macrodrip

$$\frac{21 \times 1\cancel{0}}{6\cancel{0}} = \frac{\cancel{21}}{6} = 3.5$$

```
     3.5
 6 )21.0
    18
     3 0
     3 0
```

◀ ***Learning Aid***
In a two-step IV problem, it is not necessary to show the arithmetic for microdrip because mL/hr = gtt/min.

Macrodrip at 4 gtt/min

Microdrip $\frac{21 \times \cancel{60}}{\cancel{60}} = 21 \text{ gtt/min}$

Logic: 4 gtt/min macrodrip is too slow. Choose microdrip. (See explanation for choosing the infusion set.)

Label the IV

Select a microdrip infusion set

Set the drip rate at 21 gtt/min

Practice Exercise 1

Calculate the drip factor for the following IV orders given in milliliters per hour or number of hours. Answers may be found at the end of the chapter.

1. Order: 150 mL D5 .33NS IV q8h
   Available: infusion pump

2. Order: 250 cc D5W; run at 25 cc/hr
   Available: infusion pump

3. Order: 1000 mL D5NS; run 100 mL/hr
   Available: macrodrip (20 gtt/mL); microdrip (60 gtt/mL)

4. Order: 180 mL D5 $\frac{1}{3}$ NS 12 N–6 PM
   Available: macrodrip (10 gtt/mL); microdrip (60 gtt/mL)

5. Order: 1000 mL D5 .45S IV 4 PM–12 mid
   Available: macrodrip (15 gtt/mL); microdrip (60 gtt/mL)

Choosing the Infusion Set

Experience will enable you to judge which IV tubing to use. Clinically you will be guided in making a choice. There is no problem when an electric infusion pump is used. The pump will deliver the amount programmed. There are specialized pumps in neonatal and intensive care units that can deliver 1 mL/hr and specialized syringe pumps that can deliver less than 1 mL/hr.

Some guidelines may be helpful when an IV pump is not available.

Use Microdrip When

- The IV is to be administered over a long period.
- A small amount of fluid is to be infused.
- The macrodrops per minute are too few (Why? IV fluid flows by gravity. Blood flowing in the vein exerts a pressure. If the IV is too slow, blood pressure may force blood into the tube where it clots. The IV will stop.)

Use Macrodrip When

- A large amount of fluid is ordered in a short time.
- The microdrips per minute are too many. Counting the drip rate becomes too difficult.

Table 9-2 shows a quick reference chart developed by nurses in a surgical unit for their own use. Look at microdrips per minute (60 gtt = 1 mL). The first heading is *Amount Infused.* Read across—1000 mL, 500 mL, 250 mL, 150 mL. Read down. The heading is *Total Hours for Infusion*—24, 12, 10, 8, 4. When the microdrip rate is 83 gtt/min or more, these nurses use macrodrip. Note that in the lower part of the chart, nurses use microdrip when the drip rate is below 10 gtt/min.

TABLE 9-2
Quick Reference Chart for IV Drip Factors

Total Hours for Infusion	Amount Infused: 1000 mL	500 mL	250 mL	150 mL
Microdrops/Minute (60 gtt = 1 mL)				
24	42	21	10	6
12	83/use macro	42	21	12
10	100/use macro	50	25	15
8	125/use macro	63	31	19
4	250/use macro	125/use macro	63	38
Macrodrops/Minute (10 gtt = 1 mL)				
24	7/use micro	Use micro	Use micro	Use micro
12	13	7/use micro	Use micro	Use micro
10	17	8/use micro	Use micro	Use micro
8	21	11	Use micro	Use micro
4	42	21	Use micro	Use micro

Courtesy of the Nursing Department, St. Vincent's Hospital and Medical Center of New York.

Need for Continuous Observation

Many factors may interfere with the drip rate. Do not assume that once an IV is started it will continue to flow at the rate it was set. Check the IV frequently; IVs flow by gravity. As the amount of fluid decreases in the IV bag, pressure changes occur that may affect the rate. The patient's movements may kink the tube and shut off the flow, or they may change the position of the needle or catheter in the vein. The needle may be forced against the side of the blood vessel changing the flow, or it may be forced out of the vessel, allowing fluid to enter the tissues (infiltration).

Infusion pumps have an alarm system that beeps to alert the nurse when the rate cannot be maintained or when the infusion is about to be completed.

▼ ADDING MEDICATIONS TO IVs

When a continuous IV order includes a medication, add the medication to the IV and determine the rate of flow. In some institutions, medications are added by the pharmacist; in others, nurses add the medication.

Medications Ordered Over Several Hours

EXAMPLE *Example 1:*

Order: 1000 mL D5W with 20 mEq KCl IV 10 AM–10 PM

Available: vial of KCl 40 mEq/20 mL; microdrip (60 gtt/min); macrodrip (20 gtt/min)

Logic: $\frac{D}{H} \times S = A \quad \frac{\overset{1}{\cancel{20}}\ \text{mEq}}{\underset{\underset{1}{\cancel{2}}}{\cancel{40}}\ \text{mEq}} \times \overset{10}{\cancel{20}}\ \text{mL} = 10\ \text{mL}$

Add 10 mL of KCl to the IV bag.

Use two steps to solve the drip factor.

Choose the tubing. The IV will run 12 hours.

Step 1. $\frac{\# \text{ mL}}{\# \text{ hr}} = \text{mL/hr}$ $\frac{1000}{12} = 83 \text{ mL/hr}$

Step 2. $\frac{\# \text{ mL/hr} \times \text{TF}}{\# \text{ min}} = \text{gtt/min}$

For macrodrip: $\frac{83 \times \overset{1}{\cancel{20}}}{\underset{1}{\cancel{60}}} = 28 \text{ gtt/min}$

For microdrip: mL/hr = gtt/min; hence, 83 gtt/min

Choose either drip rate.

Label the IV.

Example 2:

Order: 5 MU penicillin G potassium in 1000 mL D5W IV q8h

Available: macrodrip (10 gtt/mL); microdrip (60 gtt/mL)

Logic: MU means million units. The order is for 5 million U of penicillin G potassium. Penicillin comes in 5 MU vials of powder. Directions say that the drug must be reconstituted with a *minimum* of 100 mL. The order states to add 5 MU to 1000 mL. The order is safe because you are adding 5 MU to 1000 mL. Use a 10-cc syringe to aseptically remove fluid from the 1000-mL bag of D5W and inject into the powder to make a solution. Withdraw the solution and inject into the bag. You now have 1000 mL D5W with the medication added. The IV will run 8 hours.

Two steps are needed:

Step 1. $\frac{\# \text{ mL}}{\# \text{ hr}} = \text{mL/hr}$ $\frac{\cancel{1000}}{8} \quad 8\,\overline{)1000.}^{\,125} = 125 \text{ mL/hr}$

Step 2. $\frac{\# \text{ mL/hr} \times \text{TF}}{\# \text{ min}} = \text{gtt/min}$

Macrodrip: $\frac{125 \times \cancel{10}}{\cancel{60}} = \frac{\cancel{125}}{6} \quad 6\,\overline{)125.0}^{\,20.8} = 21 \text{ gtt/min}$

Microdrip = 125 gtt/min; macrodrip = 21 gtt/min. Choose one.

Label the IV.

Medications Ordered in mL/hr

Potent medications such as heparin and aminophylline may be added to IVs with the rate ordered in milliliters per hour. It is best to use a pump to deliver these infusions safely. If a pump is not available, a volume control set, such as a Buretrol, should be used (Fig. 9-5.)

EXAMPLE

Example 1:

Order: 10,000 U heparin in 500 mL NS; run at 10 mL/hr

Available: vial of heparin labeled 5000 U/mL; infusion pump

Logic: The vial has 5000 U/mL of heparin. Draw up 2 mL in a syringe; aseptically add this solution to 500 mL NS and label the bag. Because a pump is available, no calculation is necessary. Set the rate at 10 mL/hr.

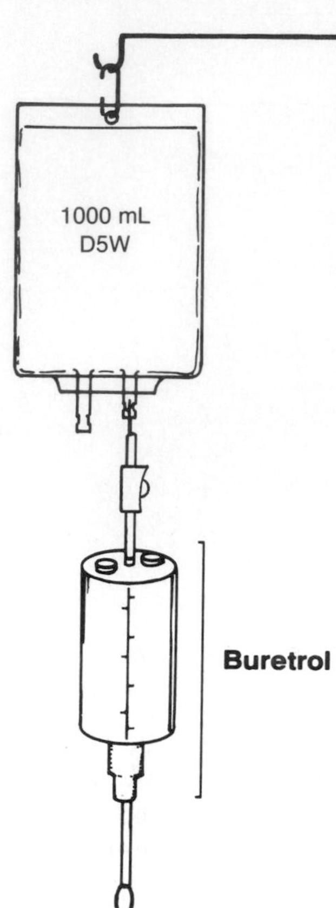

Figure 9-5
A Buretrol (*at bottom*) is an IV delivery system with tubing and a chamber that can hold 150 mL delivered as microdrip (1 mL = 60 drops). The top of the Buretrol has a port by means of which a reservoir of fluid can be added. The Buretrol is a volume control because no more than 150 mL can be infused at one time.

Example 2:

Order: aminophylline 250 mg in 250 mL D5W IV; run at 50 cc/hr

Available: Ampule of aminophylline labeled 1 g in 10 cc; Buretrol that delivers 60 gtt/mL (microdrip)

Logic: The ampule of aminophylline has 1 g in 10 mL. This is equivalent to 1000 mg in 10 mL. You want 250 mg.

$$\frac{D}{H} \times S = A$$

$$\frac{\cancel{250}^{\,1}}{\cancel{1000}_{\,4}} \times 10 = \frac{\cancel{10}}{4} \quad 4\overline{)10.0} = 2.5 \text{ mL}$$

Draw up 2.5 mL and inject into 250 mL D5W. You have 250 mg aminophylline in 250 mL D5W. Label the bag.

You want 50 cc/hr, and you have a Buretrol 60 gtt/mL.

$$\frac{\text{mL/hr} \times \text{TF}}{60} = \frac{50 \times \cancel{60}}{\cancel{60}} = 50 \text{ gtt/min}$$

Actually, since you have a microdrip Buretrol, no calculation is necessary: mL/hr = gtt/min.

Label the IV.

Practice Exercise 2

Answers may be found at the end of the chapter.

1. Order: 500 mL D5W IV with vitamin C 500 mg at 60 cc/hr
   Available: Ampule of vitamin C labeled 500 mg/2 mL
   Microdrip tubing at 60 gtt/mL

2. Order: 250 mg hydrocortisone sodium succinate in 1000 mL D5W 8 AM–12 mid
   Available: Vial of hydrocortisone sodium succinate labeled 250 mg with a 2-mL diluent
   Microdrip tubing and macrodrip tubing at 20 gtt/mL

3. Order: aminophylline 250 mg in 250 mL D5W IV. Run 50 cc/hr
   Available: Infusion pump
   Vial of aminophylline labeled 500 mg/10 mL

4. Order: 250 cc D5 $\frac{1}{2}$NS with KCl 10 mEq IV 12 N–6 PM
   Available: Microdrip tubing
   Vial of potassium chloride labeled 20 mEq/10 mL

Medications Ordered in units/hr or mg/hr

Thus far all the IV problems were solved by determining the milliliters per hour or the drops per minute. Infusion rates can also be calculated when the physician orders the IV to infuse in units per hour (U/hr) or in milligrams per hour (mg/hr). When IVs are ordered in this way, an infusion pump or a control device, such as Buretrol, is necessary to protect the patient against excessive fluid intake, since these medications are potent. Use the rule $\frac{D}{H} \times S = A$

EXAMPLE

Order: 20,000 units heparin sodium in 500 mL D5W; infusion 1000 U/hr

Available: infusion pump

Vial of heparin sodium 5000 units/mL

How will you solve these problems? See them as injections from liquid!

Step 1. Add the medication to the IV

$$\frac{D}{H} \times S = A$$

$$\frac{\overset{4}{\cancel{20,000 \text{ units}}}}{\underset{1}{\cancel{5,000 \text{ mg}}}} \times 1 \text{ mL} = 4 \text{ mL}$$

Add 4 mL heparin sodium to 500 mL D5W

Step 2. Determine the mL/hr to administer 1000 units/hr

$\frac{D}{H} \times S = A$

$\frac{\overset{25}{\cancel{1000}} \cancel{\text{units}}/\text{hr}}{\underset{\underset{1}{\cancel{40}}}{\cancel{20,000}} \cancel{\text{units}}} \times \overset{25}{\cancel{500}} \text{ mL} = 25 \text{ mL/hr}$

◀ ***Learning Aid***
Note that the units cancel out and mL/hr is left.

Set the pump at 25 mL/hr.

For patient safety in the hospital setting, these solutions are usually standardized and can be found in the procedure manual. The order then does not specify the solution. In the example above the order might read: "Infuse heparin sodium 1000 units/hr."

EXAMPLE Order: aminophylline 50 mg/hr via pump

Available: infusion pump

Procedure manual dictates the solution to be 0.5 g in 500 mL D5W.

Ampule of aminophylline labeled 1 gram/10 mL

Step 1. Add the medication to the IV bag

$\frac{D}{H} \times S = A \qquad \frac{0.5 \cancel{g}}{1 \cancel{g}} \times 10 \text{ mL} = 5 \text{ mL}$

Add 5 mL aminophylline to 500 mL D5W.

Step 2. Determine the # mL needed to give 50 mL/hr.

0.5 g = 500 mg

$\frac{D}{H} \times S = A \qquad \frac{50 \cancel{\text{mg}}/\text{hr}}{\cancel{500} \cancel{\text{mg}}} \times \cancel{500} \text{ mL} = 50 \text{ mL/hr}$

Set the pump at 50 mL/hr.

Practice Exercise 3

Answers may be found at the end of the chapter.

1. Order: heparin sodium 1400 units qh IV
Stock: Standard solution 25,000 units in 500 mL D5W
Vial of heparin sodium labeled 10,000 units/mL
Infusion pump available

2. Order: aminophylline drip 800 mg in 500 mL D5W. Run 50 mL/hr.
Stock: Vial of aminophylline labeled 1 gram in 10 mL
Infusion pump available

3. Order: diltiazem HCl 5 mL/hr IV.
Stock: Solution prepared by pharmacy of 125 mg in 125 mL
Infusion pump

Medications Ordered in mcg/min or mcg/kg/min

In intensive care units, powerful drugs are administered in minute amounts called micrograms (1 mg = 1000 mcg). The orders for these drugs differ from any we have studied:

EXAMPLE Renal dose dopamine 2 mcg/kg/min IV

Titrate levophed to maintain arterial mean pressure above 65 and below 95

lidocaine 2 mg/min IV

These drugs are administered through an infusion pump in mL/hr. They are calculated using microdrip (60 gtts/mL). Since mL/hr = microdrops per minute, once the microdrip is calculated, the mL/hr are known. These solutions are always standardized by the pharmacy for patient safety (Fig. 9-6). The rule $\frac{D}{H} \times S = A$ is used to solve these problems.

Example 1:

Order: dopamine 400 mcg/min IV

Available: infusion pump

standard solution of 200 mg/250 mL

◀ *Learning Aid*
1 mL = 60 gtt microdrip

Step 1. Reduce the standard solution to mcg per 1 mL.

The standard solution is 200 mg/250 mL.

200 mg × 1000 mcg = 200,000 mcg

$$\frac{200{,}000 \text{ mcg}}{250 \text{ mL}} = 800 \text{ mcg/mL}$$

Step 2. Substitute 60 gtt for the mL (microdrip 60 gtt = 1 mL).

The solution is 800 mcg/60 gtt.

DOPAMINE HCL

400 mg in 250 mL D5W
(1600 mcg per mL)

SINGLE-STRENGTH

INFUSION RATE	DOSE
60 mL/hr.	1600 mcg/min
55 mL/hr.	1467 mcg/min
50 mL/hr.	1333 mcg/min
45 mL/hr.	1200 mcg/min
40 mL/hr.	1067 mcg/min
35 mL/hr.	.933 mcg/min
30 mL/hr.	.800 mcg/min
25 mL/hr.	.667 mcg/min
20 mL/hr.	.533 mcg/min
15 mL/hr.	.400 mcg/min
10 mL/hr.	.267 mcg/min
5 mL/hr.	133 mcg/min

Renal dose: 0.5-2.5 mcg/kg/min
Maximum dose: 20-50 mcg/kg/min

Date: ______________ **Time:** __________

Prepared By: ______________________

Figure 9-6
A standard solution for single strength dopamine is 400 mg in 250 mL, which equals 1600 mcg per mL. Note that infusion rates for some doses are given on the label. The label is affixed to the IV bag.

Step 3. $\frac{D}{H} \times S = A$

$$\frac{\overset{1}{\cancel{400}}\ \cancel{\text{mcg}}/\text{min}}{\underset{\underset{1}{\cancel{2}}}{\cancel{800}}\ \cancel{\text{mcg}}} \times \overset{30}{\cancel{60}}\ \text{gtt} = 30\ \text{gtt/min}$$ (gtt = mL/hr; therefore, 30 gtt/min = 30 mL/hr)

Label the IV.

Set the pump:

Total # mL: 250

mL/hr: 30

Example 2:

Order: aramine 60 mcg/min IV

Available: infusion pump

standard solution 50 mg in 250 mL D5W

Step 1. Reduce the standard solution to mcg/1 mL.

50 mg × 1000 mcg = 50,000 mcg

$$\frac{50{,}000\ \text{mcg}}{250\ \text{mL}} = 200\ \text{mcg/mL}$$

Step 2. Substitute 60 gtt for 1 mL.

Solution is 200 mcg/60 gtt.

Step 3. $\frac{D}{H} \times S = A$

$$\frac{\overset{3}{\cancel{60}}\ \cancel{\text{mcg}}/\text{min}}{\underset{1}{\cancel{200}}\ \cancel{\text{mcg}}} \times 6\cancel{0}\ \text{gtt} = 18\ \text{gtt/min} = 18\ \text{mL/hr}$$

Label IV.

◀ ***Learning Aid***
1 mL = 60 gtt microdrip

Set the pump:

Total # mL: 250

mL/hr: 18

Example 3:

Order: dopamine 2 mcg/kg/min

Available: Infusion pump

Standard solution of 200 mg/250 mL D5W

Note that this order is somewhat different. We are to give 2 mcg per kilogram of body weight. First we must weigh the patient, convert pounds to kilograms if the scale is not in kilograms, then multiply the kg by 2 mcg. Once we have determined this answer, we follow the three steps given above.

The patient weighs 176 lb.

◀ ***Learning Aid***
To convert lb to kg, divide by 2.2

$$\frac{176\ \text{lb}}{2.2} \qquad 2.2\overline{)176.0} = 80. \qquad = 80\ \text{kg}$$

$$\begin{array}{r} 80\ \text{kg} \\ \times\ 2\ \text{mcg} \\ \hline 160\ \text{mcg} \end{array}$$

The order now is 160 mcg/min.

Step 1. Reduce the standard solution to mcg per 1 mL.

200 mg/250 mL =

$$200 \times 1000 \text{ mcg} = \frac{200{,}000 \text{ mcg}}{250 \text{ mL}} = 800 \text{ mcg/mL}$$

Step 2. Substitute 60 gtt for the 1 mL.

The solution is 800 mcg/60 gtt.

Step 3. $\frac{D}{H} \times S = A$

$$\frac{\overset{2}{\cancel{160}} \text{ mcg/min}}{\underset{1}{\cancel{800}} \text{ mcg}} \times \cancel{60} \text{ gtt} = 12 \text{ gtt/min} = 12 \text{ mL/hr}$$

Label the IV.

Set the pump:

Total # mL: 250

mL/hr: 12

Practice Exercise 4

Answers may be found at the end of the chapter.

1. Order: dopamine double strength 800 mcg/min
Available: Standard solution 800 mg in 250 mL D5W
Infusion pump

2. Order: norepinephrine bitartrate 12 mcg/min
Available: Standard solution of 4 mg in 250 mL D5W
Infusion pump

3. Order: dobutamine 5 mcg/kg/min
Available: Patient weight—220 lb
Standard solution of 1 gram in 250 mL D5W
Infusion pump

4. Order: dobutamine 7 mcg/kg/min
Available: Patient weight—70 kg
Standard solution of 500 mg in 250 mL D5W
Infusion pump

5. Order: nitroglycerin 10 mcg/min
Available: Standard solution of 50 mg in 250 mL D5W
Infusion pump

▼ MEDICATIONS FOR INTERMITTENT INTRAVENOUS ADMINISTRATION

Some intravenous medications are not administered continuously but only intermittently, such as q4h, q6h, or q8h. This route is termed intravenous piggyback or IVPB (refer to Fig. 9-1).

Most of these drugs are prepared in powder form. The manufacturer specifies the type and amount of diluent needed to reconstitute the drug, which is connected by IV tubing to the main IV line.

The doctor may write a detailed order: vancomycin 0.5 g IVPB in 100 mL D5W over 1 hr. More often the doctor will write only the drug, route, and time interval, relying on the nurse to research the manufacturer's directions for the amount and type of diluent and the time for the infusion to run (e.g., cefazolin 1 g IVPB q6h).

Explanation

The rule to solve IVPB problems is similar to the IV rule:

$$\frac{\#\ \text{mL} \times \text{TF}}{\#\ \text{min}} = \text{gtt/min}$$

mL—The type and amount of diluent will be stated on the label or in the package insert. Nurses' drug references and the *Physicians Drug Reference (PDR)* also contain this information.

TF—The tubing for IVPB is called a secondary administration set and has a macrodrip factor. It is shorter than main line IV tubing. To solve IVPB problems we will use the tube factor 10 gtt = 1 mL. In the clinical setting, check the label for the tube factor.

min—The manufacturer may or may not indicate the number of minutes needed for the IVPB medication to be infused. When it is not given, a general rule to follow for adults is to allow 30 minutes for every 50 mL of solution.

EXAMPLE Order: cefazolin 1 g IVPB q6h

Stock: (see Fig. 9-7 for directions)

"Piggyback" Vials
Reconstitute with 50 to 100 ml. of Sodium Chloride Injection or other I.V. solution listed under ADMINISTRATION. When adding diluent to vial, allow air to escape by using a small vent needle or by pumping the syringe. SHAKE WELL. Administer with primary I.V. fluids, as a single dose.
ADMINISTRATION
Intramuscular Administration—Reconstitute vials with Sterile Water for Injection according to the dilution table above. Shake well until dissolved. 'Ancef' should be injected into a large muscle mass. Pain on injection is infrequent with 'Ancef'.
Intravenous Administration—Direct (bolus) injection: Following reconstitution according to the above table, further dilute vials with approximately 5 ml. Sterile Water for Injection. Inject the solution slowly over 3 to 5 minutes, directly or through tubing for patients receiving parenteral fluids (see list below).
Intermittent or continuous infusion: Dilute reconstituted 'Ancef' in 50 to 100 ml. of one of the following solutions:
Sodium Chloride Injection, USP
5% or 10% Dextrose Injection, USP
5% Dextrose in Lactated Ringer's Injection, USP
5% Dextrose and 0.9% Sodium Chloride Injection, USP
5% Dextrose and 0.45% Sodium Chloride Injection, USP
5% Dextrose and 0.2% Sodium Chloride Injection, USP

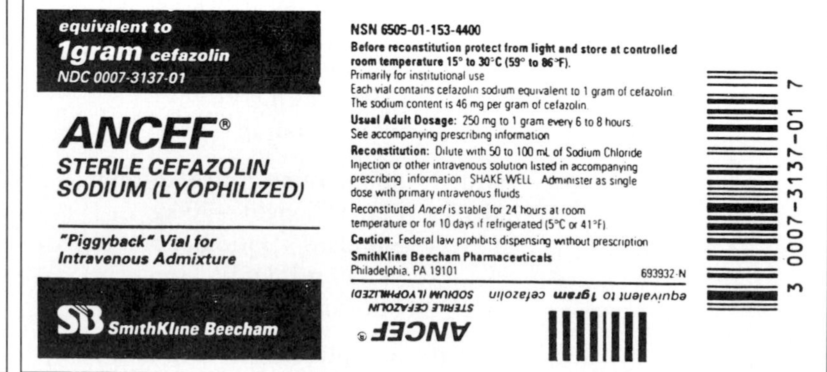

Figure 9-7
Package insert directions for IVPB dilution of cefazolin sodium (Ancef). (Courtesy of Smith Kline & Beecham Laboratories.)

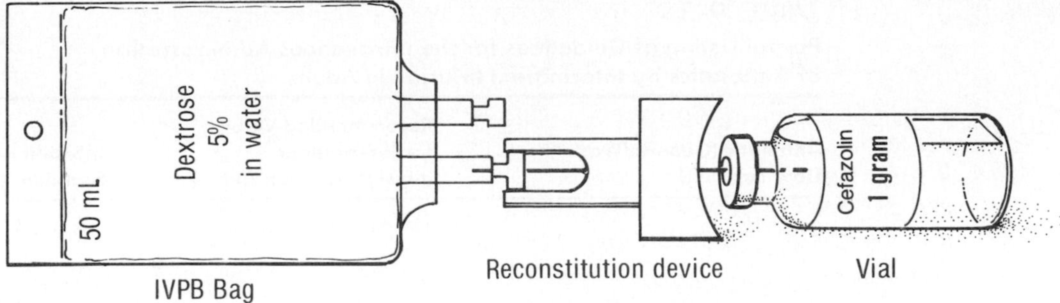

Figure 9-8
Reconstitution device. The IVPB bag is squeezed, forcing fluid into the vial of powder, which is then diluted. The three parts are turned to a vertical position—vial up, IVPB bag down. The IVPB bag is squeezed and released. This creates a negative pressure allowing the diluted medication to flow into the IVPB bag.

The label states that 1 gram can be reconstituted with 50 to 100 mL of sodium chloride or other solution and refers the reader to the package insert (refer to Fig. 9-7). Directions say that we can use D5W. Let's use 50 mL D5W. It is the most common IVPB diluent and we have 50 mL bags. (Refer to Fig. 9-2.) No time for infusion is given. Use 30 minutes for 50 mL.

$\frac{\text{\# mL} \times \text{TF}}{\text{\# min}} = \text{gtt/min}$

# mL = 50 mL D5W
TF = 10 gtt/mL (For a secondary administration set no time for administration is given. Follow the general adult rule of 30 minutes for every 50 mL.)
# min = 30

$\frac{50 \times 10}{30} = 16.6 = 17 \text{ gtt/min}$

You are ready to prepare the IVPB. You have a vial of powder labeled 1 gram. You need the whole amount. You have a 50 mL bag of D5W. You need the whole amount. Use a reconstitution device to mix the powder and the diluent. A *reconstitution device* is a sterile implement containing two needles that connect the vial and the 50 mL bag. It enables the nurse to dilute the powder and place it in the IV bag without using a syringe (Fig. 9-8). Once the powder is reconstituted, label the IV bag.

MEDICATION ADDED	
Patient Tom Smith	Room 1503-4
Drug cefazolin 1 g	Flow rate 17 gtt/min
Base solution 50 mL D5W	Initials RT
Time to run 12n – 12:30pm	Date 6/14

It is time consuming to look through package inserts for directions. Drug references will give this information in a concise manner. Table 9-3 is a set of IVPB guidelines printed by a hospital pharmacy for the convenience of nurses.

TABLE 9-3

Partial Listing of Guidelines for the Intravenous Administration of Antibiotics by Intermittent Infusion in Adults

Antibiotic (Generic/Trade)/ How Supplied	Recommended Volume for Intermittent Infusion/Infusion Fluid	Infusion Period/ Stability
Acyclovir ZOVIRAX® powder for injection 500 mg vial	100 mL/D5W,NS	1 hour/24 hours
Amikacin AMIKIN® injection, 250 mg/mL 2 mL vial	100 mL/D5W,NS	30 minutes/24 hours
Cefazolin ANCEF® KEFZOL® powder for injection 500 mg, 1 g vials	50 mL (500 mg)/D5W,NS 50 mL (1 gram)/D5W,NS 100 mL (2 grams)/D5W,NS	15–30 minutes/96 hours (REFRIGERATED)
Cefotaxime CLAFORAN® powder for injection 1 g, 2 g vials	50 mL (1 gram)/D5W,NS 100 mL (2 grams)/D5W,NS	15–30 minutes/5 days (REFRIGERATED)
Ceftazidime TAZIDIME®, FORTAZ®, TAZICEF® powder for injection 1 g, 2 g vials	50 mL (1 gram)/D5W,NS 100 mL (2 grams)/D5W,NS	15–30 minutes/7 days (REFRIGERATED)
Ciprofloxacin CIPRO I.V.® injection, 10 mg/mL 20 mL, 40 mL vials	100 mL (200 mg)/D5W,NS	60 minutes/14 days (REFRIGERATED or at room temperature)
Doxycycline VIBRAMYCIN® powder for injection 100 mg vial	250 mL (100 mg)/D5W,NS 500 mL (200 mg)/D5W,NS	1 hour (100 mg) 2 hours (200 mg)/48 hours (REFRIGERATED)
Trimethoprim-Sulfamethoxazole BACTRIM®, SEPTRA® injection 5 mL, 10 mL vials [contains 80 mg/mL (sulfamethoxazole); 16 mg/mL (trimethoprim)]	One 5 mL vial per 75 mL or 125 mL/D5W	60–90 minutes/24 hours
Vancomycin VANCOCIN®, VANCOLED® powder for injection 500 mg vial	100 mL (500 mg)/D5W,NS 250 mL (1 gram)/D5W,NS	1 hour (500 mg) 2 hours (1 gram)/7 days (REFRIGERATED)

Courtesy of the Pharmacy Department St. Vincent Hospital and Medical Center, New York.

EXAMPLE

Order: vancomycin 1 g IVPB 7 AM

Stock: 500 mg powder. For directions, see Table 9-3.

Rule:

$$\frac{\text{\# mL} \times \text{TF}}{\text{\# min}} = \text{gtts/min} \qquad \text{\# mL} = 250 \text{ mL D5W}$$

$$\text{TF} = 10$$

$$\text{min} = 2 \text{ hrs} = 120 \text{ min}$$

$$\frac{250 \times 10}{120} = \frac{250}{12} \quad 12\overline{)250.0}^{\,20.8} = 21$$

Use a reconstitution device to add 1 gram of vancomycin (2 vials of 500 mg) to 250 mL D5W. Label the IV. Set the rate at 21 gtt/min. The IVPB will run 2 hours.

Practice Exercise 5

Solve these drip factors for IVPB problems using Table 9-3. Answers may be found at the end of this chapter.

1. Order: acyclovir 500 mg IVPB q8h
   Stock: 500 mg powder
2. Order: ceftazidime 1 g IVPB q12h
   Stock: 1 gram powder
3. Order: ciprofloxacin 0.2 g IVPB q12h
   Stock: 20 mL vial labeled 10 mg/mL
4. Order: cefotaxime 1 g IVPB q6h
   Stock: 1 gram powder

▼ CHANGING THE INTRAVENOUS DRIP RATE

Setting the drip rate for an IV does not relieve the nurse of the responsibility to check the IV frequently. Many factors can interfere with the flow—kinking of the tube, movement of the client, the effect of gravity, or placement of the needle or catheter. If a discrepancy in flow exists, it may be necessary to recalculate the IV drip.

EXAMPLE

As you make rounds you check a client's IV. The label reads:

1000 mL D5W IV to run 8 AM–4 PM

The tubing is macrodrip (10 gtt/mL). Rate is set at 20 gtt/min.

It is now 1 PM. You note that there is 600 mL left in the IV. Should you change the drip?

Logic: Step 1. Calculate how many milliliters per hour.

$$\frac{1000}{8} = 125 \text{ mL/hr}$$

Step 2. It is now 1 PM. Therefore 5 hours have elapsed since the IV was started.

125 mL/hr
× 5 hr
625 mL should have been delivered.

Step 3. Because there are 600 mL left in the IV, only 400 mL were delivered.

625 mL should have been delivered
400 mL were delivered
225 mL behind

Conclusion: The nurse will have to make a judgment of whether or not to increase the IV drip on the basis of an assessment of the client's status. It may be necessary to consult with the physician.

▼ DETERMINATION OF THE HOURS THAT AN INTRAVENOUS INFUSION WILL RUN

When an IV order reads mL/hr, mg/hr, or units/hr, it is sometimes helpful for the nurse to calculate how long the IV will last so that the next IV can be prepared or new orders written.

1 soup
1 juice
1 serving

240 cc's
860 cc's
120 cc's

TIME	ORAL	ENTERAL	PARENTERAL (Type & Amount)	Amt Abs LIB	PARENTERAL (Type & Amount)	Amt Abs LIB
8a-9						
9-10						
10-11						
11-12						
12-1						
1-2						
2-3						
3-4p						
4p total			LIB		LIB	
4p-5						
5-6						
6-7						
7-8p						
8p total			LIB		LIB	
8p-9						
9-10						
10-11						
11-12						
12m total			LIB		LIB	
12a-1						
1-2						
2-3						
3-4						
4-5						
5-6						
6-7						
7-8a						
8a total			LIB		LIB	
24 hour total						

Figure 9-9
A sample flow sheet for oral, enteral, and parenteral intake.

EXAMPLE

Order: 500 mL Ringer's lactate IV; run 75 mL/hr

Divide the number of milliliters by the milliliters per hour

$$\begin{array}{r} 6.6 \text{ hr} \\ 75\overline{)500.0} \\ \underline{450} \\ 50\ 0 \end{array}$$

The IV will last approximately 6.6 hr.

Recording Intake

Fluid intake may be recorded every hour or once a shift. Figure 9-9 is a sample flow sheet for 24 hours. Liquids taken by the oral route, enterally (e.g., tube feedings) and parenterally (e.g., IV, IVPB) are noted. A record may be kept every hour or at the end of each shift. The sample sheet shows shift changes every eight hours with totals for the shift given. At the bottom of the sheet, the 24-hour intake is given. The term L.I.B. means "left in bag." A nurse beginning a shift would know how much of the IV fluid was infusing on her/his time.

Practice Exercise 6

Solve these IV infusion problems. Answers may be found at the end of the chapter.

1. 20,000 units of heparin is added to 500 mL D5W, and the order is to infuse IV at 30 mL/hr. How many hours will the IV run?
2. 900 mL of an IV solution is to infuse at 100 mL/hr. If it is 9 AM when the infusion starts, at what time will it be completed?
3. A patient is receiving an antibiotic IVPB in 75 mL q6h plus a maintenance IV of 125 mL/hr. What is the 24-hour intake parenterally?
4. An IV of 1000 mL D5NS is infusing at 10 microdrips per minute. What is the parenteral intake for 8 hours?
5. A doctor orders 500 mL aminophylline 0.5 g to infuse at 50 mL/hr. How many mg will the patient receive each hour?

Self-Test 1

Solve these problems related to intravenous and IVPB drip rates. Aim for a high degree of accuracy. Answers may be found at the end of the chapter. Review material that you find difficult.

1. Order: 1500 mL D5W 8 AM–8 PM
   Available: macrodrip tubing (10 gtt/mL)
   What is the drip rate?

(continued)

Self-Test 1 (continued)

2. Order: 250 mL D5 $\frac{1}{2}$ NS IV KVO (give over 12 hours)
   Available: microdrip tubing
   What is the drip rate?

3. Order: 150 mL D5 $\frac{1}{3}$ NS IV; run 20 mL/hr
   Available: infusion pump
   a. What is the drip rate?
   b. How long will the IV last?

4. Order: heparin 40,000 units in 1000 mL D5W; infuse 800 units/hr
   Available: infusion pump
   What is the drip rate?

5. Order: 1000 mL D5S with 15 mEq KCl IV; run 100 mL/hr
   Available: macrotubing (20 gtt/mL) and microdrip
   a. How many hours will this run?
   b. How many milliliters of KCl will you add to the IV if KCl comes in a vial labeled 40 mEq/20 mL?
   c. What tubing will you use?
   d. What are the gtt/min?

6. Order: nitroglycerin IV at 80 mcg/min
   Available: infusion pump standard solution of 50 mg in 250 mL D5W
   What is the drip rate?

Self-Test 2

1. Order: aminophylline 1 g in 500 mL D5W IV at 75 mL/hr
   Available: vial of aminophylline 1 g in 10 mL; infusion pump
   a. How many mL of aminophylline should be added to the IV?
   b. How will you set the drip rate?

2. Order: amikacin 0.4 g IVPB q8h
   Stock: 2 mL vial labeled 250 mg/mL
   See Table 9-3 for directions.

3. Order: dobutamine 250 mcg/min
   Available: Standard solution 500 mg in 500 mL D5W
   Infusion pump
   What is the drip rate?

(continued)

Self-Test 2 (continued)

4. Order: heparin sodium 800 units/hr IV
   Available: infusion pump; standard solution of 25,000 units in 250 mL D5W
   What is the rate?

5. Order: 500 mL D5 $\frac{1}{2}$ S IV q8h
   Available: microdrip tubing
   What are the gtt/min?

6. Order: bretylium 1 mg/min IV
   Available: standard solution 1 g in 500 mL D5W
   What are the gtt/min?

Proficiency Test

There are 20 questions related to IV and IVPB calculations. If you have any difficulty doing these problems, review the information in Chapter 9 which explains this information. Answers may be found at the end of this chapter.

1. Order: aqueous penicillin G 1 MU in 100 mL D5W IVPB q6h over 40 minutes (macrodrip tubing at 10 gtt/mL)
   Stock: vial labeled 5 million units of powder. Directions say to inject 18 mL of sterile water for injection to yield 20 mL of solution. Reconstituted solution is stable for 1 week.
   a. How would you prepare the penicillin?
   b. What solution will you make?
   c. What amount of penicillin solution should be placed into the bag of 100 mL D5W?
   d. What is the drip factor for the IVPB?

2. You have a 250-mL bag of D5W to which has been added 25,000 units of Liquaemin Sodium. You have an order to give the patient 1200 units IV per hour using an infusion pump.
   a. What is the drip rate?
   b. How many hours will this IV run?

3. 1000 mL of an IV solution is to infuse at 100 mL/hr. If the infusion starts at 8 AM, at what time will it be completed?

(continued)

Proficiency Test (continued)

4. Order: Gentamicin 60 mg IVPB in 50 mL D5W over 30 minutes using macrodrip (20 gtt/cc).
   Stock: vial of gentamicin 40 mg/mL; 50-mL bag of D5W. Order is correct.
   - **a.** How many mL of gentamicin will you add to the 50-mL bag of D5W?
   - **b.** What is the drip factor for the IVPB?

5. Calculate the drip factor for 1500 mL D5 $\frac{1}{2}$ NS to run 12 hours by macrodrip (10 gtt/mL).

6. Intralipid, 500 mL q6h, is ordered for a patient together with an IV that is infusing at 80 mL/hr. Calculate the 24-hour parenteral intake.

7. Order: 1000 mL D5W with 20 mEq KCl and 500 mg Vit C at 60 mL/hr. No infusion pump is available.
   - **a.** Approximately how many hours will the IV run?
   - **b.** Which tubing will you choose—macrodrip at 10 gtt/mL or microdrip at 60 gtt/mL?
   - **c.** What are the drops per minute (gtt/min) for the tubing that you choose?

8. Order: 1000 mL D5NS; run 150 mL/hr IV
   Stock: IV bag of 1000 mL D5NS
   - **a.** Approximately how many hours will the IV run?
   - **b.** Which tubing will you choose—macrodrip (10 gtt/min) or microdrip (60 gtt/min)?
   - **c.** What will be the drip rate?

9. Order: 100 mL Ringer's solution 12 noon–6 PM IV
   - **a.** What size tubing will you use?
   - **b.** What are the gtt/min?

10. Order: 150 mL NS IV over 3 hours
    Stock: bag of 250 mL normal saline for IV and macrotubing 15 gtt/mL; microtubing (60 gtt/mL)
    - **a.** What would you do to obtain 150 mL NS?
    - **b.** What IV tubing would you use?
    - **c.** What are the gtt/min?

(continued)

Proficiency Test (continued)

11. Order: Liquaemin Sodium 1500 units/hr IV
Stock: standardized solution of Liquaemin 100 units/mL. An infusion pump is available. What should be the setting on the infusion pump?

12. Order: 500 mL D5W IVKVO. Solve for 24 hours. An infusion pump is available. What should be the setting on the infusion pump?

13. Order: doxycycline 100 mg IVPB qd
Stock: 100 mg powder. See Table 9-3 for directions.
State the amount and type of IV fluid you will use and the time for infusion you will use.
What are the gtt/min?

14. Order: isoproterenol 2 mg in 250 mL D5W; titrate at 4 mcg/min
Available: ampule of isoproterenol labeled 1 mg in 5 mL
infusion pump

15. Order: aminophylline 500 mg in 250 mL D5W to run 8 hours IV
Available: vial of aminophylline labeled 1 gram in 10 mL
microdrip tubing
What is the drip rate?

16. A patient is receiving an IV at the rate of 125 mL/h. The doctor orders cefoxitin 1 g in 75 mL D5W q6h. Calculate the 24-hour parenteral intake.

17. Order: 1000 mL D5 $\frac{1}{2}$ NS to run at 90 mL/hr; infusion pump available
a. What will be the pump setting?
b. Approximately how long will the IV run?

18. Order: Aramine 50 mg IV in 250 mL D5W; titrate to 60 mcg/min
Stock: vial of Aramine 100 mg in 10 mL; infusion pump
a. How much Aramine would you add to the IV?
b. What will be the drip rate?

(continued)

Proficiency Test (continued)

19. A doctor orders 500 mL of aminophylline 0.5 g to infuse at 50 mL/hr. How many milligrams will the patient receive each hour?

20. Order: Bactrim 5 mL IVPB q6h
    Stock: vial of 5 mL. Refer to Table 9-3 for directions.
    Main IV line is connected to an infusion pump. What will you do? Refer to Figure 9-4.
    a. State the type and amount of IV fluid you would use and the time for infusion.
    b. How would you program the infusion pump?

ANSWERS

Practice Exercise 1

1. Logic: This is a continuous IV of 150 mL every 8 hours. There is a pump available. You only need Step 1.

   It will run 8 hr.

   $\frac{\# \text{ mL}}{\# \text{ hr}} = \text{mL/hr} \qquad \frac{150 \text{ mL}}{8} \qquad 8\overline{)150.0} = 18.7 \text{ mL/hr}$

   8, 70, 64, 60, 56

   Label the IV. Set the pump:

   Total # mL: 150

   mL/hr: 19

2. Logic: This is a continuous IV. A pump is available. The order states mL/hr. There is no calculation needed. Label the IV. Set the pump as follows:

   Total # mL: 250

   mL/hr: 25

3. Logic: The order gives 100 mL/hr; mL/hr = gtt per minute, so you know the microdrip is 100 gtt/min. Work out the macrodrip factor and choose the tubing. You need Step 2.

   Macrodrip

   Step 2. $\frac{\text{mL/hr} \times \text{TF}}{\# \text{ min}} = \text{gtt/min}$

   $\frac{100 \times \cancel{20}^{1}}{\cancel{60}_{3}} = \frac{100}{3} = 33.3$

   Macrodrip at 33 gtt/min

   Microdrip at 100 gtt/min

   Either drip rate could be used. Label the IV.

4. Logic: This is a small volume over several hours; use microdrip. Macrodrip would be too slow (5 gtt/min).

   Step 1. $\frac{\# \text{ mL}}{\# \text{ hr}} = \text{mL/hr} \qquad \frac{\cancel{180}^{30}}{\cancel{6}_{1}} = 30 \text{ mL/hr}$

   Step 2. $\frac{\text{mL/hr} \times \text{TF}}{\# \text{ min}} = \text{gtt/min}$

   Microdrip is 30 gtt/min because mL/hr = gtt/min

5. Logic: This is a large volume over several hours; use macrodrip. Solve using two steps and decide.

   Step 1. $\frac{\# \text{ mL}}{\# \text{ hr}} = \text{mL/hr} \qquad \frac{\cancel{1000}^{125}}{\cancel{8}_{1}} = 125 \text{ mL/hr}$

   Step 2. $\frac{\text{mL/hr} \times \text{TF}}{\# \text{ min}} = \text{gtt/min}$

   You know microdrip will be 125 gtt/min because mL/hr = gtt/min.

   Macrodrip

   $\frac{125 \times \cancel{15}^{1}}{\cancel{60}_{4}} = \frac{125}{4} \qquad 4\overline{)125.0} = 31.2$

   12, 5, 4, 10, 8

   Macrodrip at 31 gtt/min

   Microdrip at 125 gtt/min

   Use macrodrip

   Label the IV.

Practice Exercise 2

1. Logic: You want vitamin C 500 mg and the stock is 500 mg in 2 mL. Use a syringe to add the 2 mL to 500 mL D5W. You have microdrip available. The IV is to run at 60 cc/hr. Remember mL/hr = gtt/min for microdrip. No math necessary. Set the microdrip at 60 gtt/min. Label the IV.

2. Logic: You want 250 mg hydrocortisone sodium succinate, and it comes 250 mg with a 2 mL diluent. Use a syringe to reconstitute the hydrocortisone with 2 mL diluent and add it to the IV. 8 AM–12 MID is 16 hours. Microdrip tubing seems indicated. Solve using two steps.

Step 1. $\frac{\#\ \text{mL}}{\#\ \text{hr}} = \text{mL/hr}$ $\qquad \frac{\cancel{1000}}{16} \quad 16\overline{)1000.0} = 62.5 = 63\ \text{mL/hr}$

$$\begin{array}{r} 96 \\ \hline 40 \\ 32 \\ \hline 80 \\ \underline{80} \end{array}$$

Step 2. mL/hr = gtt/min for microdrip. No math for microdrip. Microdrip = 63 gtt/min

Macrodrip $\frac{\text{mL/hr}}{\text{min}} = \text{gtt/min}$

$$\frac{63 \times 20}{60} = 20.5 = 21\ \text{gtt/min}$$

Label the IV.

Microdrip 63 gtt/min; macrodrip 21 gtt/min

Choose one.

3. Logic: You want 250 mg aminophylline. Stock is 500 mg/10 mL

$\frac{D}{H} \times S = A \qquad \frac{250\ \text{mg}}{500\ \text{mg}} \times 10\ \text{mL} = 5\ \text{mL}$

Add 5 mL aminophylline to 250 mL D5W. Order is 50 cc/hr. You have an infusion pump. No math. Set the pump as follows:

Total # mL: 250

mL/hr: 50

4. Logic: You want KCl 10 mEq. Stock is 20 mEq/10 mL.

$\frac{D}{H} \times S = A \qquad \frac{10\ \text{mEq}}{20\ \text{mEq}} \times 10\ \text{mL} = 5\ \text{mL}$

Add 5 mL KCl to 250 mL D5W$\frac{1}{2}$NS. 12 N–6 PM is 6 hours. One step is needed because you have microdrip tubing.

$\frac{\#\ \text{mL}}{\#\ \text{hr}} = \text{mL/hr} \qquad \frac{\cancel{250}}{6} \quad 6\overline{)250.0} = 41.6 = 42\ \text{mL/hr}$

$$\begin{array}{r} 24 \\ \hline 10 \\ 6 \\ \hline 40 \\ \underline{36} \end{array}$$

mL/hr = gtt/min microdrip

Set the microdrip at 42 gtt/min

Label the IV.

Practice Exercise 3

1. Logic: You want 25,000 units heparin. Stock is 10,000 units/mL.

$\frac{D}{H} \times S = A \qquad \frac{\overset{5}{\cancel{25{,}000\ \text{units}}}}{\underset{2}{\cancel{10{,}000\ \text{units}}}} \times 1\ \text{mL}$

$$= \frac{\cancel{5}}{2} \quad 2\overline{)5.0} = 2.5 = 2.5\ \text{mL}$$

Add 2.5 mL heparin to 500 mL D5W
You want 1400 units/hr

$\frac{D}{H} \times S = A \qquad \frac{1400\ \text{units/hr}}{25{,}000\ \text{units}} \times 500\ \text{mL}$

$$= \frac{\cancel{140}}{5} \quad 5\overline{)140.} = 28\ \text{mL/hr}$$

Label the IV.

Set the pump as follows:

Total # mL: 500
mL/hr = 28

2. Logic: You want 800 mg aminophylline. Stock is 1 gram in 10 mL. 1 gram = 1000 mg

$\frac{D}{H} \times S = A \qquad \frac{\cancel{800}\ \cancel{\text{mg}}}{\cancel{1000}\ \cancel{\text{mg}}} \times 10\ \text{mL} = 8\ \text{mL}$

Add 8 mL aminophylline to 500 mL D5W. You have an infusion pump. No math needed. Label the IV. Set the pump as follows:

Total # mL: 500

mL/hr = 50

3. Logic: The solution is prepared by the pharmacy: 125 mg in 125 mL = 1 mg/mL. The order is 5 mL/hr and you have an infusion pump. No math necessary. Set the pump as follows:

Total # mL: 125 mL

mL/hr: 5

Practice Exercise 4

1. Logic: The standard solution is 800 mg in 250 mL D5W.

Step 1. Reduce the standard solution to mcg/1 mL

$\frac{800\text{ mg}}{250\text{ mL}} = \frac{80\text{ mg}}{25\text{ mL}} = \frac{80{,}000\text{ mcg}}{25\text{ mL}} = 3200\text{ mcg/mL}$

Step 2. Substitute 60 gtt for the mL
= 3200 mcg/60 gtt

Step 3. $\frac{D}{H} \times S = A$

$\frac{\overset{1}{\cancel{800}}\text{ mcg/min}}{\underset{\underset{1}{\cancel{800}}}{\cancel{3200}}\text{ mcg}} \times \overset{15}{\cancel{60}}\text{ gtt} = 15\text{ gtt/min};$

microgtt/min = mL/hr;

15 gtt/min = 15 mL/hr

Label the IV.

Set the pump:

Total # mL: 250

mL/hr: 15

2. The standard solution is 4 mg in 250 mL D5W

4 mg = 4000 mcg/250 mL

Step 1. Reduce the standard solution to mcg/mL

$\frac{4000\text{ mcg}}{250\text{ mL}} = 16\text{ mcg/mL}$

Step 2. Substitute 60 gtt for the mL
= 16 mcg/60 gtt

Step 3. $\frac{D}{H} \times S = A$

$\frac{\overset{3}{\cancel{12}}\text{ mcg/min}}{\underset{\underset{1}{\cancel{4}}}{\cancel{16}}\text{ mcg}} \times \overset{15}{\cancel{60}}\text{ gtt} = 45\text{ gtt/min};$

microgtt/min = mL/hr;

45 gtt/min = 45 mL/hr

Label the IV.

Set the pump:

Total # mL: 250

mL/hr = 45

3. The standard solution is 1 gram in 250 mL D5W

Convert lb to kg $\frac{220\text{ lb}}{2.2\text{ kg}}\ \ 2.2\overline{)220.0.}^{\ 100.} = 100\text{ kg}$

To obtain the order in mcg:

Multiply 100 kg
× 5 mcg/kg/min
500 mcg/min

Step 1. Reduce the standard solution to mcg/mL

1 gram = 1000 mg $\frac{1000\text{ mg}}{250\text{ mL}} = \frac{4\text{ mg}}{1\text{ mL}} = \frac{4000\text{ mcg}}{1\text{ mL}}$

Step 2. Substitute 60 gtt for the mL
= 4000 mcg/60 gtt

Step 3. $\frac{D}{H} \times S = A$

$\frac{\overset{1}{\cancel{500}}\text{ mcg/min}}{\underset{8}{\cancel{4000}}\text{ mcg}} \times 60\text{ gtt} = \frac{60}{8} = \frac{15}{2}$

= 7.5 gtt = 8 gtt/min;

microgtt/min = mL/hr;

8 gtt/min = 8 mL/hr

Label the IV.

Set the pump:

Total # mL: 250

mL/hr: 8

4. The standard solution is 500 mg in 250 mL D5W.

The patient weighs 70 kg

Multiply 70 kg
× 7 mcg/kg/min
Order in mcg/min = 490 mcg/min

Step 1. Reduce the standard solution to mcg/min

$\frac{500\text{ mg}}{250\text{ mL}} = \frac{2\text{ mg}}{1\text{ mL}} = 2000\text{ mcg/mL}$

Step 2. Substitute 60 gtt for the mL
= 2000 mcg/60 gtt

Step 3. $\frac{D}{H} \times S = A$

$\frac{\cancel{490}\text{ mcg/min}}{\underset{100}{\cancel{2000}}\text{ mcg}} \times \overset{3}{\cancel{60}}\text{ gtt} = \frac{147}{10}$

= 14.7 = 15 gtt/min;

(continued)

microgtt/min = mL/hr;

15 gtt/min = 15 mL/hr

Label the IV.

Set the pump:

Total # mL: 250

mL/hr: 15

5. The standard solution is 50 mg in 250 mL D5W.

Step 1. Reduce the standard solution to mcg/ 1 mL.

$$\frac{50 \text{ mg}}{250 \text{ mL}} = \frac{1 \text{ mg}}{5 \text{ mL}} = \frac{1000 \text{ mcg}}{5 \text{ mL}} = \frac{200 \text{ mcg}}{1 \text{ mL}}$$

Solution is 200 mcg/1 mL.

Step 2. Substitute 60 gtt for the 1 mL = 200 mcg/ 60 gtt

Step 3. $\frac{D}{H} \times S = A$

$$\frac{10 \text{ mcg/min}}{200 \text{ mcg}} \times 60 \text{ gtt} = 3 \text{ gtt/min};$$

microgtt/min = mL/hr;

3 gtt/min = 3 mL/hr

Label the IV.

Set the pump:

Total # mL: 250

mL/hr: 3

Practice Exercise 5

1. Logic: acyclovir comes in 500 mg powder. Use a reconstitution device to add the powder to 100 mL D5W; # min = 60; TF = 10 gtt/mL for IVPB

Rule: $\frac{\# \text{ mL} \times \text{TF}}{\# \text{ min}} = \text{gtt/min}$

$$\frac{100 \times 10}{60} = \frac{\cancel{100}}{6} \quad 6\overline{)100.0}^{\,16.6} = 17 \text{ gtt/min}$$

Label the IVPB.

Set the rate at 17 gtt/min.

2. Logic: ceftazidime comes in a 1 gram powder. Use a reconstitution device to add the powder to 50 mL D5W; # min = 30; TF = 10 gtt/mL for IVPB

Rule: $\frac{\# \text{ mL} \times \text{TF}}{\# \text{ min}} = \text{gtt/min}$

$$\frac{50 \times 10}{60} = \frac{50}{3} = 16.6 = 17 \text{ gtt/min}$$

Label the IVPB.

Set the rate at 17 gtt/min.

3. Logic: ciprofloxacin comes in 10 mg/mL in a 20 mL vial. You want 0.2 g = 200 mg

$\frac{D}{H} \times S = A \qquad \frac{200 \text{ mg}}{10 \text{ mg}} \times 1 \text{ mL} = 20 \text{ mL}$

Use a syringe to add 20 mL to 100 mL D5W; # min = 60; TF = 10 gtt/mL for IVPB

Rule: $\frac{\# \text{ mL} \times \text{TF}}{\# \text{ min}} = \text{gtt/min}$

$$\frac{100 \times 10}{60} = 16.6 = 17 \text{ gtt/min}$$

Label the IV.

Set the rate at 17 gtt/min.

4. Logic: cefotaxime comes as a 1 gram powder. Use a reconstitution device to add the powder to 50 mL D5W; # min = 30; TF = 10 gtt/mL for IVPB

Rule: $\frac{\# \text{ mL} \times \text{TF}}{\# \text{ min}} = \text{gtt/min}$

$$\frac{50 \times 10}{30} = 16.6 = 17 \text{ gtt/min}$$

Label the IVPB.

Set the rate at 17 gtt/min.

Practice Exercise 6

1. Logic: The IV is infusing at 30 mL/hr and the solution is 500 mL.

$$\frac{500 \text{ mL}}{30 \text{ mL/hr}} = \frac{50}{3} = 16.6 \text{ hr approximately}$$

2. Logic: 900 mL at 100 mL/hr = 9 hr to run. If the IV starts at 9 AM + 9 hr = 6 PM.

3. Logic: IVPB is 75 mL q6h or 4 times in 24 hr.

$$\begin{array}{r} 75 \\ \times 4 \\ \hline 300 \text{ mL} \end{array}$$

The patient is receiving 125 mL for 24 hours.

$$\begin{array}{r} 125 \text{ mL} \\ \times 24 \text{ hr} \\ \hline 500 \\ 250 \\ \hline 3000 \text{ mL} \end{array} \qquad \begin{array}{r} 3000 \text{ mL} \\ + 300 \text{ mL} \\ \hline 3300 \text{ mL in 24 hr} \end{array}$$

4. Logic: IV is infusing at 10 microdrips/min. It takes 60 microdrips to make 1 mL, so 1 mL in 6 min, 10 mL in 60 min

$$\begin{array}{l} 10 \text{ mL in 60 min (1 hr)} \\ \times 8 \text{hr} \\ \hline 80 \text{ mL in 8 hr} \end{array}$$

5. Logic: The IV is 0.5 g or 500 mg in 500 mL. This is equal to 1 mg/mL. The patient receives 50 mL/hr, so the patient receives 50 mg each hour.

Self-Test 1

1. $\frac{\# \text{ mL}}{\# \text{ hr}} = \text{mL/hr}$ $\qquad \frac{\cancel{1500}}{12} \quad 12\overline{)1500.} = 125. = 125 \text{ mL/hr}$

$$\begin{array}{r} 125. \\ 12\overline{)1500.} \\ 12 \\ \hline 30 \\ 24 \\ \hline 60 \\ 60 \\ \hline \end{array}$$

$\frac{\# \text{ mL/hr} \times \text{TF}}{\# \text{ min}} = \text{gtt/min}$ $\qquad \frac{125 \times \cancel{10}}{\cancel{60}} = \frac{\cancel{125}}{6}$

$$\begin{array}{r} 20.8 \\ 6\overline{)125.0} \\ 12 \\ \hline 5\,0 \\ 4\,8 \\ \hline \end{array}$$

21 gtt/min

2. $\frac{\# \text{ mL}}{\# \text{ hr}} = \text{mL/hr}$ $\qquad \frac{\cancel{250}}{12} = 21 \text{ mL/hr}$

$$\begin{array}{r} 20.8 \\ 12\overline{)250.0} \\ 24 \\ \hline 10\,0 \\ 9\,6 \\ \hline \end{array}$$

$\frac{\# \text{ mL/hr} \times \text{TF}}{\# \text{ min}} = \text{gtt/min}$ $\qquad \frac{21 \times \cancel{60}}{\cancel{60}} = 21 \text{ gtt/min}$

You could also say mL/hr = gtt/min microdrip, so 21 mL/hr = 21 gtts/min.

3. $\frac{15\cancel{0} \text{ mL}}{2\cancel{0} \text{ mL/hr}} = \frac{\cancel{15}}{2} \qquad 2\overline{)15.0} = 7.5 \text{ hr}$

a. The drip rate is 20 mL/hr. No math is necessary. Set the infusion pump.

b. The IV will last approximately $7\frac{1}{2}$ hours.

4. Step 1. Determine the solution.

$\frac{40,\cancel{000} \text{ units}}{1\cancel{000} \text{ mL}} = 40 \text{ units/mL}$

Step 2. $\frac{D}{H} \times S = A$

$\frac{\overset{20}{\cancel{800} \text{ units/hr}}}{\underset{1}{\cancel{40} \text{ units}}} \times 1 \text{ mL} = 20 \text{ mL/hr}$

5. a. $\frac{\overset{10}{\cancel{1000}} \text{ mL}}{\cancel{100} \text{ mL/hr}} = 10 \text{ hr}$

b. $\frac{D}{H} \times S = A$ $\qquad \frac{15 \cancel{\text{mEq}}}{\underset{2}{\cancel{40} \cancel{\text{mEq}}}} \times \overset{1}{\cancel{20}} \text{ mL} = \frac{15}{2} = 7.5 \text{ mL}$

c. Microdrip. Order states to run at 100 mL/hr. mL/hr = gtt/min microdrip, so microdrip at 100 gtt/min

Macrodrip. $\frac{100 \times \overset{1}{\cancel{20}}}{\underset{3}{\cancel{60}}} = \frac{100}{3} = 33 \text{ gtt/min}$

Choose either tubing.

d. 33 gtt/min macrodrip; 100 gtt/min microdrip

6. Step 1. Reduce the standard solution to mcg/mL.

50 mg = 50,000 mcg $\qquad \frac{50,000 \text{ mcg}}{250 \text{ mL}}$

= 200 mcg/min

Step 2. Substitute 60 gtt for the mL = 200 mcg/60 gtt.

Step 3. $\frac{D}{H} \times S = A$

$\frac{\overset{4}{\cancel{80}} \text{ mcg/min}}{\underset{10}{\cancel{200}} \text{ mcg}} \times 6\cancel{0} \text{ gtt} = 24 \text{ gtt/min}$

microdrip gtt/min = mL/hr

24 gtt/min = 24 mL/hr

Label the IV.

Set the pump:

Total # mL = 250

mL/hr = 24

Self-Test 2

1. a. You desire 1 g. Aminophylline comes 1 g in 10 mL. Add 10 mL to the IV of 500 mL D5W and label.
   b. You have an infusion pump; there is no math.

   Set the pump:

   Total # mL: 500

   mL/hr: 75

2. 0.4 g = 400 mg $\quad \frac{D}{H} \times S = A$

   $\frac{\overset{8}{\cancel{400}\ \cancel{mg}}}{\underset{5}{\cancel{250}\ \cancel{mg}}} \times 1\ mL = \frac{\cancel{8}}{5} \quad 5\overline{)8.0}^{\,1.6\ mL}$

   Add 1.6 mL amikacin to 100 mL D5W;
   TF = 10 gtt/mL for IVPB; # min = 30

   $\frac{\#\ mL \times TF}{\#\ min} = gtt/min \qquad \frac{100\ mL \times \cancel{10}}{\cancel{30}}$

   $= \frac{100}{3} = 33.3 = 33\ gtt/min$

   Label the IV.
   Set the rate at 33 gtt/min.

3. Step 1. Reduce the standard solution to mcg/mL.

   $\frac{500\ mg}{500\ mL} = \frac{1\ mg}{1\ mL} = 1000\ mcg/mL$

   Step 2. Substitute 60 gtt for the mL = 1000 mcg/60 gtt.

   Step 3. $\frac{D}{H} \times S = A$

   $\frac{\overset{1}{\cancel{250}\ \cancel{mcg}/min}}{\underset{\underset{1}{\cancel{4}}}{\cancel{1000}\ \cancel{mcg}}} \times \overset{15}{\cancel{60}}\ gtt = 15\ gtt/min$

   microgtt/min = mL/hr

   15 gtt/min = 15 mL/hr

   Label the IV.

   Set the pump:

   Total # mL: 500

   mL/hr: 15

4. First, determine the solution: $\frac{\overset{100}{\cancel{25,000}}\ units}{\cancel{250}\ mL}$

   = 100 units/mL

   Second, $\frac{D}{H} \times S = A$

   $\frac{\cancel{800}\ \cancel{units}/hr}{100\ \cancel{units}} \times 1\ mL = 8\ mL/hr$

   Set the rate on the pump at 8 mL/hr.

5. $\frac{\#\ mL}{\#\ hr} = mL/hr \qquad \frac{500}{8} \quad 8\overline{)500.0}^{\,62.5} = 63\ mL/hr$

   48
   20
   16
   40
   40

   You are using microdrip, so mL/hr = gtt/min.

   Set the rate at 63 gtt/min.

6. The order is in mg.

   Step 1. Reduce the standard solution to mg/mL

   1 g = 1000 mg $\quad \frac{1000\ mg}{500\ mL} = 2\ mg/mL$

   Step 2. Substitute 60 gtt for the mL = 2 mg/60 gtt

   Step 3. $\frac{D}{H} \times S = A$

   $\frac{1\ \cancel{mg}/min}{\underset{1}{\cancel{2}\ \cancel{mg}}} \times \overset{30}{\cancel{60}}\ gtt = 30\ gtt/min$

   microgtt/min = mL/hr

   30 gtt/min = 30 mL/hr

   Label the IV.

   Set the pump:

   Total # mL: 500

   # mL/hr = 30

Proficiency Test

1. a. Add 18 mL of sterile water for injection to the vial of 5 million units (5 MU).
   b. Solution is 5 MU/20 mL.
   c. You want 1 MU so $\frac{D}{H} \times S = A$

$$\frac{1\ \cancel{MU}}{\cancel{5}\ \cancel{MU}} \times \overset{4}{\cancel{20}}\ mL = 4\ ml$$

   d. $\frac{\#\ mL \times TF}{\#\ min} = gtt/min$ $\quad \frac{\overset{25}{\cancel{100}}\ mL \times \cancel{10}}{\underset{1}{\cancel{40}}}$

$= 25$ gtt/min

2. Logic: You have $\frac{25{,}000 \text{ units of drug}}{250 \text{ mL bag}} = 100$ units/mL

   a. $\frac{D}{H} \times S = A$ $\quad \frac{12\cancel{00}\ \cancel{units}/hr}{1\cancel{00}\ \cancel{units}}$

$\times$ 1 mL = 12 mL/hr

   b. If you deliver 12 mL/hr and the IV bag contains 250 mL, then

$$\frac{25\cancel{0}}{12} \quad 12\overline{)250.0}^{\,20.8} = \text{approximately 21 hours.}$$

```
      20.8
 12 )250.0
     24
     10 0
      9 6
        4
```

3. Logic: 1000 mL is infusing at 100 mL/hr, so the IV will take

$$\frac{\overset{10}{\cancel{1000}}}{\underset{1}{\cancel{100}}} = 10 \text{ hours to complete.}$$

If it starts at 8 AM, it should finish 10 hours later at 6 PM.

4. a. $\frac{D}{H} \times S = A$ $\quad \frac{\overset{3}{\cancel{60}}\ \cancel{mg}}{\underset{2}{\cancel{40}}\ \cancel{mg}} \times 1\ mL = \frac{\cancel{3}}{2} \quad 2\overline{)3.0}^{\,1.5\ mL}$

Add 1.5 mL gentamicin.

   b. $\frac{\#\ mL \times TF}{\#\ min} = gtt/min$

$$\frac{50\ mL \times 2\cancel{0}}{3\cancel{0}} = \frac{\cancel{100}}{3} \quad 3\overline{)100.00}^{\,33.3} = 33\ gtt/min$$

5. Step 1. $\frac{\#\ mL}{\#\ hr} = mL/hr$

$$\frac{\cancel{1500}}{12} \quad 12\overline{)1500.}^{\,125.} = 125\ mL/hr$$

```
      125.
 12 )1500.
     12
      30
      24
       60
       60
```

Step 2. $\frac{\#\ mL/hr \times TF}{60} = gtt/min$

$$\frac{125 \times 10}{60} = \frac{\cancel{125}}{6} \quad 6\overline{)125.0}^{\,20.8} = 21\ gtt/min$$

```
     20.8
 6 )125.0
    12
     5 0
     4 8
```

6. Logic: Intralipid 500 mL q6h means the patient is receiving 500 mL four times every 24 hours.

```
  500
 × 4
 2000 mL
```

The IV is infusing 80 mL/hr. There are 24 hr in a day so

```
   24
 × 80
 1920
```

Adding these we have

```
   2000 mL
 + 1920 mL
   3920 mL
```

7. a. You have 1000 mL running at 60 mL/hr; therefore,

$$60\overline{)1000.0}^{\,16.6} = \text{approximately } 16\tfrac{1}{2} \text{ hours}$$

```
      16.6
 60 )1000.0
      60
      400
      360
      400
```

   b. Logic: If you want 60 mL/hr and use microdrip tubing, the drip factor will be 60 gtt/min:

$$\frac{\#\ mL \times TF}{60} = \frac{60 \times \cancel{60}}{\cancel{60}} = 60\ gtt/min$$

If you use macrodrip you have $\frac{\cancel{60} \times 10}{\cancel{60}}$
$= 10$ gtt/min

(continued)

Because the IV will run over 16 hours, choose *microdrip tubing.*

c. The drip factor will be 60 gtt/min.

Note: It is not incorrect to choose the macrodrip at 10 gtt/min. However, because the IV will run so many hours, a good flow might help to keep the IV running.

8. a. You have 1000 mL running at 150 mL/hr; therefore,

$$\frac{\overset{20}{\cancel{1000}}}{\underset{3}{\cancel{150}}} = \frac{\cancel{20}}{3} = 3\,\overline{)20.0}\ \ 6.6 = \text{approximately } 6\tfrac{1}{2} \text{ hours}$$

18
20
18

b. $\frac{\#\ \text{ML} \times \text{TF}}{\#\ \text{min}} = \text{gtt/min}$

$\frac{150 \times 10}{60} = 25$ gtt/min macro

$\frac{150 \times 60}{60} = 150$ gtt/min micro

Choose macrotubing.

c. 25 gtt/min macro

9. a. Because the amount is small and will run over 6 hours, choose *microdrip tubing.*

b. Step 1.

$$\frac{\#\ \text{mL}}{\text{hr}} = \text{mL/hr} = \frac{\cancel{100}}{6} = 6\,\overline{)100.0}\ \ 16.6 = 17 \text{ mL/hr}$$

6
40
36
40
36

Step 2. $\frac{\#\ \text{mL/hr} \times \text{TF}}{\#\ \text{min}} = \frac{17 \times \cancel{60}}{\cancel{60}} = 17$ gtt/min

10. a. Because the stock bag is 250 mL NS, you would aseptically allow 100 mL to run off. This will leave 150 mL NS.

b. *Microdrip,* because:

Step 1. $\frac{\#\ \text{mL}}{\#\ \text{hr}} = \text{mL/hr}\ \frac{\overset{50}{\cancel{150}}\ \text{mL}}{\cancel{3}\ \text{hr}} = 50$ mL/hr

Step 2. $\frac{\#\ \text{mL/hr} \times \text{TF}}{\#\ \text{min}} = \text{gtt/min}$

With microdrip the # mL/hr = gtt/min; hence, microdrip would be 50 gtt/min. Proof: $\frac{50 \times \cancel{60}}{\cancel{60}}$ = 50 gtt/min

Macrodrip would be $\frac{50 \times \overset{1}{\cancel{15}}}{\underset{4}{\cancel{60}}}$

$$= \frac{\cancel{50}}{4} = 4\,\overline{)50.0}\ \ 12.5 = 13 \text{ gtt/min}$$

4
10
8
20
20

c. 50 gtt/min

Note: It would not be incorrect to choose the macrodrip. However, 50 gtt/min provides a better flow.

11. 15 mL/hr

Logic: You have to give 1500 units/hr and have a solution of 100 units/mL; therefore, $\frac{15\cancel{00}\ \cancel{\text{units}}/\text{hr}}{1\cancel{00}\ \cancel{\text{units}}/\text{mL}}$ = 15 ml/hr

12. 21 mL/hr

Logic: Step 1. $\frac{\#\ \text{mL}}{\#\ \text{hr}} = \text{mL/hr}$

$$\frac{50\cancel{0}\ \text{mL}}{24\ \text{hr}} = 24\,\overline{)500.0}\ \ 20.8 = 21 \text{ mL/hr}$$

48
20 0
19 2

Step 2 is not necessary because you have an infusion pump that delivers mL/hr.

13. Use a reconstitution device to add 100 mg powder to 250 mL D5W and give IVPB over 1 hr (60 min); TF = 10 gtts/mL

$\frac{\#\ \text{mL} \times \text{TF}}{\#\ \text{min}} = \text{gtt/min}\quad \frac{250 \times 10}{60}$

$$= \frac{\cancel{250}}{6} = 6\,\overline{)250.0}\ \ 41.6 = 42 \text{ gtt/min}$$

Label the IVPB.

Set the rate at 42 gtt/min.

14. Order is 4 mcg/min. Stock of isoproterenol is 1 mg/5 mL.

$\frac{D}{H} \times S = A \qquad \frac{2 \text{ mg}}{1 \text{ mg}} \times 5 \text{ mL} = 10 \text{ mL}$

Use 2 ampules to add 10 mL isoproterenol to 250 mL D5W to make 2 mg in 250 mL.

Step 1. Reduce the standard solution to mcg/mL

$2 \text{ mg} = 2000 \text{ mcg} \qquad \frac{2000 \text{ mcg}}{250 \text{ mL}} = 8 \text{ mcg/mL}$

Step 2. Substitute 60 gtt for the mL = 8 mcg/60 gtt

Step 3. $\frac{D}{H} \times S = A$

$$\frac{\overset{1}{\cancel{4}} \text{ mcg/min}}{\underset{2}{\cancel{8}} \text{ mcg}} \times \overset{30}{\cancel{60}} \text{ gtt} = 30 \text{ gtt/min}$$

microgtt/min = mL/hr

30 gtt/min = 30 mL/hr

Label the IV.

Set the pump:

Total # mL: 250

mL/hr: 30

15. Order is 500 mg. Stock is 1 g in 10 mL. 1 g = 1000 mg

$\frac{D}{H} \times S = A \qquad \frac{500 \text{ mg}}{1000 \text{ mg}} \times 10 \text{ mL} = 5 \text{ mL}$

Add 5 mL aminophylline to make 500 mg in 250 mL D5W.

$\frac{\# \text{ mL}}{\# \text{ hr}} = \text{mL/hr} \quad \frac{\cancel{250} \text{ mL}}{8 \text{ hr}} = 31.2 = 31 \text{ mL/hr}$

mL/hr = microgtt/min

No math necessary.

31 mL/hr = 31 gtt/min

Label IV.

Set the rate at 31 gtt/min.

16. 3300 mL

Logic: The patient gets 125 mL/hr and there are 24 hours in a day; hence,

$$\begin{array}{r} 125 \\ \times\ 24 \\ \hline 500 \\ 250 \\ \hline 3000 \text{ mL} \end{array}$$

The patient gets 75 mL q6h and, therefore, is receiving 75 mL four times in 24 hours

so
$$\begin{array}{r} 75 \\ \times\ 4 \\ \hline 300 \end{array}$$

$$\begin{array}{r} 3000 \text{ mL} \\ +\ 300 \text{ mL} \\ \hline 3300 \text{ mL} \end{array}$$

17. a. 90 mL/hr

b. $\frac{\text{total \# mL}}{\text{mL/hr}} = \text{hr}$

$$\begin{array}{r} \cancel{1000} \quad 11.1 \\ 90\ \overline{)1000.0} \\ 90 \\ \hline 100 \\ 90 \\ \hline 100 \end{array}$$

Approximately 11 hours

18. a. 5 mL

$\frac{D}{H} \times S = A \qquad \frac{\overset{1}{\cancel{50} \text{ mg}}}{\underset{\underset{1}{\cancel{2}}}{\cancel{100} \text{ mg}}} \times \overset{5}{\cancel{10}} \text{ mL} = 5 \text{ mL}$

Add 5 mL aramine to 250 mL D5W.

b. Step 1. Reduce the solution to mcg/min

$\frac{50 \text{ mg}}{250 \text{ mL}} = \frac{1 \text{ mg}}{5 \text{ mL}} = \frac{1000 \text{ mcg}}{5 \text{ mL}} = 200 \text{ mcg/mL}$

Step 2. Substitute 60 gtts for the mL = 200 mcg/60 gtt

Step 3. $\frac{D}{H} \times S = A$

$$\frac{\overset{3}{\cancel{60}} \text{ mcg/min}}{200 \text{ mcg}} \times \cancel{60} \text{ gtt} = 18 \text{ gtt/min}$$

microgtt/min = mL/hr

18 gtt/min = 18 mL/hr

Label the IV.

Set the pump:

Total # mL: 250

mL/hr: 18

19. 50 mg

Logic: Have 0.5 g in 500 mL. Substitute milligrams for grams: 0.5 g = 500 mg. The solution is 500 mg in 500 mL. Reducing this means 1 mg in 1 mL. As the patient is receiving 50 mL/hr, he is receiving 50 mg of aminophylline per hour.

20. a. Need 75 mL D5W. Take a 100 mL bag of D5W and aseptically remove 25 mL. Add 5 mL Bactrim to the 75 mL. Time is 60 min. The order is 75 mL/hr. No math is necessary.

Label the IVPB.

b. Set the pump:

Secondary volume (mL): 75 (refer to Fig. 9-4)

Secondary rate (mL/hr): 75

---

10 Dosage Problems for Infants and Children

CONTENT TO MASTER

Dosage based on mg/kg of body weight

Converting pounds to kilograms

Determinating a safe dose

Calculating pediatric doses

In previous chapters we have discussed calculations for adult medications administered orally and parenterally. This chapter considers dosage for infants and children. Wide variations in age, weight, growth and development within this group require special care in computation. Pediatric doses are often minute, and a slight error can result in serious harm.

Before preparing and administering a pediatric medication, the nurse determines that the dose is safe for the child. *Safe* means that the amount ordered is not an overdose or an underdose. An overdose can produce toxic effects; underdose may lead to therapeutic failure. When a discrepancy is noted the nurse consults the physician who ordered the drug.

Children's medications are usually given by mouth in a liquid form or intravenously. Injections are not common except for immunizations. Pediatric injections are calculated to the nearest hundredth and administered using a 1 mL precision (tuberculin) syringe. For IV therapy microdrip, Buretrols or other volume control sets and infusion pumps are used. Most institutions will have guidelines for pediatric infusions; when these are not available the nurse must consult a reliable *pediatric* reference. Adult guidelines are not safe for children.

Recall these equivalents as you begin this chapter:

1 g = 1000 mg	16 oz = 1 lb
1 kg = 2.2 lb	microdrip = 60 gtt/mL
1 mg = 1000 mcg	> = greater than
1 tsp = 5 mL	< = less than
1 oz = 30 mL	q4° = every four hours

▼ DOSAGE BASED ON MG/KG OF BODY WEIGHT

The most common way to assess the safety of a pediatric dose is to determine the weight of a child in kilograms, and then compare the dose ordered with a reference which indicates mg/kg body weight. This information can be found in a pediatric drug reference, package insert, label, the *PDR*, the *USPDI*, and other reliable sources. Consider this problem:

A child weighing 33 lb is ordered amoxicillin oral suspension 150 mg po q8h. Figure 10-1 shows the label for amoxicillin, which comes as a dry powder. The label states that children should receive 20 to 40 mg/kg/day. You don't know if the dose ordered for the child is safe. Several steps are needed:

1. Convert lb to kg.
2. Determine the safe dose range in mg/kg.
3. Decide if the ordered dose is safe.
4. Calculate the dose needed.

Step 1. Convert lb to kg. Divide lb by 2.2.

$$\begin{array}{r} 15. \\ 2.2\overline{)33.0} \\ \underline{22} \\ 11\,0 \\ \underline{11\,0} \end{array}$$

The child weighs 15 kg.

◀ ***Learning Aid***

2.2 lb = 1 kg

$$\frac{2.2 \text{ lb}}{1 \text{ kg}} = \frac{33 \text{ lb}}{x \text{ kg}}$$

$2.2\,x = 33$

$$x = \frac{33}{2.2}$$

Therefore, to obtain kg divide lb by 2.2.

Step 2. Determine the safe dose range in mg/kg. In Figure 10-1, the label states that children should receive 20–40 mg/kg/day in divided doses every 8 hours.

Lower Range

$$\begin{array}{r} 20 \text{ mg} \\ \times\, 15 \text{ kg} \\ \hline 100 \\ 20 \\ \hline 300 \text{ mg/kg/day} \end{array}$$

Upper Range

$$\begin{array}{r} 40 \text{ mg} \\ \times\, 15 \text{ kg} \\ \hline 200 \\ 40 \\ \hline 600 \text{ mg/kg/day} \end{array}$$

The safe range for the child is 300–600 mg/day.

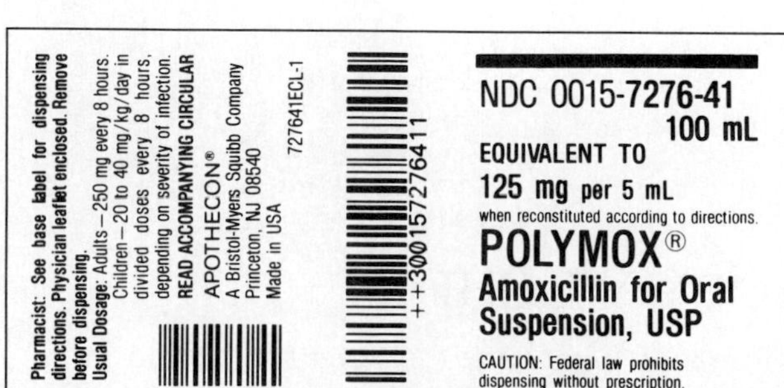

Figure 10-1
Label for amoxicillin for oral suspension (Polymox). (Courtesy of Apothecon, a Bristol Meyers Squibb Company)

Step 3. Decide if the ordered dose is safe. The order is 150 mg q8h. The child will receive 3 doses in 24 hours.

◀ ***Learning Aid***
There are 24 hours in a day. The child is to receive a dose every 8 hours

$$8 \overline{)24.} = 3.$$

150 mg
× 3 doses
450 mg

The ordered dose of 450 mg in 24 hours is in the range between 300–600 mg/day. It is a safe dose.

Step 4. Calculate the dose needed. Directions say to add a total of 59 mL in two portions. Shake well after each dilution. Stock is 125 mg/5 mL.

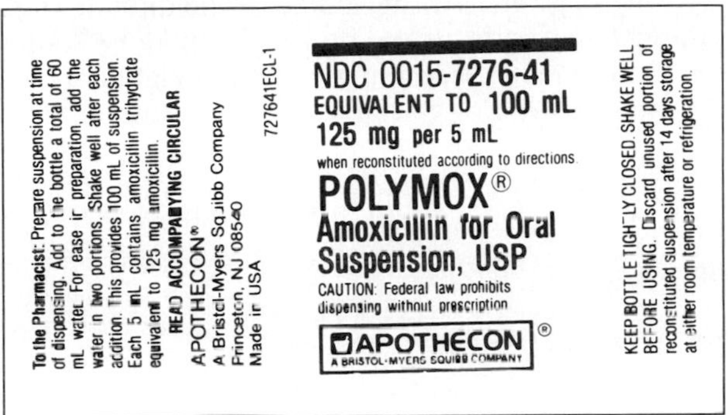

Rule: $\frac{D}{H} \times S = A$ $\qquad \frac{\overset{6}{\cancel{150}\text{ mg}}}{\underset{\cancel{25}}{\cancel{125}\text{ mg}}} \times \overset{1}{\cancel{5}}\text{ mL} = 6 \text{ mL}$

Give 6 mL.

RULE

DETERMINING A PEDIATRIC DOSE USING THE FOLLOWING STEPS

Step 1. Convert lb to kg by dividing by 2.2.

Step 2. Determine the safe dose range in mg/kg using a reference.

Step 3. Decide if the ordered dose is safe by comparing the order with the safe dose range listed in the reference.

Step 4. Calculate the dose needed.

EXAMPLE

Order: Lasix 15 mg po bid

Stock: See Figure 10-2.

Child weighs 16 lb 10 oz.

Step 1. Convert lb to kg.
a. Change the oz to part of a lb

◀ ***Learning Aid***
Equivalent is 16 oz = 1 lb. Change oz to a part of a lb by dividing by 16. Carry arithmetic out to two places and round off.

$$\begin{array}{rl} \frac{10 \text{ oz}}{16} & \overset{.62 \text{ lb}}{\overline{)10.00}} \\ & \underline{9\ 6} \\ & 40 \\ & \underline{32} \end{array}$$

Child's weight is 0.6 lb + 16 lb = 16.6 lb

b. Change lb to kg.

$$\frac{16.6 \text{ lb}}{2.2} \qquad 7.54 = 7.54 \text{ kg}$$

```
         7.54
2.2 )16.6 00
     15 4
      1 2 0
      1 1 0
        1 00
          88
          12
```

Step 2. Determine the safe dose range in mg/kg.

The package insert states: The initial dose of oral Lasix (furosemide) in infants and children is 2 mg/kg body weight, given as a single dose. If the diuretic response is not satisfactory after the initial dose, dosage may be increased by 1 or 2 mg/kg no sooner than 6 to 8 hours after the previous dose. Doses greater than 6 mg/kg body weight are not recommended.

Single Dose

$$\begin{array}{r} 7.54 \text{ kg} \\ \times\ 2 \text{ mg} \\ \hline 15.08 \text{ mg/day} \end{array}$$

High Range

$$\begin{array}{r} 7.54 \text{ kg} \\ \times\ 6 \\ \hline 45.24 \text{ mg/day} \end{array}$$

Step 3. Decide if the ordered dose is safe. The order is 15 mg po bid. The 15 mg meets the requirement for a single dose. The order is bid which means twice in a day, so 15 mg × 2 = 30 mg. The child will receive 30 mg in a day. The high range is 45 mg, so the dose is safe.

Step 4. Calculate the dose needed. The stock is 10 mg/mL.

$$\frac{D}{H} \times S = A \qquad \frac{\overset{3}{\cancel{15}\text{ mg}}}{\underset{2}{\cancel{10}\text{ mg}}} \times 1 \text{ mL} = \frac{3}{2} = 1.5 \text{ mL}$$

The label states that Lasix comes with a calibrated safety dropper. The dropper can be used to obtain the dose of 1.5 mL. Techniques and procedures to administer pediatric medications are beyond the scope of this workbook. Please consult a pediatric nursing textbook.

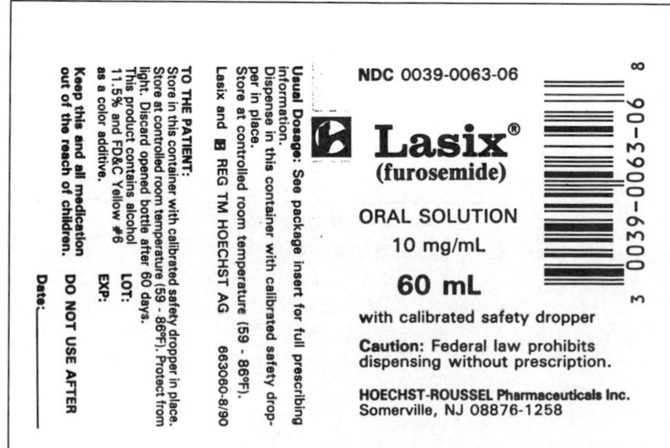

Figure 10-2
Label for furosemide (Lasix). (Courtesy of Hoechst-Roussel Pharmaceuticals)

NDC 0015-7941-64
NSN 6505-01-017-0340

Pharmacist: See base label for dispensing directions. Physician leaflet enclosed. Remove before dispensing.
Usual Dosage: Adults — 250 mg q. 6h. • Children — 50 mg/kg/day in equally divided doses at 6-hour intervals.
READ ACCOMPANYING CIRCULAR

Tegopen®
(CLOXACILLIN SODIUM FOR ORAL SOLUTION, USP)
EQUIVALENT TO
125 mg per 5 mL
CLOXACILLIN 200 mL
when reconstituted according to directions.
CAUTION: Federal law prohibits dispensing without prescription.
©1977, Bristol-Myers Company

BRISTOL LABORATORIES®
Bristol-Myers U.S. Pharmaceutical and Nutritional Group, Evansville, Indiana 47721 Made in U.S.A.
N 3 0015-7941-64 6
79416AFF-01

Figure 10-3
Label for cloxacillin (Tegopen). (Courtesy of Bristol Laboratories)

EXAMPLE

Order: cloxacillin 250 mg po q6h. Child weighs 44 lb.

Stock: See Figure 10-3.

Step 1. Convert lb to kg

$$\frac{44}{2.2} \qquad 2.2\overline{)44.0} = 20. = 20 \text{ kg}$$

44

Step 2. Determine the safe dose range. The label states: 50/mg/kg/day in equally divided doses at 6-hour intervals.

20 kg
× 50 mg
1000 mg in 4 equal doses

Step 3. Decide if the ordered dose is safe. The order is 250 mg po q6h. 250 mg × 4 doses = 1000 mg. The order is safe.

Step 4. Calculate the dose needed.

$$\frac{D}{H} \times S = A \qquad \frac{\overset{2}{\cancel{250}\text{ mg}}}{\underset{1}{\cancel{125}\text{ mg}}} \times 5 \text{ mL} = 10 \text{ mL}$$

Give 10 mL.

Exercise 1

Convert pounds to kilograms. Answers will be found at the end of the chapter.

1. 30 lb = ________ kg
2. 15 lb 5 oz = ________ kg
3. $7\frac{1}{4}$ lb = ________ kg
4. 22 lb = ________ kg
5. 54 lb 8 oz = ________ kg

Self-Test 1

In these practice problems, determine if the doses are safe and calculate the amount needed. Answers may be found at the end of the chapter. You may find it helpful to use a calculator.

1. Order: Amoxil 60 mg po q8h
   Stock: See Figure 10-4.
   Child weighs 20 lb.

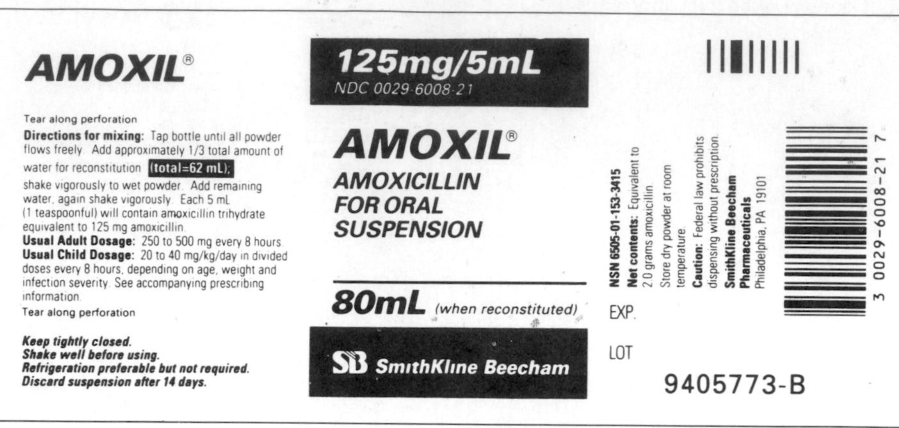

Figure 10-4
Label for (Amoxil) amoxicillin. (Courtesy of SmithKline Beecham)

2. Order: Augmentin 175 mg po q8h
   Patient: child weighing 29 lb
   Literature states: 40 mg/kg/day in divided doses

3. Order: Ferrous sulfate 200 mg po tid
   Stock: bottle of 125 mg/5 mL
   Child is 9 years old and weighs 30 kg.
   Literature states: children 6–12 years old, 600 mg divided doses tid.

   a. Is the dose safe?
   b. How many milliliters would you pour?

4. Order: Tylenol 80 mg po q4° prn for temp 100.9° and above
   Stock: chewable tablets 80 mg
   Child is 6 years old; weighs 20.5 kg.
   Literature states for child 6–8 years give four chewable tablets. May repeat four or five times daily. Not to exceed five doses in 24 hours.

   Is dose safe?

5. Order: Slo-Phyllin 110 mg po q8h
   Stock: 80 mg/15 mL
   Child is 6 years old; weighs 28 kg.
   Literature states: child po 50–100 mg q6h not to exceed 12 mg/kg/24 hour.

   a. Is the dose safe?
   b. How much will you prepare?

(continued)

Self-Test 1 (continued)

6. Order: diazepam 1 mg IM q3–4h prn
   Stock: vial 5 mg/1 mL
   Infant 30 days old
   Literature states: child < 6 mo IM 1–2.5 mg tid or qid.

   a. Is dose safe?
   b. How much will you prepare?

7. 10-kg boy with otitis media
   Order: amoxacillin 125 mg po q8h for 10 days
   Stock: bottle labeled amoxacillin 125 mg/5 mL
   Safe range: 20–40 mg/kg/day in divided doses q8h

   a. Is the dose safe?
   b. How much will you prepare?

8. Order: meperidine HCl 20 mg IM stat.
   Stock: 50 mg/mL
   Child weighs 35 lb.
   Literature states: Children: usual dose is 0.5 mg/lb to 1 mg/lb.

   a. Is the dose safe?
   b. How much will you prepare?

9. 15-year-old boy, 58 kg, with a urinary tract infection
   Order: prophylactic Septra (160 mg TMP/800 mg SMZ) tabs; double-strength 1 tab q12h po
   Stock: tablets labeled Septra Double-Strength
   Therapeutic dose: The usual adult dose in the treatment of urinary tract infection is one Septra DS tablet, two Septra tablets, or 4 teaspoonsful (20 mL) Septra Suspension every 12 hours for 10–14 days.

10. 8-year-old boy, 26 kg, with rheumatic fever
    Order: prophylactic penicillin benzathine 1.2 MU q28d IM
    Stock: vial labeled 600,000 units/mL
    Therapeutic dose: IM 1.2 million units in a single dose q month or 600,000 units q2wk

    a. Is the dose safe?
    b. How many milliliters will you administer?

▼ DOSAGE FOR PARENTERAL MEDICATIONS

Intravenous medications are administered when a child cannot maintain an oral fluid intake, has a fluid electrolyte imbalance, or requires IV medication. Buretrols or other volume control units are used to administer IV fluids; they are calibrated and hold no more than 100 to 150 mL at a time. This reduces the possibility of fluid overload. Infusion pumps are also used to provide a second safeguard. In neonatal areas, syringe pumps can deliver IV fluid ranging from 1 to 60 mL.

Dosages for IV medications are calculated in mg/kg. In pediatrics, drugs are administered in small amounts of diluent; a pediatric reference must be consulted to determine the minimum safe amount (Table 10-1). Institutions may provide guidelines to aid the nurse in preparing IVs.

Drugs for IVPB must be initially diluted following the manufacturer's directions. Once the initial dilution is made, the amount of drug required to obtain the dose is withdrawn from the vial and then diluted further. IV solutions in pediatrics usually range from 10 to 20 mL for smaller children and infants requiring IVPB medications. This amount of fluid will fill the tubing from the Buretrol to the patient. When the Buretrol is empty of the IV medication, most of the drug will be in the tubing. For this

TABLE 10-1

Sample of a Table Listing the Safe Dosage Range for Pediatric Medications

Drug	Dose and Route
Amoxicillin	Child: 20–40 mg/kg/24h po
Ampicillin	Neonate <7 days: 50–150 mg/kg/24h q8–12h IM or IV >7 days: 75–200 mg/kg/24h q9–8h IM or IV Child—moderate, mild infections 50–100 mg/kg/24h given q6h po
Cefotaxime	Neonate <1 wk: 100 mg/kg/24h given q12h IM or IV 1–4 wk: 150 mg/kg/24h given q8h IM or IV Infant and child (<50 kg) 50–200 mg/kg/24h given q4–6h IV or IM
Chloral hydrate	Children Sedative: 5–15 mg/kg/dose q8h po or pr Hypnotic: 50–75 mg/kg/dose po or pr
Meperidine HCl	po, IM, IV, SC Children: 1–1.5 mg/kg/dose q 3–4h prn Max. dose 100 mg
Penicillin G	Newborn: 50,000 units/kg × 1 IM
Benzathine	Infants/children: 50,000 units/kg × 1 IM Max. 2.4 MU Rheumatic fever prophylaxis 600,000 units q2 weeks or 1.2 MU q month IM

reason an IV flush of 15 to 20 mL must be added to the Buretrol *after* the medication is infused to ensure that the patient receives the drug.

In this section we will consider the calculation of pediatric doses for IV and IVPB administration. These problems may seem complex. However, their solution requires a step-by-step analysis that is easily learned and applied.

Steps to Solve Parenteral Pediatric Medications

1. Decide if the dose is safe; check a pediatric reference.
2. Decide if the dilution ordered meets the minimum pediatric safety standard (Table 10-2).

TABLE 10-2

Sample of a Dilution Table for Pediatric Antibiotics

Antibiotic	Recommended Final Concentration IV	Recommendation Duration of IV
Ampicillin	50 mg/mL	10–30 min
Cefotaxime	50 mg/mL	10–30 min
Clindamycin	6–12 mg/mL	15–30 min
Gentamicin	2 mg/mL	15–30 min
Penicillin G	Infants: 50,000 units/mL Large child: 100,000 units/mL	10–30 min
Pentamidine	2.5 mg/mL	1 hr

3. Prepare the medication according to directions.
4. Draw up the dose and dilute further as needed.
5. Set the pump in mL/hr. If the infusion time is 30 minutes, set the pump for double the amount because the pump delivers mL/hr.

EXAMPLE The order is 10 mL over 30 minutes. Set the pump for 20 mL/hr. It will deliver 10 mL in 30 minutes.

6. When the IV is completed, add a flush of 15 mL to the Buretrol to clear the tubing of the medication. Be sure to chart the flush as fluid intake.

EXAMPLE ***Example 1:***

Child 4 years old; 17 kg

Order: Tazicef 280 mg IV q8h in 10 mL D5$\frac{1}{3}$NS (Fig. 10-5)

Reference: Safe dose 30–50 mg/kg/day
Concentration for IV use: 50 mg/mL over 30 minutes

Stock: 1 gram powder. Directions: dilute with 10 mL sterile water for injection to make 95 mg/mL; stable for 7 days if refrigerated.

1. Safe dose is 30 to 50 mg/kg/day.

Low Range

$$\begin{array}{r} 30 \text{ mg} \\ \times\ 17 \text{ kg} \\ \hline 510 \text{ mg/day} \end{array}$$

High Range

$$\begin{array}{r} 50 \text{ mg} \\ \times\ 17 \text{ mg} \\ \hline 850 \text{ mg/day} \end{array}$$

Order is 280 mg q8h (3 doses).
280 mg × 3 = 840 mg. Dose falls within the range and is safe.

2. Minimum safe dilution is 50 mg/mL. Dose is 280 mg.

$$\begin{array}{r} 5.6 \\ 50\overline{)280.} \\ \underline{250} \\ 300 \\ \underline{300} \end{array}$$

5.6 = 6 mL is the minimum dilution. The order of 10 mL is safe since it is more than the minimum.

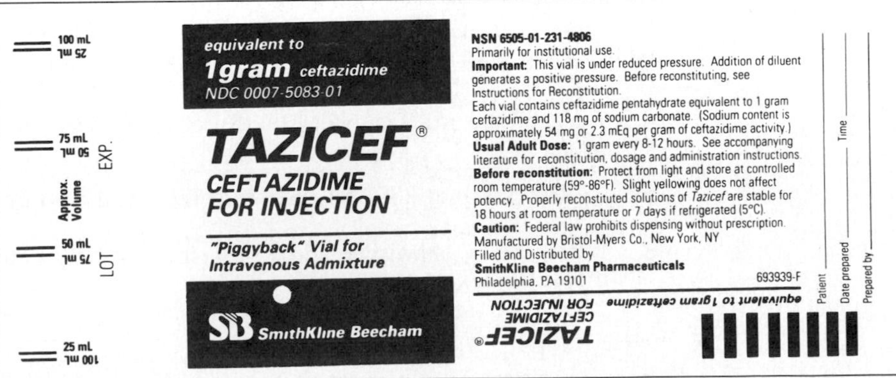

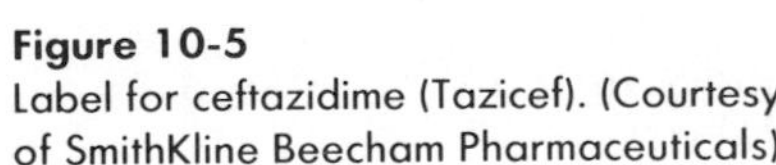
Figure 10-5
Label for ceftazidime (Tazicef). (Courtesy of SmithKline Beecham Pharmaceuticals)

3. Dilute 1 g with 10 mL sterile water to make 95 mg/mL.

$\frac{D}{H} \times S = A \qquad \frac{280 \text{ mg}}{95 \text{ mg}} \times 1 \text{ mL}$

= 2.9 mL. Withdraw 2.9 mL; label the vial and store in the refrigerator.

4. Run about 5 mL D5$\frac{1}{3}$NS into the Buretrol. Add the 2.9 mL drug. Add more D5$\frac{1}{3}$NS to make 10 mL.

5. Set the pump at 20. This is 20 mL/hr; the pump will deliver 10 mL in 30 minutes.

6. When the IV is completed add a 15 mL flush of D5$\frac{1}{3}$NS to clear the IV tubing of medication.

Example 2:

Infant 4.3 kg

Order: ampicillin 100 mg IV q6h in 10 cc D5$\frac{1}{3}$NS

Reference: Safe dose 75–200 mg/kg/24h given q6–8h IV
Concentration for IV use: 50 mg/mL over 10–30 min

Stock: vial of powder labeled 500 mg. Directions: add 1.8 mL of sterile water for injection to make 250 mg/mL; use within 1 hr.

1. Safe dose is 75 to 200 mg/kg/24h given q6–8h.

Low Range

$$\begin{array}{r} 75 \text{ mg} \\ \times\ 4.3 \text{ kg} \\ \hline 322.5 \text{ mg/24hr} \end{array}$$

High Range

$$\begin{array}{r} 200 \text{ mg} \\ \times\ 4.3 \text{ kg} \\ \hline 860 \text{ mg/24h} \end{array}$$

Order is 100 mg q6h (4 doses)
100 mg × 4 doses = 400 mg. This is within the range. The dose is safe.

2. Minimum safe dilution is 50 mg/mL (see Table 10-2). Dose is 100 mg.

$50\overline{)100}$ = 2 mL is the minimum dilution; 10 mL is safe.

3. Add 1.8 mL sterile water for injection to 500 mg powder to make 250 mg/mL.

$\frac{D}{H} \times S = A \qquad \frac{10\not{0} \not{\text{mg}}}{25\not{0} \not{\text{mg}}} \times 1 \text{ mL} = \frac{2}{5} = 0.4 \text{ mL}$

Withdraw 0.4 mL from the vial. Discard the remainder (directions say to use within 1 hr).

4. Add about 5 mL D5$\frac{1}{3}$NS to the Buretrol. Add 0.4 mL drug. Add more D5$\frac{1}{3}$NS to make 10 cc.

5. Set the pump at 20. This means 20 mL/hr; the pump will deliver 10 mL in 30 min.

6. When the IV is finished add 15 mL flush of D5$\frac{1}{3}$NS to the Buretrol to clear the tubing of medication.

Example 3:

Infant 3 mo; 6 kg

Order: nafcillin 150 mg IV q8h in 10 mL D5$\frac{1}{3}$NS

Reference: Safe dose 100–200 mg/kg/24h given q6h
Concentration for IV use: 6 mg/mL over 30–60 min

Stock: 500 mg vial of powder. Directions: Add 1.7 mL sterile water for injection to make 500 mg/2 mL. Stable for 48 hours if refrigerated.

1. Safe dose is 100 to 200 mg/kg/24h given q6h.

Low Range

100 mg
× 6 kg
600 mg/24h

High Range

200 mg
× 6 kg
1200 mg/24h

Order is 150 mg q8h (3 doses) = 450 mg/24h

The dose is below range and is q8h. Reference states q6h.

2. Minimum safe dilution is 6 mg/mL. Order is 150 mg.

$6\overline{)150}$ mg = 25 = 25 mL The dilution of 10 mL does not meet concentration requirements.

Consult with the physician regarding the dose, the times of administration, and the dilution. Do not prepare the dose.

Self-Test 2

In these practice problems determine if the dose is safe, calculate the amount needed and state how the order will be administered. Answers may be found at the end of this chapter. Follow the steps used in the examples.

1. Infant 6 mo; 8 kg

Order: cefuroxime 200 mg IV q6h in 10 mL D5$\frac{1}{4}$NS

Reference: Safe dose 50–100 mg/kg/24h given q6–8h
Concentration for IV use: 50 mg/mL over 30 min

Stock: 750 mg vial of powder. Directions: dilute with 8 mL sterile water for injection to make 90 mg/mL; stable for 3 days if refrigerated.

2. Child 3 years; 15 kg

Order: Bactrim (as TMP/SMX) 75 mg IV q12h in 75 mL D5W over 1 hr

Reference: Safe dose for a child 8–10 mg/kg/24h given q12h
Concentration for IV use: 1 mL in 15–25 mL (stock is a liquid)

Stock: vial labeled 80 mg/5 mL

(continued)

Self-Test 2 (continued)

3. Child 8 yr; 25 kg

   Order: erythromycin 300 mg IV q6h in 75 mL D5$\frac{1}{3}$NS

   Reference: Safe dose 20–50 mg/kg/24h given q6h
   Concentration for IV use: 5 mg/mL over 20–30 min

   Stock: 1 gram powder. Directions: Add 20 mL sterile water for injection. Makes 50 mg/mL. Stable in the refrigerator 7 days.

4. Child 12 yr; 40 kg

   Order: tobramycin 100 mg IV q8h in 50 mL D5$\frac{1}{3}$NS

   Reference: Safe dose 6–7.5 mg/kg/24h given q8h
   Concentration for IV use: 2 mg/mL over 15–30 min
   Stock: Vial 80 mg/2 mL

5. Child 5 yr; 18 kg

   Order: cefotaxime 900 mg IV q6h in 25 mL D5$\frac{1}{3}$NS

   Reference: Safe dose 50–200 mg/kg/24h given q6h
   Concentration for IV use: 50 mg/mL; give over 30 min.

   Stock: 1 g powder. Directions: Dilute with 10 mL sterile water for injection to make 95 mg/mL. Stable in the refrigerator 10 days.

Proficiency Test

Here is a mix of oral and parenteral pediatric orders. For each problem, determine the safe dose and calculate the amount to be given. If you experience any difficulty, review the content. Answers may be found at the end of this chapter.

1. Newborn; weighs 4 kg
   Order: vitamin K 1 mg IM × 1 dose
   Reference: Prophylaxis and treatment: 0.5–1 mg/dose IM, SC, IV × 1
   Stock: Vial 10 mg/mL

2. Infant 1 yr; 10 kg
   Order: Augmentin 125 mg po q8h
   Reference: Safe dose amoxicillin-clavulanic acid:
   20–40 mg/kg/24h given q8h po
   Stock: 125 mg/5 mL

3. Infant 10 mo; 10 kg
   Order: benzathine penicillin 500,000 units IM × 1 dose
   Reference: Safe dose 50,000 units/kg × 1 IM. Max. 2.4 MU
   Stock: Vial labeled 600,000 units/mL

4. Infant 3.6 kg

   Order: gentamicin 9 mg IV q8h in 10 mL D5$\frac{1}{4}$NS
   Reference: Safe dose 2.5 mg/kg/dose q8h
   Concentration for IV 2 mg/mL given over 15–30 min
   Stock: Vial 40 mg/mL

5. Infant 6.7 kg
   Order: Colace Syrup 10 mg po bid
   Reference: Infants and children under 3: 10 to 40 mg
   Stock: 20 mg/5 mL

(continued)

Proficiency Test (continued)

6. Infant 5.5 kg
   Order: vancomycin 54 mg IV q8h in 12 mL D5$\frac{1}{4}$NS
   Reference: Safe dose 10 mg/kg q8h IV
   Concentration for IV 5 mg/mL; infuse over 1 hr
   Stock: 500 mg powder. Directions: add 10 mL sterile water for injection to give 50 mg/mL. Stable in the refrigerator 14 days.

7. Infant 6.7 kg
   Order: chloral hydrate 350 mg po prior to electroencephalogram (EEG)
   Reference: Hypnotic for children: 50–75 mg/kg/dose po
   Stock: 500 mg/5 mL

8. Child 3 yr; 9.9 kg
   Order: theophylline 65 mg qid via ngt
   Reference: 22 mg/kg/24h given q6h
   Stock: bottle labeled 80 mg/15 mL

9. Child 8 yr; 24 kg
   Order: Fortaz 2 g IVPB q8h in 50 mL D5$\frac{1}{3}$NS
   Reference: Safe dose 2–6 g/24h given q8–12h IV
   Concentration for IV 50 mg/mL over 15–30 min.
   Stock: 2 g vial of powder. Dilute initially with 10 mL sterile water for injection.

10. Child 35 lb
    Order: meperidine HCl 20 mg IM stat
    Reference: Children: usual dose 0.5 mg/lb to 1 mg/lb
    Stock: 50 mg/mL

ANSWERS

Exercise 1

1.
```
       1 3.636
2.2 )30.0 000  = 13.64 kg
     22
      8 0
      6 6
      1 4 0
      1 3 2
          80
          66
         140
```

2. $\frac{5 \text{ oz}}{16 \text{ oz}} = 16\overline{)5.000}^{\,.312} = 0.31$ lb

Weight is 15.31 lb.

Change to kilogram.

```
        6.95 8
2.2 )15.3 1000  = 6.96 kg
     13 2
      2 1 1
      1 9 8
        1 30
        1 10
         200
         176
```

3. $\frac{1}{4} = 0.25$ lb

7.25 lb ÷ 2.2

```
        3.295
2.2 )7.2 500  = 3.3 kg
     6 6
       6 5
       4 4
       2 10
       1 98
        120
        110
```

4.
```
        1 0.
2.2 )22.0  = 10 kg
     22
```

5. $\frac{8 \text{ oz}}{16 \text{ oz}} = \frac{1}{2} = 0.5$ lb

54.5 lb ÷ 2.2

```
        2 4.772
2.2 )54.5 000  = 24.77 kg
     44
     10 5
      8 8
      1 7 0
      1 5 4
        1 60
        1 54
          60
          44
```

Self-Test 1

1. Step 1. $\frac{9.0 \text{ kg}}{2.2\,)20.0.0}$; 20, 19 8, 2 0

Step 2. *Low range:* 9.0 kg × 20 mg = 180 mg/day

High range: 9.0 kg × 40 mg = 360.0 mg/day

Step 3. 60 mg × 3 doses = 180 mg/day
The order is safe.

Step 4. $\frac{60 \text{ mg}}{125 \text{ mg}} \times 5 \text{ mL} = \frac{12}{5}$; $5\,)12.0 = 2.4$ (10, 20, 20)

Give 2.4 mL.

2. Step 1. 29 lb – 13.18 kg (calculator)

Step 2. 40 mg × 13.18 kg = 527 mg (calculator) = safe dose

Step 3. 175 mg × 3 = 525 mg = child's dose

Step 4. Order is safe. Give 7 mL po q8h.

3. a. It was not necessary to use a rule. The literature was clear. Children 6–12 years should receive 600 mg divided into three doses, which equals 200 mg/dose; the ordered dose is safe.

b. $\frac{D}{H} \times S = A$ $\quad \frac{200}{125} \times 5 = \frac{1000}{125}$; $125\,)1000. = 8.0$ mL

Give 8 mL.

4. Tylenol 80 mg seems low. Literature says a child of 6 should receive four chewable tablets. This would be 320 mg. Check with the physician.

5. a. Literature states dose should not exceed 12 mg/kg/24 hour.

Literature 28 kg × 12 mg = 336 mg = safe dose

Child 110 mg × 3 doses = 330 mg

Dose is safe.

b. $\frac{D}{H} \times S = A$

$\frac{110 \text{ mg}}{80 \text{ mg}} \times 15 \text{ mL} = \frac{165}{8}$; $8\,)165.0 = 20.6 = 21$ mL (16, 50, 48, 2)

Give 21 mL.

6. a. The literature states that children under 6 months can receive 1–2.5 mg IM three to four times a day. The individual dose for the infant is 1 mg. This is safe, but the physician wrote q3–4h prn for the time. This would allow six to eight doses per 24 hours. The nurse can give the first dose but should clarify the times with the doctor.

b. $\frac{D}{H} \times S = A$ $\quad \frac{1 \text{ mg}}{5 \text{ mg}} \times 1 \text{ mL} = 0.2$ mL IM

7. a. Range is

20 mg/kg × 10 kg = 200 mg/day to 40 mg/kg × 10 kg = 400 mg/day

The baby is receiving 125 mg × 3 doses = 375 mg/day. The dosage is safe.

b. No math is necessary. Pour 5 mL.

8. a. The literature states the range in lb. No need to convert.
Range is

0.5 mg × 35 lb = 17.5 mg to 1 mg × 35 lb = 35 mg

The dose is safe.

b. $\frac{D}{H} \times S = A$ $\quad \frac{20 \text{ mg}}{50 \text{ mg}} \times 1 \text{ mL} = \frac{2}{5}$; $5\,)2.0 = .4 = 0.4$ mL

Give 0.4 mL IM stat.

9. No calculation is necessary. A 15-year-old receives an adult dose. The literature is clear. The dose is safe. Give Septra DS 1 tab po q12h.

10. a. The literature is clear—1.2 million units IM q month. The dose is safe.

b. $\frac{D}{H} \times S = A$ $\quad \frac{1{,}200{,}000 \text{ units}}{600{,}000 \text{ units}} \times 1 \text{ mL} = 2$ mL

Self-Test 2

1. Step 1. Safe dose is 50–100 mg/kg/24h.

Low Range

$$\begin{array}{r} 50 \text{ mg} \\ \times\ 8 \text{ kg} \\ \hline 400 \text{ mg/24h} \end{array}$$

High Range

$$\begin{array}{r} 100 \text{ mg} \\ \times\ 8 \text{ kg} \\ \hline 800 \text{ mg/24h} \end{array}$$

Order is 200 mg q6h (4 doses).
200 mg × 4 = 800 mg/24h. Dose is safe.

Step 2. Minimum safe dilution is 50 mg/mL.

$$50\overline{)200 \text{ mg}}^{\;4 \text{ mL}}$$ is the minimum dilution; 10 mL is safe.

Step 3. Dilute 750 mg with 8 mL sterile water to make 90 mg/mL.

$\frac{D}{H} \times S = A \qquad \frac{200 \text{ mg}}{90 \text{ mg}} \times 1 \text{ mL} = 2.2 \text{ mL (calculator)}$

Withdraw 2.2 mL of the drug into a syringe. Label the remainder and store in the refrigerator.

Step 4. Add about 5 mL D5$\frac{1}{4}$NS to the Buretrol.

Add the 2.2 mL of drug. Add more D5$\frac{1}{4}$NS to make 10 mL.

Step 5. Set the pump at 20. This means 20 mL/hr. The pump will deliver 10 mL in 30 min.

Step 6. When the IV is finished add a 15 mL flush of D5$\frac{1}{4}$NS to clear the tubing of medication.

2. Step 1. Safe dose is 8–10 mg/kg/24h given q12h.

Low Range

$$\begin{array}{r} 8 \text{ mg} \\ \times\ 15 \text{ kg} \\ \hline 120 \text{ mg/24h} \end{array}$$

High Range

$$\begin{array}{r} 10 \text{ mg} \\ \times\ 15 \text{ kg} \\ \hline 150 \text{ mg/24h} \end{array}$$

Order is 75 mg q12h (2 doses) = 150 mg/24h. Dose is safe.

Step 2. Minimum safe dilution is 1 mL in 15–25 mL. The drug comes as a liquid 80 mg/5 mL.

$\frac{D}{H} \times S = A$

$$\frac{75 \text{ mg}}{80 \text{ mg}} \times 5 \text{ mL} = \begin{array}{l} 4.7 \text{ mL (calculator)} \\ \times\ 15 \text{ mL (minimum dilution factor)} \\ \hline 70.5 \text{ mL is the safe dilution.} \end{array}$$

Step 3. 75 mL D5W is a safe concentration (more than 70.5 mL).

Step 4. Draw up 4.7 mL drug into a syringe. Discard the remainder.

Step 5. Add about 50 mL D5W to the Buretrol. Add the 4.7 mL medication. Now add D5W until 75 mL is reached. Order is to administer over 1 hr. Set the pump at 75.

Step 6. When the IV is completed, add a 15 mL flush of D5W to clear the tubing of medication.

3. Step 1. Safe dose range is 20–50 mg/kg/24h given q6h.

Low Range

$$\begin{array}{r} 20 \text{ mg} \\ \times\ 25 \text{ kg} \\ \hline 500 \text{ mg/24h} \end{array}$$

High Range

$$\begin{array}{r} 50 \text{ mg} \\ \times\ 25 \text{ kg} \\ \hline 1250 \text{ mg/24h} \end{array}$$

Order is 300 mg q6h (4 doses).
300 mg × 4 = 1200 mg/24h. Dose is safe.

Step 2. Minimum safe dilution is 5 mg/mL.

$$5 \text{ mg}\overline{)300 \text{ mg}}^{\;60 \text{ mL}}$$ 60 mL is the safe minimum dilution. 75 mL is safe.

Step 3. Dilute 1 g powder with 20 mL sterile water to make 50 mg/mL.

$\frac{D}{H} \times S = A \qquad \frac{\overset{6}{\cancel{300 \text{ mg}}}}{\underset{1}{\cancel{50 \text{ mg}}}} \times 1 \text{ mL} = 6 \text{ mL.}$

Withdraw 6 mL of drug into a syringe. Label the vial and refrigerate.

Step 4. Add about 50 mL D5W into the Buretrol. Add 6 mL medication. Add more D5W to make 75 mL.

Step 5. Set the pump at 150. This means 150 mL/hr. The pump will deliver 75 mL in 30 min. (Some nurses would set the pump at 75 to deliver the 75 mL over an hour.)

Step 6. When the IV is finished, add a 15 mL flush of D5W to clear the tubing of medication.

4. Step 1. Safe dose range is 6–7.5 mg/kg/24h given q8h.

Low Range

$$\begin{array}{r} 6 \text{ mg} \\ \times\ 40 \text{ kg} \\ \hline 240 \text{ mg/24h} \end{array}$$

High Range

$$\begin{array}{r} 7.5 \text{ mg} \\ \times\ 40 \text{ kg} \\ \hline 300 \text{ mg/24h} \end{array}$$

Order is 100 mg q8h (3 doses).
100 mg × 3 = 300 mg. Dose is safe.

Step 2. Minimum safe dilution is 2 mg/mL.

$$2 \text{ mg } \overline{)100 \text{ mg}} \quad = 50 \text{ mL}$$

is the safe minimum dilution. Order is 50 mL.

Step 3. $\frac{D}{H} \times S = A$

We need 100 mg of tobramycin. Stock is 80 mg per 2 mL. We will need two ampules. Use the first ampule (2 mL) and 20 mg from the second ampule.

$\frac{20 \text{ mg}}{80 \text{ mg}} \times 2 \text{ mL} = \frac{1}{2} = 0.5 \text{ mL} + 2 \text{ mL} = 2.5 \text{ mL}$

Step 4. Draw up 2.5 mL tobramycin into a syringe. Add about 30 mL D5$\frac{1}{3}$NS into the Buretrol. Add the 2.5 mL medication. Now add more D5$\frac{1}{3}$NS to make a total of 50 mL.

Step 5. Set the pump at 100. The pump will deliver 50 mL over 30 min.

Step 6. When the IV is finished, add a 15-mL flush of D5$\frac{1}{3}$NS to clear the tubing of medication.

5. Step 1. Safe dose is 50–200 mg/kg/24h given q6h.

Low Range

$$\begin{array}{r} 50 \text{ mg} \\ \times\ 18 \text{ kg} \\ \hline 900 \text{ mg/24h} \end{array}$$

High Range

$$\begin{array}{r} 200 \text{ mg} \\ \times\ 18 \text{ kg} \\ \hline 3600 \text{ mg/24h} \end{array}$$

Order is 900 mg q6h (4 doses).
900 mg × 4 = 3600 mg/24h. Dose is safe.

Step 2. Minimum safe dilution is 50 mg/mL.

$$50 \text{ mg } \overline{)900 \text{ mg}} \quad = 18$$

18 mL is the minimum safe dilution.
25 mL is safe.

Step 3. 1 g powder. Dilute with 10 mL to make 95 mg/mL.

$\frac{D}{H} \times S = A$

$\frac{900 \text{ mg}}{95 \text{ mg}} \times 1 \text{ mL} = 9.5 \text{ mL}$ drug (calculator)

Draw up the 9.5 mL in a syringe. Discard the remainder. Too small to keep.

Step 4. Add about 10 mL of D5$\frac{1}{3}$NS to the Buretrol. Add the 9.5 mL medication. Add D5$\frac{1}{3}$NS to make a total of 25 mL.

Step 5. Set the pump at 50. The pump will deliver 25 mL in 30 min.

Step 6. When the IV is finished add a flush of 15 mL D5$\frac{1}{3}$NS to clear the tubing of medication.

Proficiency Test

1. Safe dose 0.5 mg to 1 mg/dose IM. The order is safe.

   $\frac{D}{H} \times S = A$

   $\frac{1 \text{ mg}}{10 \text{ mg}} \times 1 \text{ mL} = 0.1 \text{ mL IM.}$

   Use a precision syringe.

2. Safe dose is 20–40 mg/kg/24h given q8h.

   Low Range

   $$\begin{array}{r} 20 \text{ mg} \\ \times\ 10 \text{ kg} \\ \hline 200 \text{ mg/24h} \end{array}$$

   High Range

   $$\begin{array}{r} 40 \text{ mg} \\ \times\ 10 \text{ kg} \\ \hline 400 \text{ mg/24h} \end{array}$$

   Order is 125 mg q8h (3 doses).
   125 mg × 3 doses = 375 mg. Dose is safe.

   No math necessary. Stock is 125 mg/5 mL. Give 5 mL.

3. Safe dose: 50,000 units/kg × 1 dose.

   $$\begin{array}{r} 50{,}000 \text{ units} \\ \times\ 10 \text{ kg} \\ \hline 500{,}000 \text{ units} \end{array}$$

   The order is safe.

   $\frac{D}{H} \times S = A \qquad \frac{500{,}000 \text{ units}}{600{,}000 \text{ units}} \times 1 \text{ mL} = \frac{5}{6} = 0.83 \text{ mL}$

   Give 0.83 mL IM. Use a precision syringe.

4. Step 1. Safe dose: 2.5 mg/kg/dose q8h

   $$\begin{array}{r} 2.5 \text{ mg} \\ \times\ 3.6 \text{ kg} \\ \hline 9 \text{ mg} \end{array}$$

   Order is safe.

   Step 2. Minimum safe dilution: 2 mg/mL

   $$2 \text{ mg} \overline{)9 \text{ mg}} = 4.5 \text{ mL}$$

   is the minimum safe dilution. 10 mL is safe.

   Step 3. $\frac{D}{H} \times S = A$

   $$\frac{9 \text{ mg}}{40 \text{ mg}} \times 1 \text{ mL} = \frac{9}{40} \quad 40 \overline{)9.000} = .225 = 0.23 \text{ mL}$$

   Use a precision syringe to draw up 0.23 mL.

   Step 4. Add about 5 mL D5$\frac{1}{4}$NS to the Buretrol.

   Add the 0.23 mL drug. Add more D5$\frac{1}{4}$NS to make 10 mL.

   Step 5. Set the pump at 20 because 20 mL in an hr will deliver the 10 mL in 30 min.

   Step 6. When the IV is completed add a flush of 15 mL D5$\frac{1}{4}$NS to the Buretrol to clear the tubing of medication.

5. Safe dose: infants and children under 3 yr: 10–40 mg. The dose is safe.

   $\frac{D}{H} \times S = A \qquad \frac{10 \text{ mg}}{20 \text{ mg}} \times 5 \text{ mL} = \frac{5}{2} = 2.5 \text{ mL po}$

6. Step 1. Safe dose: 10 mg/kg q8h IV

   $$\begin{array}{r} 10 \text{ mg} \\ \times\ 5.5 \text{ kg} \\ \hline 55 \text{ mg q8h} \end{array}$$

   Dose is safe.

   Step 2. Minimum safe dilution: 5 mg/mL; infuse over 1 hr.

   $$5 \text{ mg} \overline{)54 \text{ mg}} = 10.8 = 11 \text{ mL; 12 mL is safe.}$$

   Step 3. To the 500 mg powder add 10 mL sterile water for injection to make 50 mg/mL.

   $\frac{D}{H} \times S = A$

   $$\frac{54 \text{ mg}}{50 \text{ mg}} \times 1 \text{ mL} = \frac{54}{50} = 50 \overline{)54.00} = 1.08 = 1.1 \text{ mL}$$
   $$\underline{4\ 00}$$

   Withdraw 1.1 mL of the drug; label the vial; refrigerate.

   Step 4. Add about 5 mL D5$\frac{1}{4}$NS to the Buretrol.

   Add 1.1 mL drug. Add more D5$\frac{1}{4}$NS to make 12 mL.

   Step 5. Set the pump for 12 (12 mL over 1 hr)

   Step 6. When the IV is completed add 15 mL D5$\frac{1}{4}$NS as a flush to the Buretrol to clear the tubing of medication.

7. Safe dose: 50–75 mg/kg/dose

Low Range

$$\begin{array}{r} 50 \text{ mg} \\ \times\ 6.7 \text{ kg} \\ \hline 335 \text{ mg/dose} \end{array}$$

High Range

$$\begin{array}{r} 75 \text{ mg} \\ \times\ 6.7 \text{ kg} \\ \hline 502.5 \text{ mg/dose} \end{array}$$

Order of 350 mg is safe.

$\frac{D}{H} \times S = A \qquad \frac{\overset{35}{\cancel{350}} \text{ mg}}{\underset{100}{\cancel{500}} \text{ mg}} \times \overset{1}{\cancel{5}} \text{ mL} = \frac{35}{10} = 3.5 \text{ mL}$

8. Safe dose: 22 mg/kg/24h given q6h

$$\begin{array}{r} 22 \text{ mg} \\ \times\ 9.9 \text{ kg} \\ \hline 217.8 \text{ mg/24h} \end{array}$$

Order is 65 mg qid (4 doses).
65 mg × 4 = 260 mg
The dose does not meet safe requirements. Do not prepare the medication. Consult with the physician who ordered the drug.

9. Step 1. Safe dose is 2 g to 6 g in a 24-hr period divided into either q8h or q12h.
The order is 2 g q8h (3 doses).
2 g × 3 doses = 6 g. The order is safe.

Step 2. Minimum safe dilution is 50 mg/mL over 30 min.

$$50 \text{ mg} \overline{\smash{)}2000 \text{ mg}} = 40 \text{ mL}$$

is the minimum safe dilution; 50 mL is safe.

Step 3. Order is 2 g. Stock is a 2-g powder. Directions say to dilute initially with 10-mL sterile water for injection. Draw the total amount into a syringe.

Step 4. Add about 20 mL D5$\frac{1}{3}$NS to the Buretrol. Add the medication from the syringe. Then add more D5$\frac{1}{3}$NS to make 50 mL.

Step 5. Set the pump for 100. It will deliver 50 mL in 30 min.

Step 6. When the IV is completed, add 15 mL D5$\frac{1}{3}$NS as a flush to the Buretrol to clear the tubing of medication.

10. Usual dose is 0.5 mg/lb to 1 mg/lb.

Low Range

$$\begin{array}{r} 35 \text{ lb} \\ \times\ 0.5 \text{ mg} \\ \hline 17.5 \text{ mg} \end{array}$$

High Range

$$\begin{array}{r} 35 \text{ lb} \\ \times\ 1 \text{ mg} \\ \hline 35 \text{ mg} \end{array}$$

20 mg is a safe dose.

$\frac{D}{H} \times S = A \qquad \frac{2\cancel{0} \text{ mg}}{5\cancel{0} \text{ mg}} \times 1 \text{ mL} = \frac{2}{5} = 0.4 \text{ mL IM.}$

Use a precision syringe.

11 Information Basic to Administering Drugs

CONTENT TO MASTER

Generic and trade names

Pregnancy categories

Basic knowledge essential for safe drug administration

Legal considerations: criminal and civil

Ethical principles in drug administration

Tips for safe pouring and administration and accurate charting of medications

Key terms

Drug Metabolism	*Ethical Principles*
Absorption	Nonmaleficence
Distribution	Justice
Biotransformation	Beneficence
Excretion	Confidentiality
Tolerance	Autonomy
Cumulation	Truthfulness

In previous chapters we have learned drug forms and preparations, how to read prescriptions, and how to calculate dosages. This chapter provides the opportunity to focus on some of the nurse's responsibilities for drug therapy—drug knowledge, legal and ethical considerations, and, finally, specific points that may prove helpful in giving medications.

▼ DRUG KNOWLEDGE

Although a current *Physician's Desk Reference* (*PDR*) and the package insert are the best references for dosage, nursing drug handbooks are the best references for the nurse practitioner who needs a variety of information specifically designed to help assess, manage, evaluate, and teach the patient. The following headings represent the type of information found in a nursing handbook.

Generic and Trade Names

The generic name is the official name given a drug. A drug has only one generic name in the United States. It may have different generic names in other countries. The letters USP (United States Pharmacopeia) following a generic name indicate that the drug meets government standards for purity and assay.

A trade name is the brand name under which a company manufactures a generic drug. A drug may have several trade names, but still only one generic name.

Consumer groups have advocated that drugs be prescribed by generic name only so that the pharmacist may dispense the least expensive drug available on the market. The nurse should understand that generic drugs, manufactured by different companies, are not exactly the same. The active ingredient in the drug meets standards of uniformity and purity, but manufacturers use different fillers and dyes. These substances can cause adverse effects (e.g., severe nausea caused by the dye used in coloring). Additionally, when a different trade name is prescribed a patient may become confused and distressed about receiving medication that appears unlike previous doses. The active ingredient is the same, but size, shape, or color may vary.

Drug Class

The class of drug is a quick reference to the therapeutic action, use, and adverse effects of a drug. As the nurse develops a knowledge base, the drug class will identify general nursing implications and precautions in administering a drug, such as an antihypertensive agent, immunosuppressant, or anticonvulsant.

Pregnancy Category

The Federal Drug Administration (FDA) has established the following categories:

A. No risk to the fetus in any trimester.

B. No adverse effect demonstrated in animals; no human studies available.

C. Animal studies have shown adverse reactions. No human studies are available. Given only after risks to the fetus have been considered.

D. Definite fetal risk exists; may be given in spite of risk to the fetus if needed for a life-threatening condition.

X. Absolute fetal abnormality; not to be used anytime in pregnancy.

A nurse administering a drug to a woman of childbearing age should be aware of the pregnancy category of a drug to teach the patient and protect the fetus. In addition, this knowledge will aid in discussing the use of over-the-counter (OTC) drugs in pregnancy.

Dosage and Route

Information about the dosage and route of administration is crucial to protect against medication error. Most handbooks give a dosage range for the adult, the elderly, and the child.

Action (Pharmacokinetics)

The nurse should understand how the drug is absorbed into the bloodstream, distributed to the cells, metabolized, and excreted. Some drugs should be taken between meals; some with food; some may not be combined because of incompatibility or interaction; some may not be taken orally.

Patients with liver or kidney disease may not be able to metabolize or excrete certain drugs. The drug accumulates in the body, leading to adverse effects. The nurse who knows the pharmacokinetics of a drug can better assess, manage, and evaluate drug therapy.

Uses

One of the most common questions asked of nurses is, "Why am I getting this drug?" The nurse relates the use of the drug to the expected therapeutic outcome. This information aids in observing for expected effects and in patient teaching.

Side Effects or Adverse Effects

Side effects are transient, nontherapeutic reactions to a drug. *Adverse effects* are untoward, nontherapeutic effects that may be harmful to the patient and that require lowering the dosage or discontinuing the drug. An example of a side effect is drowsiness, which occurs with some antihistamines. An example of an adverse effect is a serious decrease in white blood cells that results in lowered resistance to infection. The nurse must observe for these effects, know how to manage them, and teach the patient necessary information.

Contraindications and Precautions

These refer to conditions in which a drug should be given with caution or not given at all. For example, patients who have exhibited a previous reaction to penicillin should be cautioned against taking it again. Certain antibiotics must be administered with caution to patients who have poor kidney function. The nurse has a responsibility to know this information in order to safeguard the patient and carry out effective nursing care.

Interactions and Incompatibilities

When more than one drug is administered at a time, unexpected or nontherapeutic responses may occur. Some interactions are desirable. For example, naloxone (Narcan) is a narcotic antagonist that reverses the effects of a morphine overdose. Other interactions, however, are undesirable. For example, aspirin should not be taken with an oral anticoagulant because the possibility of an adverse effect is increased.

Some drugs may be incompatible and should not be mixed. This information is especially important when medications are combined for injection in IV administration. Chemical incompatibility is usually indicated by a visible sign, such as precipitation or color change. Physical incompatibility can occur without any visible sign; therefore, the nurse should check a suitable reference before combining drugs. A good rule of thumb is: when in doubt, do not mix.

Interactions may also occur between drugs and certain foods. Calcium present in dairy products interferes with the absorption of tetracycline. Foods high in vitamin B_6 can decrease the effect of an antiparkinson drug. Foods high in tyramine, such as wine and cheese, can precipitate a hypertensive crisis in patients taking monoamine oxidase inhibitors.

Cigarette smoke can increase liver metabolism of drugs and decrease drug effectiveness. Even individuals who are passively exposed to cigarette smoke may require higher doses of medication.

Nursing Implications

This is information the nurse needs to administer the drug safely and to assess, manage, and teach the patient. This is not found in the *PDR*.

Evaluation of Effectiveness

Few drug references actually list this heading, yet the nurse is expected to evaluate the drug regimen and to record and report observations. Knowledge of the drug's class, its action, and its use leads to an understanding of expected therapeutic outcomes.

For example, ampicillin sodium is a broad-spectrum antibiotic that is used for urinary, respiratory, and other infections. Signs of effectiveness might include: normal temperature; the laboratory report of the white blood cell (WBC) count indicating a normal result; clear urine; no pain on urination; no WBC in urine; decreased pus in an infected wound; wound healing; a patient who is more alert and interested in surroundings; improved appetite.

Patient Teaching

The patient has a right to know the name and dose of the drug, why the drug is ordered, and what effects to expect or watch for. In addition, the patient who is to take a drug at home needs specific information. This is a professional responsibility shared by the physician and the nurse.

Drug Action (Pharmacokinetics)

When a drug is taken orally, it is absorbed through the villi of the small intestine, distributed to the cells by the blood stream, metabolized to a greater or lesser extent, and then excreted from the body.

Absorption

Absorption of an oral drug depends upon the degree of stomach acidity, the time it takes for the stomach to empty, whether or not food is present, the amount of contact with villi in the small intestine, and blood flow to the villi.

Absorption of a drug may be affected in many ways. Enteric-coated (EC) tablets are not meant to dissolve in the acidic stomach. They ordinarily pass through the stomach to the duodenum. When an antacid is administered with an EC tablet, the pH of the stomach is raised, and the tablet may dissolve prematurely. The drug may become less potent, or it may irritate the gastric lining. Timed-release EC capsules that dissolve prematurely can deliver a huge dose of drug, causing adverse effects.

Laxatives increase gastrointestinal movement and decrease the time a drug is in contact with the villi of the small intestine where most absorption occurs. The presence of food in the stomach can impair absorption. Penicillin is a good example of a drug that should be taken on an empty stomach. Foods that contain calcium, such as milk and cheese, form a complex with some drugs and inhibit absorption.

Distribution

Distribution is the movement of a drug through body fluids, chiefly the bloodstream, to cells. Drugs do not travel freely in the blood. Most travel attached to plasma proteins, especially albumen. Drugs that are free can attach to cells, on which they produce an effect.

When more than one drug is present in the bloodstream, they may compete for protein-binding sites. One drug may displace another. The displaced drug is now free to act with the cells, and its effect will be more pronounced. Aspirin is a common drug for displacement; it should not be given with oral anticoagulants, which are 99% bound to albumin. Aspirin displaces the anticoagulant; more is free to act at the cellular level, and a toxic effect may occur—bleeding.

Metabolism

Metabolism refers to the chemical biotransformation of a drug to a form that can be excreted. Most biotransformation occurs in the liver. Because oral drugs are carried first to the liver, this process begins once the drug is absorbed. Here, too, one drug can interfere with the effects of another. Barbiturates increase the activity of the liver enzymes. Because drugs are metabolized more quickly, their effect is reduced. Conversely, acetaminophen (Tylenol) will block the breakdown of penicillin in the liver, thereby increasing its activity.

Excretion

Excretion refers to the removal of a drug from the body. The major organ of excretion is the kidney. Drug interactions may also occur at this level; for example, probenecid inhibits the excretion of penicillin and increases its length of action, and furosemide (Lasix), a diuretic, blocks the excretion of aspirin and can lead to adverse effects by aspirin.

Drug interactions are not necessarily harmful. For example, narcotic antagonists are used to reverse the adverse effects of general anesthetics. This action is termed *antagonism*. *Synergism* is a term used when a second drug increases the intensity or prolongs the effect of a first drug. For example, a narcotic and a minor tranquilizer produce more pain relief than the narcotic alone. The nurse administering medications needs to be aware of possible interactions and evaluate the patient's response.

To minimize adverse interactions, the nurse should know the patient's drug profile, give as low a dose as possible, know the actions and adverse effects of the drugs administered, and monitor the patient. Some drug interactions may take several weeks to develop.

Tolerance

When a pain or sleeping medication is given frequently, the liver enzymes become skilled in biotransforming more quickly. Less drug is available, and thus the drug is less effective in relieving pain or in aiding sleep. Some nurses call this reaction "addiction," because the patient complains that the drug is not working and asks for more. In fact, it is a physiologic response. The patient requires more of the drug or a drug with a different molecular structure.

Cumulation

When biotransformation or excretion is inhibited, as can occur in liver or kidney disease, the drug accumulates in the body and an adverse effect can occur. Cumulation can also result from taking too much drug or from taking a drug too frequently.

Other factors that affect drug action include:

- Weight: larger individuals need a higher dose.
- Age: extremes of life respond more strongly. The livers and kidneys of infants are not well developed; in the aged, systems are less efficient.
- Pathologic conditions: especially of liver and kidney.
- Hypersensitivity to a drug: allergic reaction.
- Psychological and emotional state: depression or anxiety can decrease or increase body metabolism and affect drug action.

Adverse reactions may occur in any system or organ. Drug knowledge will enhance the nurse's observational skills and lead to responsible and appropriate intervention.

▼ LEGAL CONSIDERATIONS

There are two types of law that affect nursing practice—criminal and civil.

Criminal Law

Criminal law relates to offenses against the general public that are detrimental to society as a whole. Criminal actions are prosecuted by governmental authorities. If the defendant is judged guilty, the penalty may be a fine, imprisonment, or both.

Nurses must know the scope of nursing practice in the state in which they function. They should be familiar with government regulations—federal, state, and local—that affect nursing. The policies and procedures of the agency in which they practice also have legal status. Failure to follow guidelines or lack of knowledge can lead to liability.

Criminal charges include unlawful use, possession, or administration of a controlled substance. The Comprehensive Drug Abuse, Prevention and Control Act of 1970 classified drugs that are subject to abuse into one of five schedules according to their medical usefulness and abuse potential.

Schedule I drugs have no valid use and are not available for prescription use (e.g., LSD).

Schedule II drugs have a valid medical use and are available for prescriptions, but exhibit a high abuse potential. Misuse can lead to physical and psychological dependence. Labels for these drugs are marked with the symbol CII (Fig. 11-1). Controlled drugs are counted each shift, and discrepancies are

CONTROLLED DRUG REQUISITION FORM

II

III -V

____
NURSING UNIT

QUANTITY	UNIT OF ISSUE	CONTROLLED DRUG	DOSAGE FORM	STRENGTH	QUANTITY	UNIT OF	CONTROLLED DRUG	DOSAGE FORM	STRENGTH
	10	Alfentanil	Ampule	500ug/2ml		25	Alprazolam	Tablet	0.25mg 0.5mg
	1	Amobarbital	Vial	500mg		5	Buprenorphine	Ampule	0.3mg
	10	Amobarbital	Capsule	200mg		10	Chloral Hydrate	Capsule	500mg
	1	Cocaine 4%	Solution	4ml		10	Chloral Hydrate	Syrup	500mg (5ml Cup)
	10	Codeine	Tablet	15mg 30mg		10	Chlordiazepoxide	Capsule	5mg 10mg 25mg
	10	Codeine	Syringe	30mg 60mg		10	Clonazepam	Tablet	0.5mg 1mg
		Fentanyl	Ampule	5ml 20ml		10	Diazepam	Tablet	2mg 5mg 10mg
	10	Hydromorphone	Tablet	2mg 4mg		1	Diazepam	Vial	10mg/ml (1ml)
	10	Hydromorphone	Syringe	2mg		10	Fiorinal	Capsule	
	10	Levorphanol	Tablet	2mg		10	Guaifenesin/Codeine	Syrup	(5ml Cup)
	10	Levorphanol	Ampule	2mg		10	Hycodan	Tablet	5mg
	10	Meperidine	Tablet	50mg		10	Hycodan	Syrup	5mg (5ml Cup)
	10	Meperidine	Syringe	25mg 50mg		10	Lomotil	Tablet	
	10	Meperidine	Syringe	75mg 100mg		10	Lomotil	Liquid	(10ml Cup)
	25	Meperidine	Ampule	50mg		10	Lorazepam	Tablet	1mg 2mg
	1	Methadone	Vial	10mg/ml (20ml)		10	Lorazepam	Syringe	2mg
	10	Methadone	Tablet	5mg 10mg		10	Midazolam	Ampule	10mg
	10	Methadone	Solution	10mg (10ml Cup)		10	Paregoric	Elixir	(5ml Cup)
	10	Methylphenidate	Tablet	5mg 10mg		1	Pentothal 5 GM Kit		
	10	Methylphenidate SR	Tablet	20mg		25	Phenobarbital	Tablet	15mg 30mg
	10	Morphine	Solution	10mg (5ml Cup)		10	Phenobarbital	Elixir	20mg (5ml Cup)
	1	Morphine	Suppository	10mg 20mg		1	Phenobarbital	Vial	65mg 130mg
	10	Morphine	Syringe	4mg 10mg 15mg		10	Propoxyphene	Capsule	65mg
	25	Morphine SA (MS Contin)	Tablet	30mg 60mg		25	Temazepam	Capsule	15mg
	10	Pentobarbital	Capsule	50mg 100mg		25	Triazolam	Tablet	0.125mg .25mg
	10	Pentobarbital	Syringe	100mg		25	Tylenol #3	Tablet	
	10	Percodan	Tablet			10	Tylenol/Codeine	Elixir/Cup	
	25	Percocet	Tablet						
	10	Secobarbital	Capsule	50mg 100mg					
	10	Sufentanil	Ampule	100ug/2ml					
	1	Tincture of Opium	Solution	5ml/bottle					

Ordered By: ______________________ Date: ______________
Print name and sign--Nurse

Received By: ______________________ Date: ______________
Print name and sign--Nurse

Dispensed By: ______________________ Date: ______________
Print name and sign--Pharmacist

Figure 11-1
Nursing Controlled Drug Requisition Form for Schedule II, III, IV, and V drugs. (Courtesy of Pharmacy Department, St. Vincent Hospital and Medical Center, New York City)

reported. Government and institutional regulations specify how these drugs are stored and protected. For example, an order for a narcotic in a hospital setting might be valid for 3 days. When the 3 days have elapsed, the order must be rewritten. A nurse who administers a controlled drug after the order has expired commits a medication error. Figure 11-2 is an example of a hospital policy on controlled drugs.

Schedule III, IV, and V drugs are classed as having less abuse potential than Schedule II drugs, but they can cause some physical and psychological dependence. Figure 11-1 lists some generic and trade names of controlled drugs in Schedules III, IV, and V. Note that CIII, CIV, and CV symbols identify these drugs.

Nurses who become impaired (unable to function) owing to alcohol or drug abuse leave themselves open to criminal action, as well as to disciplinary action by the state board of nursing. Many states have laws requiring mandatory reporting of impaired nurses.

Civil Law

Civil law is concerned with the legal rights and duties of private persons. When an individual believes that a wrong was committed against him or her personally, that individual can sue for damages in the form of money.

The legal wrong is called a *tort. Malpractice* refers to negligence on the part of the nurse. There are four elements of negligence:

1. A claim that the nurse owed the patient a special duty of care, that is, a nurse–patient relationship existed.
2. A claim that the nurse was required to meet a specific standard of care in carrying out the action or function. To prove or disprove this element, both sides bring in expert witnesses to testify.

Nursing Responsibilities

1. Count will be done each shift by two (2) registered nurses.
   a. The oncoming nurse should handle and physically count the controlled drugs.
   b. The off-going nurse should verify the count and record the number on hand on the controlled drug sheets.
   c. Both nurses should sign the controlled drug sheets.
2. All controlled drugs will be stored in a double-locked cabinet specifically designated for this purpose.
3. At all times, the narcotic keys must be in the possession of a staff nurse who is physically present on the unit.
4. A written physician's order must precede administration of any controlled substance, except in a dire emergency (emergency intubation, acute control of seizures, etc.), in which case the order will be written as soon as the emergency is over.
5. All controlled substances must be signed for by the nurse administering the medication at the time it is removed from the cabinet. The name of the prescribing physician should be inserted in the appropriate space.
6. If a controlled substance is removed from the cabinet in preparation for administration and is not used, or if part is wasted, the waste should be witnessed by another nurse and recorded as such on the controlled substance sheet. The signatures of both nurses are required.
7. In the event of a discrepancy at the time of count, the Nursing Care Coordinator or Divisional Nursing Coordinator is notified, and the loss section of the controlled drug order form is completed.
8. Controlled substances delivered by Pharmacy will not be accepted if the bag is opened or tampered with in any manner.
9. Upon receipt of the drugs, the nurse will verify the count/delivery and complete the addition to the controlled drug sheet.
10. Narcotics must be reordered every seventy-two (72) hours. Barbiturates must be ordered every seven (7) days.

Figure 11-2
A hospital policy for signing and counting controlled drugs. (Courtesy of Nursing Department, St. Vincent's Hospital and Medical Center, New York City)

3. A claim that the nurse failed to meet the required standard.
4. A claim that harm or injury resulted for which compensation is sought.

The nurse–patient relationship is a legal status that is created the moment a nurse actually provides nursing care to another person.

For administration of medications, *a nurse is required by law to exercise the degree of skill and care that a reasonably prudent nurse with similar training and experience, practicing in the same community, would exercise under the same or similar circumstances.* When a nursing student performs duties that are customarily performed by a registered nurse, the courts have held the nursing student to the higher standard of care of the registered nurse.

Mistakes in administering medications are among the most common causes of malpractice. Liability may result from administering the wrong dose, giving a medication to a wrong patient, giving a drug at the wrong time, or failing to administer a drug at the right time or in the proper manner.

A frequent cause of medication errors is misreading the physician's order or failing to check with the physician when the order is questionable. Faulty technique in administering medications, especially injections that result in injury to the patient, is another common medication error.

Not all malpractice is a result of negligence. Malpractice claims are also founded upon the daily interaction between the nurse and the patient; consequently, the nurse's personality plays a major role in the fostering or prevention of malpractice claims. All nurses should be familiar with the principles of psychology. The surest way to prevent claims is to recognize the patient as a human being who has emotional, as well as physical, needs and to respond to these needs in a humane and competent manner.

Should an error occur, primary consideration must be given to the patient. The nurse notifies the physician and the immediate nursing supervisor; students notify the instructor. Error-in-medication forms are filled out and appropriate action is taken under the direction of the physician.

To prevent malpractice claims, the nurse must render, as consistently as possible, the best possible care to patients. Every nurse involved in direct care should regard prevention of malpractice claims as an integral part of daily nursing responsibilities for two fundamental reasons:

1. Such measures result in higher quality care.
2. All affirmative measures taken to minimize malpractice will minimize the nurse's exposure to personal liability.

How can liability claims be avoided?

- Know and follow institutional policies and procedures.
- Look up what you do not know.
- Do not leave medicines at the bedside.
- Chart carefully.
- Listen to the patient: "I never took that before," and the like.
- Check.
- *Double check* when a dose seems high. Most oral tablet doses range from $\frac{1}{2}$ to 2 tablets.
- Most injections are less than 3 mL.
- Label any powder you dilute. Label any IV bag you use.
- When necessary, seek advice from competent professionals.
- Do not administer drugs poured by another nurse.
- Keep drug knowledge up to date—attend continuing education programs; update nursing skills.

It is possible to render high-quality nursing care and never commit a medication error. Safe, effective drug therapy is a combination of knowledge, skill, carefulness, and caring.

▼ ETHICAL PRINCIPLES IN DRUG ADMINISTRATION

A moral as well as legal dimension is involved in the administration of medications. Nurses are responsible for their actions.

The American Nurses Association Code of Ethics contains several statements that apply to drug therapy. Briefly stated, they are:

1. The nurse provides services with respect for the human dignity and the uniqueness of the patient.
2. The nurse safeguards the patient's right to privacy.
3. The nurse acts to safeguard the patient from incompetent, unethical, or illegal practice.
4. The nurse assumes responsibility and accountability for nursing judgments and actions.
5. The nurse maintains competence in nursing.

Several principles can be used as guides when an ethical decision must be made. These principles are autonomy, truthfulness, beneficence, nonmaleficence, confidentiality, and justice.

Autonomy

Autonomy is a form of personal liberty in which an individual has the freedom to decide, knows the facts and understands them, and acts without outside force, deceit, or constraint. For the patient, this implies a right to be informed about drug therapy and a right to refuse medication. For the nurse, autonomy brings a responsibility to discuss drug information with the patient and to accept the patient's right to refuse. Autonomy also gives the nurse the right to refuse to participate in any drug therapy deemed to be unethical or unsafe.

Truthfulness

The nurse has an obligation to tell the truth. Some ethicists hold that this is not an absolute obligation and argue that it may be more beneficial not to give all the facts or, sometimes, even to deliberately deceive. In drug therapy, this principle can lead to a dilemma when a *placebo* is ordered.

A placebo is a nondrug or a dummy drug that produces a therapeutic effect, not because of any chemical property but because of the positive relationship that exists between the patient who receives it and the nurse who administers it. Placebos are sometimes ordered in place of pain medication. The nurse administers the placebo, stating that it will relieve pain. "Cooperative" patients are said to produce *endorphins,* chemical mediators that block pain impulses. Patients who do not have a positive relationship with the nurse experience no relief. The dilemma is that some nurses see the use of a placebo as lying to the patient, whereas others see it as a benevolent way of providing relief without pharmacologic intervention. To act in an ethical manner, the nurse who administers a placebo should respect the patient and believe that this therapy can be effective. The nurse should not use the placebo with the intent of tricking or punishing the patient.

The principle of truthfulness also applies when giving drug information to a patient. It is generally held that patients should be informed about drug therapy. There is disagreement about the extent of disclosure.

Beneficence

This concept holds that the nurse must contribute to the good health and welfare of the patient. Every action has both benefits and costs. Do the benefits outweigh the cost? Relative to disclosure of drug information, do the principles of autonomy and veracity outweigh the possible negative effects of revealing all the consequences of taking a drug? Might the patient refuse a drug that, in the end, would be beneficial? In the use of chemotherapy (for cancer), informed consent is required, and the patient is given detailed information. Disclosure is not so complete in other areas of medical care.

Nonmaleficence

Nonmaleficence holds that the nurse must not inflict harm on the patient and must prevent harm whenever possible. Doing something good may lead to a secondary effect that is harmful. For example, giving morphine may relieve pain—a good effect—but may hasten death. It is moral to act for the benefit and to permit the harm, provided the intent is the benefit.

Confidentiality

Confidentiality is respect for information learned from professional involvement with patients. A patient's drug therapy and responses should be discussed only with those individuals who have a right to know, that is, other professionals caring for the patient. To what extent the family or significant others have a right to know depends on the specific situation and wishes of the patient and sometimes may cause conflict.

Justice

Justice refers to the patient's right to receive the right drug, the right dose, by the right route, at the right time. In addition, the patient has a right to the nurse's careful assessment, management, and evaluation of drug therapy and to those nursing actions that promote the patient's safety and well-being. The nurse's obligation is to maintain a high standard of care.

▼ SPECIFIC POINTS THAT MAY BE HELPFUL IN GIVING MEDICATIONS

Medication Orders

A correct medication order has the patient's name and room number, the date, the name of the drug (generic or trade), the dose of the drug, the route of administration, and the times to administer the drug. It ends with the physician's signature.

There are several types of orders:

1. Standing order with termination

   EXAMPLE thyroxin 4 mg qd × 5 days

2. Standing order without termination

   EXAMPLE digoxin 0.5 mg po qd

3. A prn order

   EXAMPLE demerol 50 mg IM q4h prn

4. Single-dose order

   EXAMPLE atropine SO_4 0.3 mg SC 7:30 AM on call to OR

5. Stat order

   EXAMPLE morphine sulfate 10 mg SC stat

Hospital guidelines provide for an automatic stop time on some classes of drugs; for example, narcotic orders may be valid for only 3 days, antibiotics for 10 days. When the nurse first picks up and transfers the order, care must be taken to note the expiration time so that all staff who pour medications are alerted. State laws and hospital policies vary.

- Medical students may write orders on charts, but they must be countersigned by a house physician before they are legal. Medical students are not licensed.
- In states that allow nurses or paramedical personnel to prescribe drugs, hospital guidelines must be followed in carrying out orders.
- Do not carry out an order that is not clear or that is illegible. Check with the physician who wrote the order. Do not assume anything.
- Do not carry out an order if a conflict exists with nursing knowledge; for example, Demerol 500 mg IM is above the average dose.
- Nursing students should not accept oral or telephone orders. They should refer the physician to the nurse manager.
- Professional nurses may take oral or telephone orders in accord with institutional policy. These orders must be written and signed by the physician within 24 hours. Two nurses should listen to and verify the order.

Knowledge Base

- Nurses should know generic and trade names of drugs to be administered, class, average dose, routes of administration, use, side and adverse effects, contraindications, and nursing implications in administration. Nurses should also know what signs of effectiveness to look for and what drug interactions are possible. New or unfamiliar drugs should be researched.
- The nurse should be aware of the patient's diagnosis and medical history, especially relative to drugs taken. Be especially alert to over-the-counter (OTC) drugs, which the patient often does not consider important. Check for allergies.
- Assess the patient's need for drug information. Be prepared to implement and evaluate a nursing care plan in drug therapy.

Pouring Medications

- The patient has a right to considerate and respectful care and the right to refuse a medication. The patient also has a right to know the name of the medication, what it is supposed to do, any side effects that may occur, and what to do should these occur.
- In the ticket system, the Kardex is the main check against the medication ticket. If the ticket does not agree with the Kardex, go to the chart and find the original order. Check through every order to the current date to identify changes in orders.
- In the unit-dose, mobile cart system, the nurse has the medication sheets of each patient together in a folder or on a computer printout. If unsure of an order, take the sheet to the patient's chart and check from the date ordered to the current date.
- Do not pour and administer a drug about which any doubt exists. Check further with the physician, the pharmacist, or a supervising nurse.
- Quiet and concentration are needed to pour drugs. Follow a routine in pouring. *Methodology is the best safeguard in preventing error.*
- Keys are needed to obtain controlled drugs (e.g., narcotics) and to prevent others' access to medications.
- Pour oral medications first, then injections. Medical asepsis (clean technique) is used for oral administration. Injections require sterile technique.

- Read labels three times: (1) when removing the drug from storage, (2) when calculating the dose, and (3) after pouring the drug.
- Orders issued as "stat" take precedence and must be carried out immediately.
- Perform indicated nursing actions before administering certain medications; for example, digitalis preparations require an apical heart rate, whereas antihypertensives require a blood pressure reading.
- Medications should be administered within 30 minutes of the time given. They may be prepared before then in the ticket system. When the mobile cart is used, medications are prepared at the patient's bed and administered.
- Keep medications within sight at all times. Never leave medications unattended. The mobile cart or the medication tray must be kept in view.
- Administer irritating oral drugs with meals or a snack to decrease gastric irritation.
- Break a tablet only if it is scored.
- Never open capsules or break enteric-coated tablets. If the patient cannot swallow them, ask the physician to order a liquid, or check with the pharmacist.
- Check tablets in a stock container. Are they the same size? Same color? If not, return them to the pharmacy.
- It is a fallacy that the nurse is no longer required to calculate or prepare drugs dispensed as unit-dose. Fractional doses may still be necessary. The pharmacy may not have the exact dose. Antibiotics must be prepared for IM or IV use. The label must still be read three times.
- Labels must be clear. If not, return them to the pharmacy.
- Never return any poured drug to a stock bottle once the drug has been taken from the preparation room.
- Never combine medications from two stock bottles. Return both bottles to the pharmacy. It is the responsibility of the pharmacists to combine drugs.
- Hydrophilic capsules are not medications. They are labeled DO NOT EAT and are placed in stock containers of tablets and capsules to absorb dampness and maintain the drug in a solid state.
- If the patient is nauseous or vomiting, hold oral medications and notify the physician or the immediate superior. Be sure to chart this action.
- A medication should not be administered if it is assessed that the drug is contraindicated or that an adverse effect may have occurred as a result of a previous dose.
- Some liquid medications require dilution. Check references for directions.
- Some liquids may have to be administered through a straw; for example, liquid iron preparations discolor teeth and should not come in contact with them.
- Liquids are poured at eye level using a medicine cup. Measure at the *center* of the meniscus—pour with the label up to prevent soiling.
- After the patient has taken a liquid antacid, add 5–10 mL of water to the cup, mix, and have patient drink it as well. Antacids are thick and medication often remains in the cup.
- The nurse who pours medications is responsible for administering and charting.
- Do not give drugs that another nurse has poured.

Giving Medications

- Follow the universal safeguards in administration of medications. (See Chapter 12.)
- *Always* check the patient's ID band before administering medications. If the patient does not have

an ID band, have a responsible person identify the patient for you and be sure to notify the ward clerk to obtain an ID band for the patient.

- Listen to the patient's comments and act on them, for example, "Not mine" or "Never took this before." Check carefully, then return to the patient with the result of your investigation. Failure to do this will result in loss of the patient's trust and confidence and may also result in a medication error.
- If a patient refuses a drug, find out why. Then implement nursing action to correct the situation. Chart the reason for refusal.
- Watch to make sure the patient takes the drugs. Stay until oral drugs are swallowed.
- Keep drugs within view at all times.
- Never leave any drug at the bedside stand unless hospital policy permits this. If a medication is left, inform the patient why the drug is ordered, how to take it, and what to expect. Check to determine if the drug was taken and record findings.

Charting

- Chart single doses, stat doses, and prn medications immediately and use the *exact time* when administered.
- Chart standing orders using *standard time* (e.g., tid).
- If it was necessary to hold a drug or the drug was refused, write the reason on the nurse's notes.
- Chart any nursing actions preliminary to administering drugs, for example, apical heart rate or blood pressure.

Evaluation

- Check for the expected effect of the drug. Did side effects or adverse effects occur? Perform indicated nursing actions. Record observations.

Error in Medication

- Report an error immediately to the charge nurse and the physician.
- Primary concern must be given to the patient.
- Error-in-medication forms should be filled out. Follow the physician's directions in caring for the patient.

Self-Test 1 *Give the information requested. Answers may be found at the end of the chapter.*

1. List at least ten kinds of information the nurse needs to know to give drugs safely.

____________________	____________________
____________________	____________________
____________________	____________________
____________________	____________________
____________________	____________________

(continued)

Self-Test 1 (continued)

2. List the five pregnancy categories used to identify the safety of drugs for the fetus and briefly define each.

3. Name the major organ for these drug activities.
   a. Absorption ______ c. Biotransformation ______
   b. Distribution ______ d. Excretion ______

4. Define:
   a. Tolerance ______
   b. Cumulation ______

5. List the four elements of negligence.
   ______, ______, ______, and ______

6. What is the standard by which a tort is judged?

7. List at least five positive actions to avoid liability.

(continued)

Self-Test 1 (continued)

8. List and briefly describe five ethical principles in drug therapy.

9. What are the seven elements of a correct medication order?

10. What action should a nurse take when an order is not clear?

Self-Test 2

Choose the correct answer. Answers will be found at the end of the chapter.

1. Two drugs are given for different reasons, but drug Y interferes with the excretion of drug X. The effect of drug X would be
   a. increased
   b. decreased
   c. unchanged
   d. stopped
2. Major biotransformation of drugs occurs in the
   a. lungs
   b. kidney
   c. liver
   d. urine
3. Toxicity to a drug is more likely to occur when
   a. elimination of the drug is rapid
   b. the drug is bound to the plasma protein, albumen
   c. the drug will not dissolve in the lipid layer of the cell
   d. the drug is free in the blood circulation
4. The term USP after a drug name indicates that the drug
   a. is made only in the United States
   b. meets official standards in the United States
   c. cannot be made by any other pharmaceutical company
   d. is registered by the U.S. Public Health Service
5. When an order is written to be administered "as needed" it is called a
   a. standing order
   b. prn order
   c. single order
   d. stat order

(continued)

Self-Test 2 (continued)

6. Signs of effectiveness of a drug are based on what information?
   a. Action and use
   b. Untoward effects
   c. Generic and trade names
   d. Drug interaction

7. Drug classification is an aid in understanding
   a. use of the drug
   b. drug idiosyncrasy
   c. the trade name
   d. the generic name

8. Names of many drugs include
   a. several generic, several trade names
   b. several generic, one trade name
   c. one generic, one trade name
   d. one generic, several trade names

9. Which pregnancy category is considered safe for the fetus?
   a. A
   b. B
   c. C
   d. D

10. What is the primary purpose of enteric-coating medications?
    a. Improve taste
    b. Delay absorption
    c. Code the drug for identification
    d. Make the drug easier to swallow

11. Which of the following drug preparations does *not* have to be shaken before pouring?
    a. Emulsion
    b. Gel
    c. Suspension
    d. Aqueous solution

12. Most oral drugs are absorbed in the
    a. mouth
    b. stomach
    c. small intestine
    d. large intestine

13. Nursing legal responsibilities associated with controlled substances include
    a. storage in a locked place
    b. assessing vital signs
    c. evaluating psychological response
    d. establishing automatic 24-hour stop orders

14. Characteristics of a Schedule II drug include
    a. accepted medical use with a high abuse potential
    b. medically accepted drug with low-dependence possibility
    c. no accepted use in patient care
    d. unlimited renewals

(continued)

Self-Test 2 (continued)

15. The responsibilities of the medication nurse in the hospital include

a. prescribing drugs
b. teaching patients
c. regulating automatic expiration times of drugs
d. preparing solutions

16. Under what condition does a nurse have a right to refuse to administer a drug?

a. The pharmacist ordered the drug.
b. The drug is manufactured by two different companies.
c. The drug is prescribed by a licensed physician.
d. The dose is within the range given in the *PDR*.

17. When administering medication in the hospital, the nurse should

a. chart medications before administering them
b. chart only those drugs that she or he personally gave the patient
c. chart all medications given for the day at one time
d. determine the best method for giving the drugs

18. Which of the following illustrates a medication error?

a. Administering a 10 AM dose at 10:20 AM
b. Giving 2 tablets of Gantrisin 500 mg when 1 g is ordered
c. Pouring 5 mL of cough syrup when 1 tsp is ordered
d. Giving digoxin IM when digoxin 0.25 mg is ordered

19. A nurse reads a medication order that is not clear. What action is indicated?

a. Ask the charge nurse to explain the order.
b. Ask a doctor at the nurses' station for help.
c. Check the *PDR* on the unit.
d. Check with the doctor who wrote the order.

20. Which nursing action is illegal?

a. Pouring medication from one stock bottle into another
b. Counting control drugs in the narcotic closet each shift
c. Labeling a vial of powder after dissolving it
d. Refusing to carry out an order that is confusing

ANSWERS

Self-Test 1

1. Generic/trade name; class; pregnancy category; dose and route; action; use; side/adverse effects; contraindications/precautions; interactions/incompatibilities; nursing implications; evaluation of effectiveness; patient teaching
2. **A.** No risk to fetus
   B. No adverse effects in animals, but no human studies
   C. Animals show adverse effects; calculated risk to fetus
   D. Fetal risk exists
   X. Absolute fetal abnormality
3. **a.** Small intestines
   b. blood
   c. liver
   d. kidney
4. **a.** Repeated administration of a drug increases microsomal enzyme activity in the liver. The drug is broken down more quickly and its effectiveness is decreased.
   b. Biotransformation is inhibited and the drug level remains high. Adverse effects are more likely to occur.
5. A claim that a nurse–patient relationship existed

   The nurse was required to meet a standard of care

   A claim that the nurse failed to meet that standard

   A claim that this resulted in injury
6. Whether the nurse exercised the degree of skill and care that a reasonably prudent nurse with similar training and experience, practicing in the same community, would exercise under the same or similar circumstances
7. Know policies and practices of the institution.

   Research unfamiliar drugs.

   Do not leave medicines at the bedside.

   Chart carefully.

   Listen to the patient's complaints.

   Check yourself (e.g., read labels three times).

   Label anything you dilute.

   Keep up to date.
8. Autonomy: freedom to decide based on knowledge with no constraint

   Truthfulness: truth telling that can create a dilemma. Is it absolute or is there a beneficient deceit?

   Beneficence: obligation to help others

   Nonmaleficence: do no harm

   Confidentiality: keep secrets

   Justice: rights of an individual
9. Patient's name and room; date; name of drug; dose; route; times of administration; doctor's signature
10. The nurse does not administer the drug and checks with the physician who wrote the order.

Self-Test 2

1. a	**5.** b	**9.** a	**13.** a	**17.** b
2. c	**6.** a	**10.** b	**14.** a	**18.** d
3. d	**7.** a	**11.** d	**15.** b	**19.** d
4. b	**8.** d	**12.** c	**16.** a	**20.** a

12 Administration Procedures

CONTENT TO MASTER

Universal precautions

Systems of administration

Guidelines for administration of drugs:

- Oral
- Parenteral—IM, SC, IV, IVPB, intradermal
- Topical—skin, mucous membranes

Throughout this text we have calculated dosages and studied information related to drug therapy. Finally, we arrive at the "how to" chapter—methods of administering drugs orally, parenterally, and topically. The adages "practice makes perfect" and "one picture is worth a thousand words" apply. Learning to administer medications is a skilled activity that requires practice, with supervision, to ensure correct technique.

Every institution has a standard procedure for administering medications, which depends on the way the drugs are dispensed—unit-dose, multidose containers, or a combination of the two. Institutional procedure may call for the use of a tray and medication tickets or for a mobile cart with medication sheets or the use of a computer printout.

Whatever the procedure is, follow it carefully. Do not look for shortcuts. *Methodology*—a step-by-step attention to detail—is the best safeguard to assure the patient's five rights. Research has proved time after time that most medication errors occur because the nurse violated procedural guidelines.

▼ UNIVERSAL PRECAUTIONS APPLIED TO ADMINISTRATION OF MEDICATIONS

In administering drugs, there is a risk of potential exposure to hepatitis B virus (HBV) and the human immunodeficiency virus (HIV) through contact of the nurse's skin or mucous membranes with patient blood, body fluids, or tissues. The Centers for Disease Control (CDC) in Atlanta advocate that *Universal Precautions be employed in caring for all patients and when handling equipment contaminated with blood or blood-streaked body fluids.*

The following points that are based on CDC guidelines are offered to aid in determining appropriate safeguards in giving medications. These points are *dependent upon the type of contact you have with patients.*

General Safeguards in Administering Medications

1. Oral medications: Handwashing is adequate unless there is a possibility of exposure to blood or body secretions.
2. Injections: Handwashing is adequate. If there is a possibility of exposure to blood or body secretions, gloves may be worn. Use nursing judgment. Carefully dispose of used sharps in a puncture-proof container. Never take your eyes from the sharp during the disposal process!
3. Heparin locks, intravenous catheters, and intravenous needles: Wear gloves when inserting or removing intravenous needles and catheters. The use of a clamp is recommended to hold contaminated IV needles and catheters being carried to a puncture-proof container.
4. Secondary administration sets or intravenous piggyback sets: Handwashing is adequate after removing this equipment from the main IV tubing because there is no direct exposure to blood or body secretions. Used needles should be placed in a puncture-proof container.
5. Application of medication to mucous membranes: Gloves should be worn (see the following guidelines in using gowns, masks, goggles).
6. Applications to skin: Exercise nursing judgment. Handwashing may be sufficient protection when applying such drug forms as transdermal patches. Use gloves when the patient's skin is not intact. Use gloves when applying lotions, ointments, or creams to areas of rash or to skin lesions.

Hands

1. Hands must be washed before preparing medications and after administering medications to each patient.
2. Hands must be washed *after* removing gloves, gowns, masks, goggles, and *before* leaving the room of any patient for whom they are used.
3. Hands must be washed immediately when soiled with patient blood or body fluids.
4. Hands must be washed *after* handling equipment soiled with blood or body fluids.

Gloves

1. Gloves must be worn for any direct ("hands-on") contact with patient's blood, bodily fluids, or secretions while administering medications.
2. Gloves must be worn when handling materials or equipment contaminated with blood or body fluids.
3. When gloves are used, they must be changed upon completion of procedures for each patient *and* between patients.

Gowns

When administering medications, gowns are required *only* if the nurse's clothing may become contaminated with a patient's blood or body fluids.

Masks

Masks *are not required* except in the following instances:

1. The patient is placed on *strict* or *respiratory* isolation precautions.
2. Carrying out a medication procedure may cause blood or body fluids to splash directly onto the nurse's face.

Goggles (Protective Eyewear)

Goggles should be worn during the performance of any medication procedure in which the nurse would be in *extremely close contact* with the patient and there is possibility of splashing or aerolization of blood or blood-tinged fluids into the nurse's eyes or mucous membranes (e.g., use of power spray apparatus).

Management of Used Needles and Sharps

1. All used needles, syringes, sharps, and IV catheters must be placed in appropriate, labeled, puncture-proof containers.
2. Do not break, bend, or recap needles after use. Place needles immediately into a puncture-proof container.
3. Exercise caution in removing heparin locks, intravenous catheters, and intravenous needles. Gloves should be worn. The use of a clamp is advisable to hold the used IV needle being transported to a puncture-proof container. *Do not remove the IV needle from the IV tubing by hand; use a clamp or use the needle unlocking device on the sharps container.*
4. If *reusable* needles and syringes are employed, the needle should be separated from the syringe with a clamp. *Never manipulate a used needle by hand.* Place the needle and syringe in appropriate puncture-proof containers for sterilization. *It is strongly recommended that disposable needles and syringes be used.*
5. Never take your eyes from the sharps container during the disposal process.

Management of Materials Other Than Needles and Sharps

Paper cups, plastic cups, and other equipment not contaminated with blood or body fluids may be discarded according to routine hospital procedure. In cases of *strict* or *respiratory* isolation precautions, follow the protocol established by the institution.

Management of Nurse Contaminated With Blood or Body Fluids

The nurse who is exposed to blood or blood-streaked body fluids of any patient through a personal needlestick or injury or through laceration of the skin should immediately squeeze the area if this is indicated, wash the area with soap and water, and scrub the area with povidone–iodine (Betadine), alcohol 70%, or another acceptable antiseptic. If mucous membrane exposure occurs, flush the exposed areas with copious amounts of warm water. The protocol established by the health care institution for management of needlestick injury or accidental exposure to blood or body fluids should be followed.

▼ SYSTEMS OF ADMINISTRATION

The ticket system is used when drugs are dispensed in multidose containers. Drugs are prepared in a medication room and carried to the patient on a tray. When unit-dose packaging is available, drugs are placed in individual patient drawers on a mobile cart. The cart is wheeled into the patient's room and medications are prepared at the bedside for administration.

Ticket System

In this system, a medication order is transferred to three places: a medication ticket, the patient's medication sheet, and the patient's Kardex file, which contains the nursing care plan.

Tickets for all patients are kept in a central location. The nurse sorts them according to time of administration. Each ticket is compared with the Kardex entry. If there is a discrepancy, the nurse checks the original order on the patient's chart. When all tickets have been verified, the nurse obtains the keys to the medication room, washes his/her hands, and enters the room. Quiet and concentration are essential.

The first patient's tickets are separated and placed together in a pile one on top of another, so that only one ticket is visible at a time. The ticket is read, the medication is located, and the label is verified with the ticket (first check).

The dose on the ticket is compared with the label, and the amount of drug is calculated and poured (second check).

Before discarding the unit dose packet or returning the container to the shelf, the order and the label are read again, and the poured dose is verified (third check).

EXAMPLE I want digoxin 0.125 mg. I have a stock of scored tablets of digoxin 0.25 mg. I pour ½ tablet.

The medication is placed on a tray with the ticket in front to identify it (Fig. 12-1). When all medications have been prepared, the nurse locks the door to the medication room and proceeds to each patient.

The patient is greeted and the tray is placed on a flat surface within the nurse's view. The tray must never be out of sight.

The nurse picks up the patient's tickets and medicines. The name on the ticket is compared with the patient's ID band. Any required nursing assessment is carried out. For example, an apical heart rate is required before digoxin can be administered. The nurse will make a decision to withhold or to give the drug on the basis of this assessment. The nurse administers the drugs, watches to be sure the patient has taken them, carries out comfort measures as necessary, washes his/her hands, picks up the tray, and moves to the next patient.

When all medications have been given, the tray is cleaned and put away and the medication tickets are brought to the nurse's station and used to record doses on each patient's chart.

There are several disadvantages to this system. Every order must be transcribed to three different places. Each time the order is rewritten an error is possible. Tickets may be lost or misplaced. An error may occur in choosing the stock. The tickets may become mixed, so that the wrong patient receives a medication. Medications that require assessment must be tagged in some way to identify them. It is time-consuming to locate the chart of each patient.

Mobile-Cart System

Compared with the ticket system, the mobile-cart system has many advantages. The pharmacist dispenses unit-dose medications directly to the patient's drawer (Fig. 12-2). Each drawer is labeled with the patient's name. The cart contains all the equipment the nurse might require to administer medications.

When a drug is ordered, the nurse transcribes the order to one place—the patient's medication sheet, found in a medication book on the cart. This book contains the medication sheets for every patient on the unit.

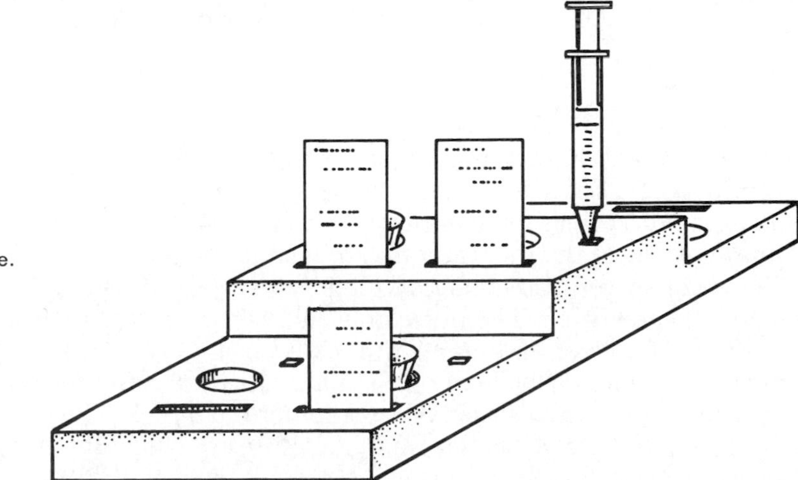

Figure 12-1
A medication tray with tickets and drugs in place.

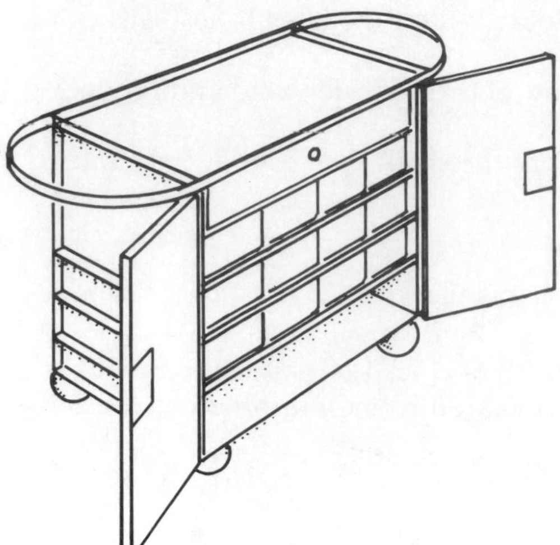

Figure 12-2
A mobile cart: Each drawer is labeled with a patient's name. Unit-dose drugs are placed in the drawers by the pharmacist. The nurse administers the drugs.

When it is time to administer medications, the nurse washes his/her hands and rolls the cart to the bedside of the first patient, unlocks the cart, and opens the medication book to the first patient's medication sheet.

The sheet is checked for special nursing actions required before giving medication. These are carried out, the results are recorded, and the decision is made to withhold or to administer the medication.

The patient's drawer is placed on the top of the cart. The nurse reads each medication order, starting with the first medication listed. When a dose is to be given, the nurse chooses the unit dose from the drawer and compares the label with the order (first check).

The dose is computed after comparing the order with the unit measure, the unit dose is opened, and the amount is poured (second check).

The unit-dose label and the order are again read and the dose is verified (third check). The unit-dose package is then discarded in a waste receptacle on the cart. When all the patient's medications have been prepared, the nurse reads the name on the medicine sheet, checks the patient's ID band, and administers the drugs. The nurse remains with the patient until the medications are taken, provides any comfort measures, washes his/her hands, and returns to the cart to chart the drugs administered. The patient's drawer is replaced and the cart is rolled to the next patient. When all medications have been administered, the mobile cart is returned to its designated area.

This system has several advantages. There are two professionals involved in checking the medication in the drawer—the pharmacist and the nurse. All the medication sheets are together on the cart. This is time-saving. Nursing assessment can be carried out and results charted before any medication is poured. The drugs can be signed for immediately after administration.

Note, however, that in both systems, the nurse checks the label three times—when choosing the drug, when calculating and pouring the dose, and before replacing the stock.

Computer Printouts

Institutions may have computerized medication procedures. Doctors input orders directly on the computer. The order is received in the pharmacy, where it is added to the patient's drug profile. The nursing unit receives the computer printout listing the medications and times of administration. The printout replaces the medication administration record (MAR).

There are several advantages to this system. Neither the nurse nor the pharmacist has to interpret the doctor's handwriting. The nurse does not have to transfer the written orders to an MAR, thus reducing the chance for error and saving time. Moreover, a computer check will identify possible interactions among the patient's medications and alert the nurse and the pharmacist.

Figure 12-3 is an example of a computerized MAR. The patient's name, ID number, room, date of admission, age, diagnosis, sex, and attending physician are printed at the top. The administration period

```
Continental Healthcare Sys: JONES, SALLY            436-1  4RED : Diagnosis: HYPERTENSION
  Medication              : Patient ID: 345673        Age:64 :            CHF
Administration            : Admitted: 2/21/94         Sex: F : Allergies  PCN
    Record                : Physician: MARSHANE              :
                          : Patient Ref. #                   : Note:
________________________________________________________________________________________
ADMINISTRATION PERIOD   07:00 2/21/94 to 06:59 2/22/94:
________________________________________________________________________________________
No.:Medication                     :START    :STOP    : 07:00 to 15:00: 15:01 to 23:00: 23:01 to 06:59
________________________________________________________________________________________
SCH: LASIX 40 MG/UD 1 TABLET       :09:00    :  :     :0900           :               :
  1: 1 TAB             QD   PO     :02/21/94:  / /                                
FIL:                               :         :        :               :               :
________________________________________________________________________________________
SCH: LANOXIN 0.25 MG/UD 1 TABLET   :09:00    :12:00   :0900
  2: 1 TAB             QD   PO  PUL:02/21/94:2/26/94:
FIL:
________________________________________________________________________________________
SCH: ALDOMET 259 MG/UD 1 TABLET    :19:00    :  :     :               :               :
  3: 1 TABLET          QID  PO     :02/21/94:  / /    :               :1900           :2400
FIL:                               :         :        :               :               :
________________________________________________________________________________________
SCH: APRESOLINE 25 MG UD 1 TABLET  :21:00    :  :     :               :2100           :
  4: 1 TAB             BID  PO     :02/21/94: / /     :               :               :
FIL:                               :         :        :               :               :
________________________________________________________________________________________
SCH: GARAMYCIN OPH SOLN 5 ML BOTTLE:09:00    :17:50   :0900
  6: 5 ML BOTTLE          OPHTHAL  :02/21/94:2/21/94:                 :               :
FIL: 2 DROPS QD                    :         :        :               :               :
________________________________________________________________________________________


________________________________________________________________________________________
PRN: TYLENOL E.S. 500 MG/UD 1 CAPULE:16:00   :  :     :               :               :
  5: 1 CAP             Q4H   PO    :02/21/94:         :               :               :
FIL:                               :         : / /    :               :               :
________________________________________________________________________________________
PRN: VASELINE(USE:PETROLATUM) REF. :09:00    :        :               :               :
  7: APPLY TO CHAPPED  PRN  TOPICAL:02/21/94: / /     :               :               :
FIL: AREAS
________________________________________________________________________________________
SIGNATURE                 :INITIALS : SIGNATURE      : INITIALS  : SIGNATURE     :INITIALS: SIGNATURE
__________________________:_________:________________:___________:_______________:________:__________

__________________________:_________:________________:___________:_______________:________:__________
          JONES, SALLY                   345678
```

Figure 12-3
A sample 24-hour computerized medication record. Scheduled drugs are listed at the top of the sheet and PRN orders at the bottom. Military time is used. The nurse initials the boxes to indicate the drug was administered and signs at the bottom of the sheet. (Courtesy of Continental Healthcare System)

for this record covers 24 hours using military time. Note that the order for Aldomet was written at 7 PM (19:00). Although it is a qid order, only two doses can be administered because of the lateness of the time. Apresoline was ordered at 9 PM (21:00). One dose will be given. There are two prn orders that have no time indicated; the nurse will exercise judgment whether to administer. The bottom of the printout has places for the nurses' signatures.

▼ ROUTES OF ADMINISTRATION

Oral Route

Regardless of the system used to pour the medications, the procedure for administering drugs contains specific steps. The nurse greets the patient orally and checks the ID band. The patient is assisted to a sitting position. The patient should be alert and able to swallow. Oral solids are given first, together with a full glass of water whenever possible, followed by oral liquid medications. The nurse watches to be sure the patient has swallowed all of the drugs before leaving. The paper and plastic cups may be discarded according to routine hospital procedure, unless the patient is on strict or respiratory isolation. For this, special isolation bags are utilized. The nurse makes the patient comfortable, washes his/her hands, and charts the doses given.

Special considerations for oral administration include the following:

- If the patient is NPO (nothing by mouth), check with the doctor to determine if oral medication can be administered with a small amount of water. The doctor may not wish to withhold certain drugs (for example, an anticonvulsant for a patient with epilepsy).
- When a patient refuses a drug, find out why, chart the reason, and initiate action to correct the situation.
- Solid stock medications are poured first into the container lid and then into a paper cup, using medical asepsis. The medication is not touched. Several solids may be combined in the cup, but each medication should first be poured into a separate cup until the third check is completed. Unit dose medications should be checked three times before the package container is discarded.
- Medical asepsis is followed to break a scored tablet. This means that clean, not sterile, technique is required. One method is to place the tablet in a paper towel, fold the towel over and, with thumbs and index fingers in apposition, break the tablet along the score line. Tablets that are not scored should not be broken.
- Check expiration dates on all labels.
- If the patient has difficulty swallowing solids, first determine if the medication is available in a liquid form. Enteric- and film-coated tablets should not be crushed. Ordinarily, capsules should not be opened. Check with the pharmacist for alternative forms. If a capsule can be opened, mix the drug with a small amount of applesauce, custard, or other vehicle which will make the medication more palatable and easy to swallow.
- If a medication can be crushed, it is best to use a "pill" crusher, with the medication placed between two paper cups. If a mortar and pestle is used, be sure it is cleaned before and after crushing so there is no residue. If no equipment is available, place the tablet in a paper towel and use the edge of a bottle or other hard surface to crush the drug. A crushed drug may be mixed with water or semisolids, such as applesauce or custard, for ease in swallowing.
- Some drugs are best taken on an empty stomach; others may be taken with food. The nurse should be aware of foods or fluids that may be ingested with the drug and of those that are contraindicated.
- Check patients for allergies to drugs. This should be a routine procedure.
- The nurse should be knowledgeable about food–drug and drug–drug interactions and act to safeguard the patient.
- Failure to shake some liquid medications can result in a wrong dose. The drug settles to the bottom, and only the weak diluent is poured.
- Pour liquids at eye level, with the thumb indicating the meniscus. In pouring liquids, the label should be up so it will not be stained. Wipe the lip of the bottle with a paper towel before recapping.
- Note the presence of an unusual color change or precipitate in a liquid. If such a change is present, do not use. Send the container to the pharmacy with a note indicating your observation.
- Check references to determine how to disguise liquids that are distasteful or irritating. Two possibilities are to mix with juice or give through a straw after diluting well. Liquid iron preparations stain the teeth and are taken through a straw placed in the back of the mouth. Tinctures are always diluted.
- Liquid cough mixtures are not diluted. They have a secondary soothing (demulcent) effect on the mucous membranes in addition to the antitussive action.
- The oral route is the least expensive, the safest, and the easiest to take.

Parenteral Route

Medications may be given by the IM, SC, IVPB, or IV route or intradermally. The parenteral route is used when a drug cannot be given orally, when it is necessary to obtain a rapid systemic effect, or when a drug would be rendered ineffective or destroyed by the oral route.

Choosing the Site

The following areas should be avoided: bony prominences, large blood vessels, nerves, sensitive areas, bruises, hardened areas, abrasions, and inflamed areas. The site for IM injections should be able to accept 3 mL, rotate sites when repeated injections are given.

Preparation of the Skin

Cleanse the site with an alcohol pad while using a circular motion from the center out. Grasp the area firmly between the thumb and forefinger and insert the needle with a dartlike motion (Fig. 12-4). If the area is obese, the skin may be spread rather than pinched together.

Syringes for Injection

The most common syringe used for injections is a standard 3-mL size, marked in minims and in milliliters (mL or cc) to the nearest tenth. The precision (tuberculin) syringe is marked in half-minims and milliliters to the nearest hundredth. There are two insulin syringes: a regular 1-mL size marked to the U 100, and a 0.5-mL size (low-dose) insulin syringe marked to U 50.

Needles for Injections

Needles are chosen for their gauge and their length. *Gauge* is the diameter of the needle opening. The principle is: the higher the gauge number, the finer the needle.

The 28-gauge needle on the insulin syringe is the finest needle currently available for routine injections. Numbers 25, 26, 28 are used for SC injections for adults and for IM injections for children and emaciated patients. Numbers 23 and 22 are used for IM injections; 20 and 21 for IV therapy; and 15 and 18 for blood transfusions.

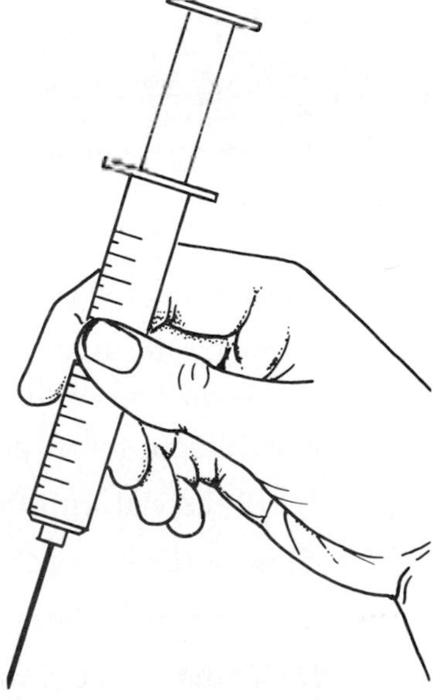

Figure 12-4
An injection is administered with a quick dartlike motion into taut skin that has been spread or bunched together.

Angle of Insertion

Intramuscular. For IM injection the syringe should be held at a right angle to the skin and the injection given at a 90-degree angle.

Subcutaneous. For SC injections the syringe should be held at a 45-degree angle when the needle is inserted. Some SC injections may be administered at a 90-degree angle if the subcutaneous layer of fat is thick and the needle is short. Care must be exercised to reach the correct site. When in doubt use the 45-degree angle. Intramuscular sites have a good blood supply and absorption is rapid; subcutaneous sites have a poor blood supply, and absorption is prolonged.

Intradermal. A 26-gauge or other fine needle is used for skin testing for allergy and tuberculosis.

Preparing the Dose

Ordinarily, to prevent incompatibility of drugs only one medication should be drawn up in a syringe. When two drugs are given in one syringe, follow the procedure for mixing after determining that the drugs are compatible.

Adding Air to a Syringe

Some nurses add 0.1 to 0.2 mL air to the syringe after the dose is obtained and before giving the injection. The air bubble rises to the top of the barrel and is injected last. The air acts as a seal to prevent medication oozing to the skin from the injection tract and empties the needle of medication. This procedure is required in giving a Z tract injection; otherwise it is optional. Institutional policy should be followed.

Drugs That Are Liquids in Vials

1. Cleanse the top of the vial with an alcohol sponge.
2. Draw the amount of air equivalent to the amount of solution desired into the syringe.
3. Inject the needle through the rubber diaphragm into the vial.
4. Expel air from the syringe into the vial. This increases the pressure in the vial and makes it easier to withdraw medication.
5. The medication can be drawn up in one of two ways (Fig. 12-5). Invert the vial and draw up the desired amount into the syringe, or leave the vial on the table and pull up the medication.
6. Withdraw the needle quickly from the vial.
7. The rubber diaphragm will seal.

Drugs That Are Powders in Vials

1. Cleanse the top of the vial with an alcohol sponge.
2. Draw up the amount of calculated diluent from a vial of distilled water or normal saline for injection. Follow pharmaceutical directions if another solvent is indicated.
3. Add diluent to the powder and roll the vial between your hands to dissolve the powder.
4. Label the vial with the solution made, your initials, and the date.
5. Cleanse the top of the vial again.
6. Draw up the amount of air equivalent to the amount of solution you desire into the syringe.
7. Inject the needle through the rubber diaphragm into the vial.

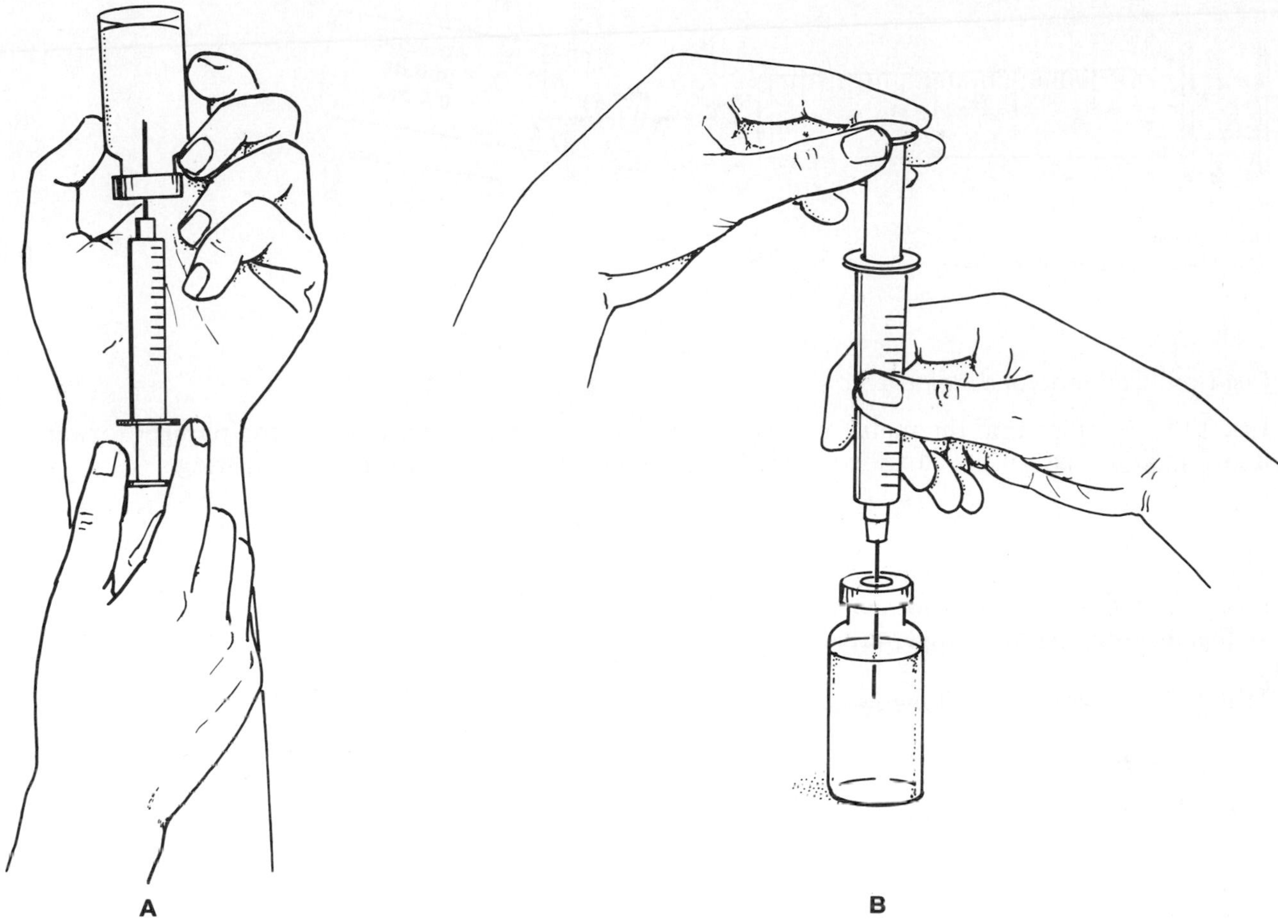

Figure 12-5
Two methods of withdrawing medication from a vial: **(A)** Invert the vial and draw up the desired amount into the syringe. **(B)** Leave the vial on the table and pull up the medication.

8. Expel the air into the vial. Invert the vial and draw up the desired amount of medication into the syringe.
9. Check directions for storage of any remaining drug.

Note: When the whole amount of powder contained in a vial is needed for an IVPB medication, a reconstitution device may be used to dilute the powder without using a syringe (see Chapter 9, Figure 9-8).

Drugs in Glass Ampules

1. Tap the top of the ampule with your finger to clear out any drug.
2. Place an opened alcohol pad around the neck of the ampule.
3. Hold the ampule sideways.
4. Place thumbs in apposition above and index fingers in apposition below the ampule neck.
5. Press down with thumbs to break the ampule.
6. Insert the syringe needle into the solution, tilt the ampule, and withdraw the dose (Fig. 12-6). *Important: Do not add air before removing dose.* This will cause medication to spray from the ampule.

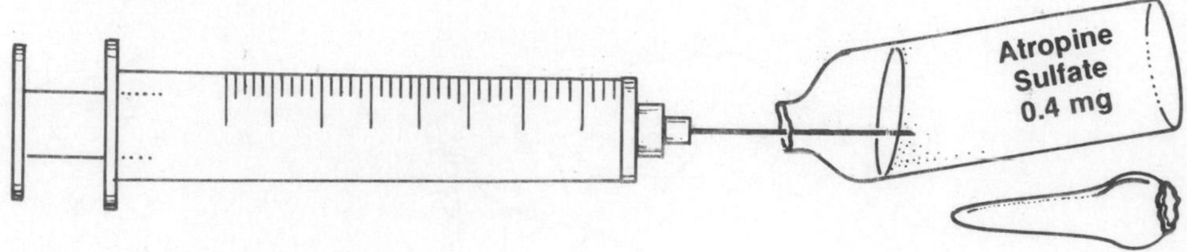

Figure 12-6
Withdrawing medication from an ampule.

Unit-Dose Cartridge and Holder

Insert the cartridge into the metal or plastic holder and screw into place. Move the plunger forward until it engages the shaft of the cartridge. Twist the plunger until it is locked into the cartridge.

Unit-Dose Prefilled Syringes

The medication is in the syringe. Some prefilled syringes are simple and require no action other than removing the needle cover; others are packaged for compactness and directions are given to prepare the syringe for use. These syringes are disposable.

Mixing Two Medications in One Syringe

General Principles

1. Determine that the drugs are compatible by consulting a standard reference.
2. When in doubt about compatibility, prepare medications separately and administer into different injection sites.
3. When medications are in a vial and an ampule, draw up the medication from the vial first, then add the medication from the ampule. Discard any medication left in the ampule.
4. In preparing two types of insulin in one syringe, the vial containing *regular insulin must be drawn first* into the syringe. Regular insulin has not been adulterated with protein as have other insulins such as protamine zinc insulin.

Method

1. Clean both vials with an alcohol pad.
2. Choose one vial as *primary.* For example, with vials of a narcotic and a nonnarcotic, the narcotic is primary. With two insulins, regular insulin is primary.
3. Inject air into the *second* vial equal to the medication to be withdrawn. Do not permit the needle to touch the medication.
4. Inject air into the *primary* vial equal to the amount to be withdrawn and withdraw medication in the usual way. Be sure there are no air bubbles.
5. Insert the needle into the *second* vial. Do not touch the plunger while doing this, to avoid pushing the primary medication into the second vial.
6. *Slowly* withdraw the needed amount of drug from the second vial. The two medications are now combined.
7. Remove the needle from the second vial and cap it. *Note:* Some authorities suggest that the needle be changed after withdrawing medication from the primary vial. Since this may result in air bubbles, be careful in withdrawing the second medication to obtain an accurate dose.

Identifying the Injection Site—Adults

Intramuscular

Common sites are dorsogluteal, ventrogluteal, vastus lateralis, and deltoid.

Dorsogluteal Site. The dorsogluteal site is composed of the thick gluteal muscles of the buttocks.

Position: The patient may be prone or in a side-lying position with both buttocks fully exposed.

Location of injection site: The area must be chosen very carefully to avoid striking the sciatic nerve, major blood vessels, or bone. The landmarks of the buttocks are the crest of the posterior ilium as the superior boundary and the inferior gluteal fold as the lower boundary. The exact site can be identified in either of two ways:

1. *Diagonal landmark* (Fig. 12-7): Find the posterior superior iliac spine and the greater trochanter of the femur. Draw an imaginary diagonal line between these two points, and give the injection lateral and superior to that line 1 to 2 inches below the iliac crest to avoid hitting the iliac bone. Should you hit the bone, withdraw the needle slightly and continue the procedure. This method is preferred since all the landmarks are bony prominences.
2. *Quadrant landmark* (Fig. 12-8): Divide the buttocks into imaginary quadrants. The vertical line extends from the crest of the ilium to the gluteal fold. The horizontal line extends from the medial fold of the buttock to the lateral aspect of the buttock. Locate the upper aspect of the upper-outer quadrant. The injection should be given in this area, 1 to 2 inches below the crest of the ilium, to avoid hitting bone. The crest of the ilium must be palpated for precise site selection.

Ventrogluteal Site. The ventral part of the gluteal muscle has no large nerves or blood vessels and less fat. It is identified by finding the greater trochanter, anterior superior iliac spine, and the iliac crest. The nurse should be standing by the patient's knee. Use the hand opposite to the patient's leg (e.g., left leg, right hand). Open an alcohol pad. Place the palm of the hand on the greater trochanter. Point the index finger toward the anterior superior iliac spine. Point the middle finger toward the iliac crest. The injection is given in the center of the triangle between the middle finger and the index finger (Fig. 12-9). Place the alcohol pad over the site. Remove the hand and proceed with the injection in the usual manner. Use the alcohol pad to prep the area from the center out.

Position: The patient may be supine, lying on the side, sitting, or standing.

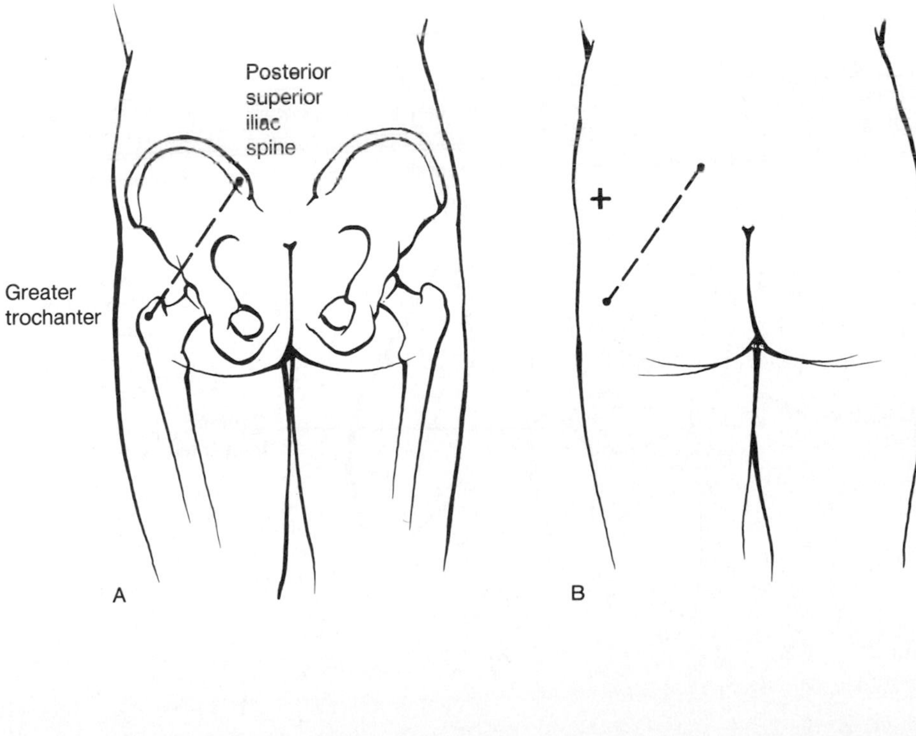

Figure 12-7
Identification of the dorsogluteal site using a diagonal between bony prominences **(A)**. The cross indicates the injection area **(B)**.

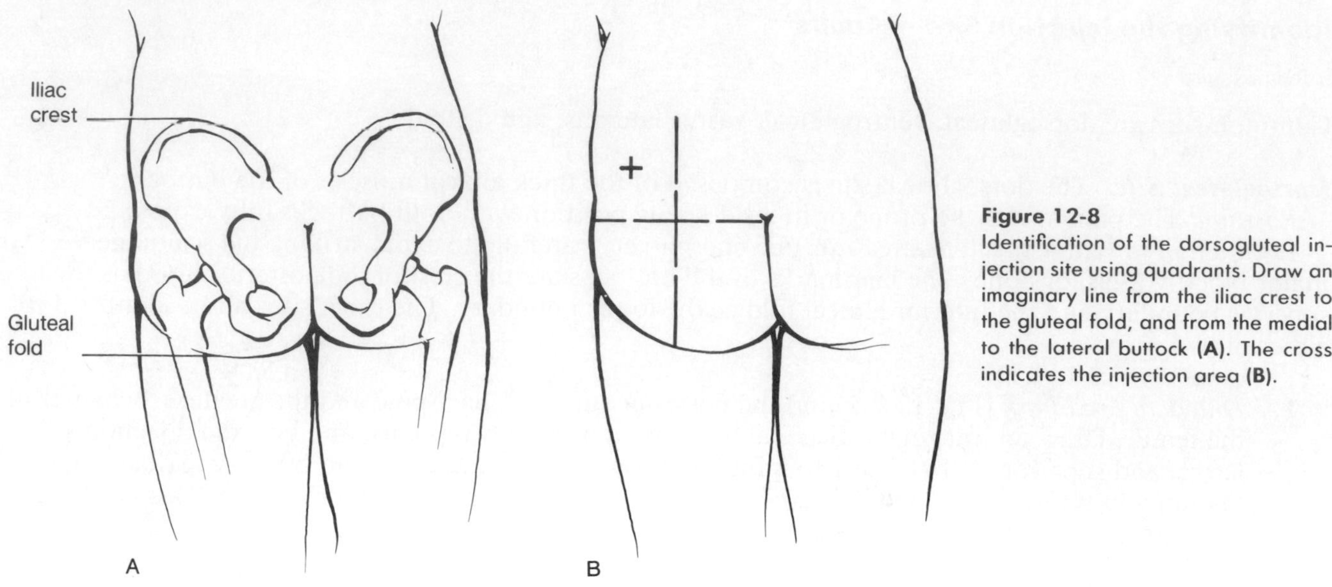

Figure 12-8
Identification of the dorsogluteal injection site using quadrants. Draw an imaginary line from the iliac crest to the gluteal fold, and from the medial to the lateral buttock **(A)**. The cross indicates the injection area **(B)**.

Vastus Lateralis Site: Lateral Thigh. Measure one hand's width below the greater trochanter and one hand's width above the knee (Fig. 12-10). Give the injection in the lateral thigh. Ask the patient to point the big toe to the center of his body. This relaxes the vastus muscle.

Position: The patient may be supine, lying on the side, or standing.

Deltoid Site. The deltoid muscle on the lateral aspect of the upper arm is a small muscle close to the radial and brachial arteries. *It should be used for IM injections only if specifically ordered,* and no more than 2 mL should be injected. The boundaries are the lower edge of the acromion process (shoulder bone) and the axilla (armpit) (Fig. 12-11). Give the injection into the lateral arm between these two points and about 2 inches below the acromion process.

Position: The patient may be sitting or lying down.

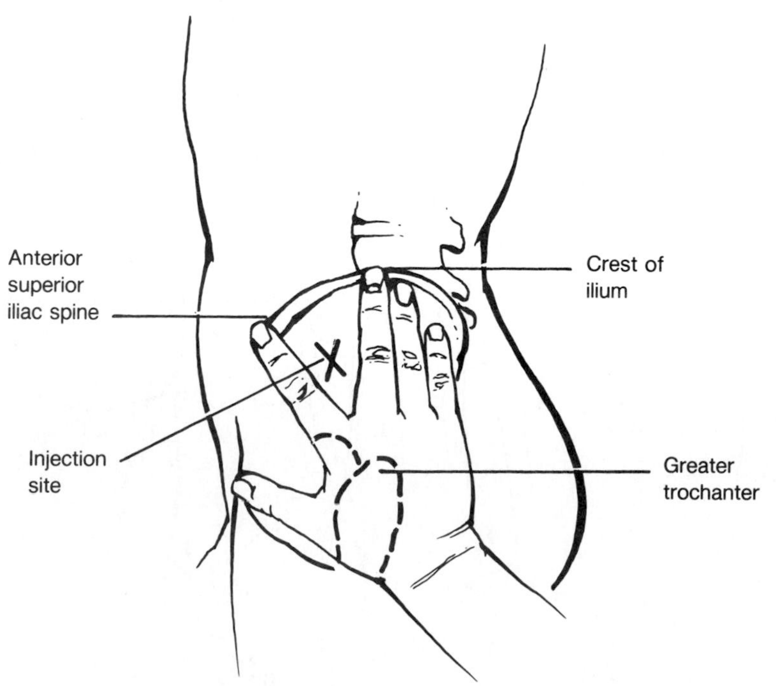

Figure 12-9
The ventrogluteal site for IM injections. The cross indicates the injection site.

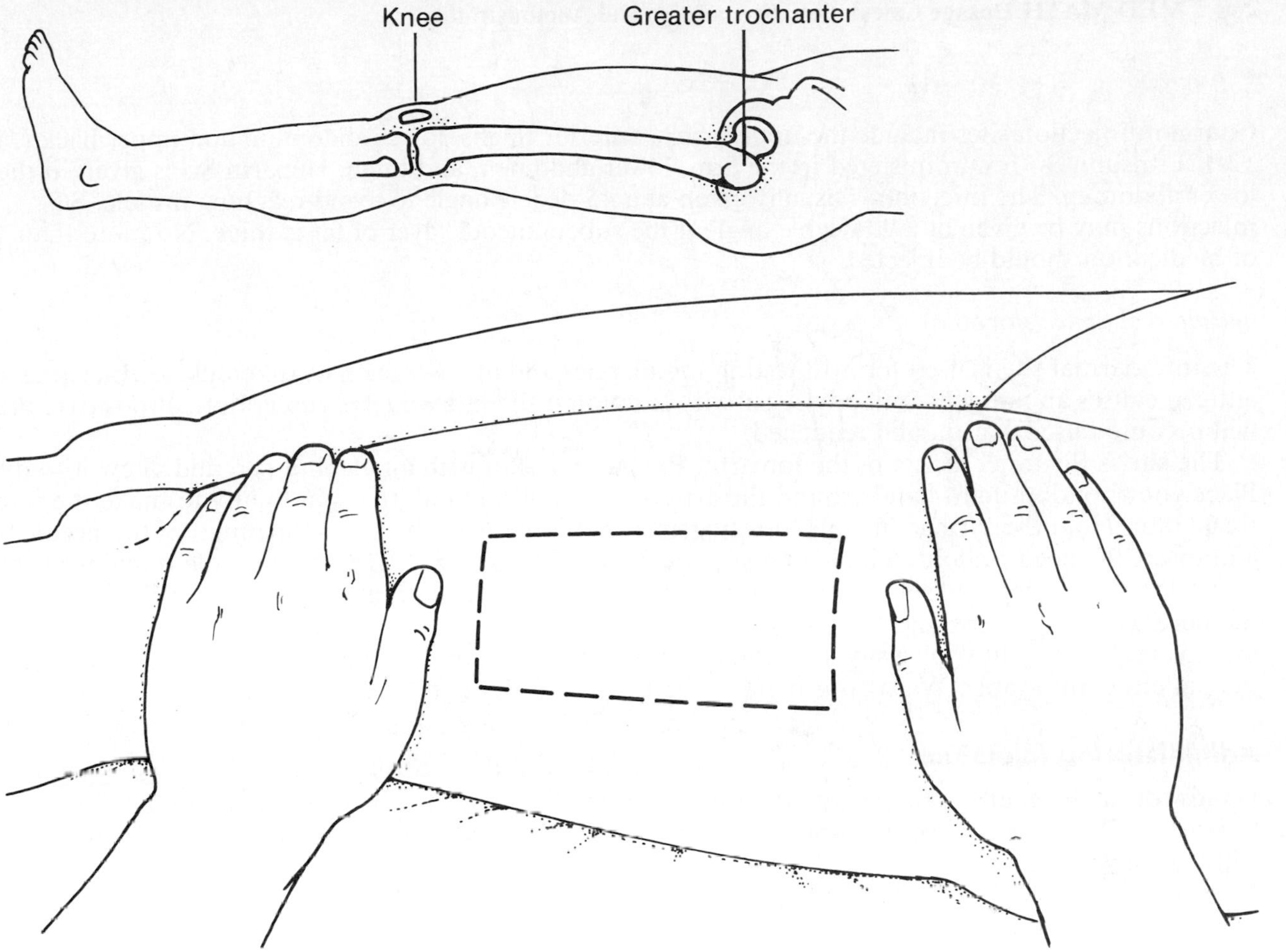

Knee
Greater trochanter

Figure 12-10
Vastus lateralis injection site.

Acromion
process
Axilla

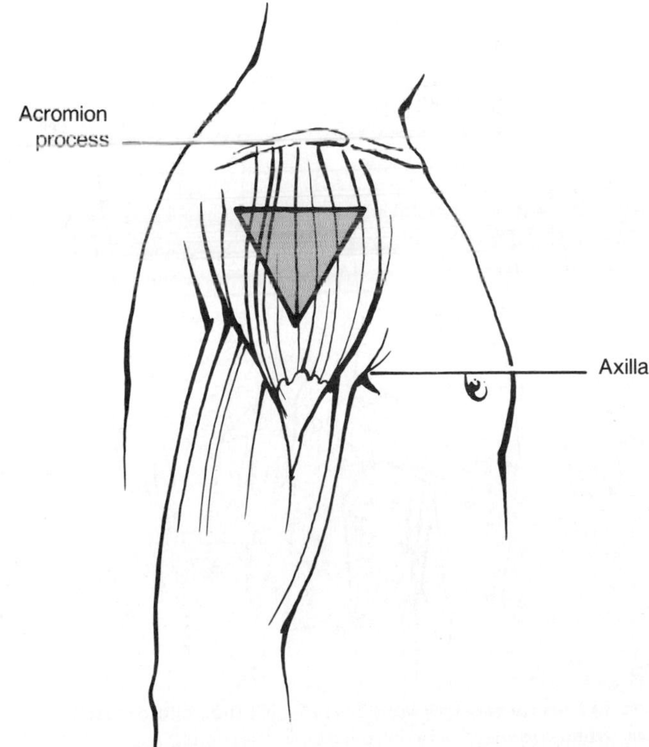

Figure 12-11
The deltoid muscle site for IM injections. The triangle indicates the injection site.

Subcutaneous

Common injection sites include the upper arms, anterior thighs, lower abdomen, and upper back (Fig. 12-12). Insulin SC is administered in the arm, lower abdomen, and thigh. Heparin SC is given in the lower abdomen. The injection is usually given at a 45-degree angle to avoid reaching muscle. SC injections may be given at a 90-degree angle if the subcutaneous layer of fat is thick. No more than 1 mL of medication should be injected.

Intradermal (Intracutaneous)

The intradermal site is used for skin testing for allergies and diseases such as tuberculosis. Injecting an antigen causes an antigen–antibody sensitivity reaction if the individual is susceptible. If positive, the area will become raised, warm, and reddened.

The site is the inner aspect of the forearm. Prepare the skin with an alcohol pad and allow it to dry. Place your nondominant hand around the arm from below and pull the skin tightly to make the forearm tissue taut. Hold the syringe in your four fingers and thumb, with the bevel (opening) of the needle up, and insert the needle about 1/8 inch almost parallel to the skin (Fig. 12-13). The needle remains visible under the skin. Inject the solution such that it raises a small wheal (a raised bump or a blister). Remove the needle and allow the injection site to dry. *Do not massage the skin.* An alcohol pad or dry gauze pad may be used gently to wipe away any residue. Place the needle and syringe in a sharps container. Make the patient comfortable. Wash your hands. Chart the procedure.

Administering Injections

Handwashing is an adequate safeguard. Gloves are optional and may be worn. The Centers for Disease Control (CDC) does not require gloves as long as an alcohol pad is used as a barrier to prevent contact with blood.

1. Identify the patient verbally.
2. Check ID band.

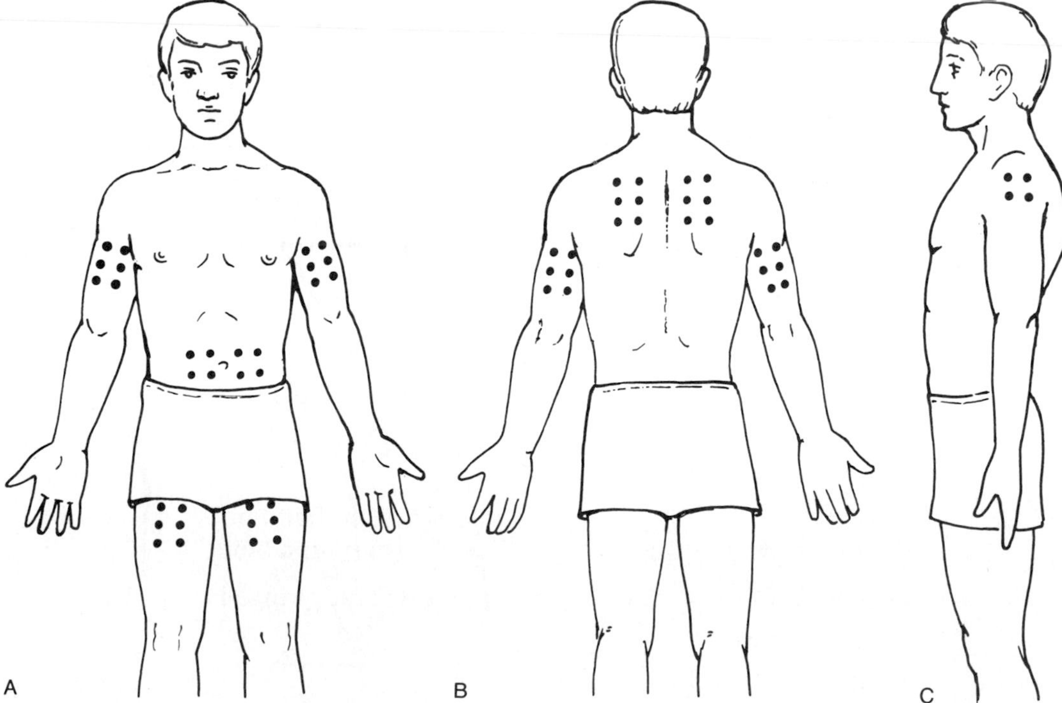

Figure 12-12
(A, B) Sites for subcutaneous injection. **(C)** The deltoid muscle may be used for subcutaneous injections or, when ordered, small intramuscular injections.

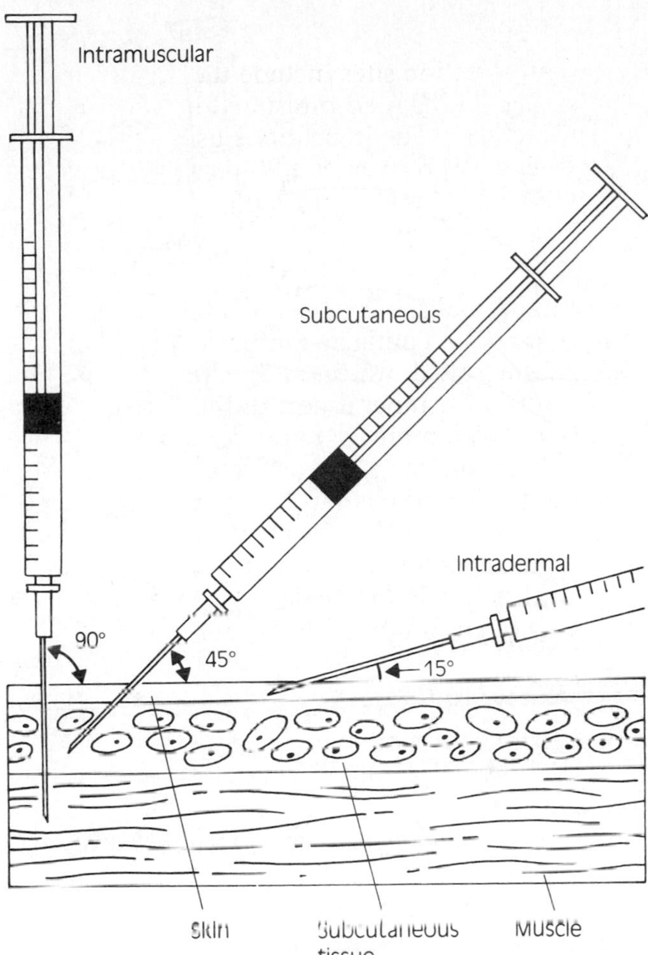

Figure 12-13
Comparison of angles of insertion for intramuscular, subcutaneous, and intradermal injection. (Taylor C, Lilles C, LeMone P. *Fundamentals of Nursing, ed 2.* Philadelphia: J. B. Lippincott, 1993, p. 1233)

3. Perform any assessment before injection (e.g., vital signs, apical rate, site integrity).
4. Explain the procedure to the patient.
5. Ask the patient where the last injection was given. The sites should be rotated.
6. Prepare the area with an alcohol pad, using a circular motion from the center out.
7. Place the alcohol pad between your fingers or lay it on the patient's skin above the site.
8. Remove the needle cover.
9. Make the skin taut by mounding the tissue between thumb and index finger or by spreading it firmly.
10. Dart the needle in quickly (Fig. 12-14).
11. Hold the barrel with your nondominant hand and with your dominant hand pull the plunger back. This is termed *aspiration* and is done to be sure the needle is not in a blood vessel.
12. If blood enters the syringe, withdraw the needle, discard the needle and syringe into a sharps container, and prepare another injection.
13. If no blood is aspirated, inject the medication slowly.
14. Remove the needle quickly.
15. Press down on the area with the alcohol pad or a dry gauze pad to inhibit bleeding.

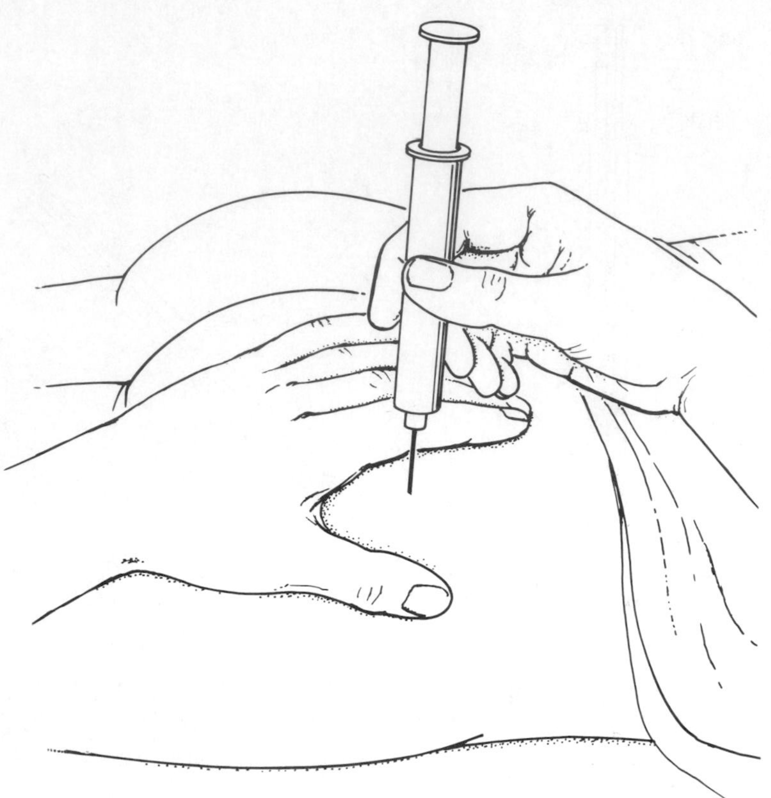

Figure 12-14
Darting an IM injection at the dorsogluteal site.

16. *Do not recap the needle.* Dispose of needle and syringe in a sharps container. Make the patient comfortable. Wash hands. Chart the medication.

Special Injection Techniques

Subcutaneous Heparin

Heparin is an anticoagulant, and care must be taken to minimize tissue trauma. Slow bleeding at the site of the injection can cause bruising. Several changes in routine injection technique are indicated. The injection is given with a fine (25-gauge) ½-inch needle into the lower abdominal fold at least 2 inches from the umbilicus.

1. Change the needle after drawing up the dose to prevent leakage along the tract.
2. Allow the skin to dry after prepping with an alcohol pad.
3. Bunch the tissue with the nondominant hand to a depth of at least ½ inch.
4. Inject the needle at a 90-degree angle.
5. *Do not aspirate.* This minimizes tissue damage.
6. Inject the medication slowly.
7. Hold the needle in place for 10 seconds.
8. Remove the needle quickly.
9. *Do not massage the area.* If bleeding is noted, apply pressure with a dry gauze pad or alcohol pad for 1 to 2 minutes.

Z-Track Technique for Intramuscular Injections

Some medications, such as iron dextran (Imferon) and hydroxyzine (Vistazine), are irritating to the tissues and can stain the skin. The Z-track method may be used at the dorsogluteal site to prevent seepage of the medication into the needle tract and onto the skin.

1. After preparing the medication, change the needle to prevent leakage along the tract.
2. Add 0.2 mL of air to the syringe. As medication is injected the air will rise to the top of the syringe and will be administered last. This will seal off the medication and prevent its leakage to the skin.
3. Prepare the patient and the site in the usual manner.
4. Use the fingers of your nondominant hand to retract the tissue to the side. *Hold this position during the injection* (Fig. 12-15).
5. Inject as usual at a 90-degree angle. Be sure to aspirate before giving this injection.
6. Count 10 seconds after giving the injection.
7. Remove the needle quickly.
8. Remove the hand that has been retracting the tissue.
9. *Do not massage the site.*
10. Using an alcohol pad or dry gauze pad, press down on the site to inhibit bleeding.

Application to Skin and Mucous Membrane

Drug preparations are administered for their local effect or to act systemically. To achieve a systemic effect the drug must be absorbed into the circulation.

Buccal Tablet (Universal Safeguard: Handwashing)

Identify the patient orally. Check the ID band. Explain the procedure and give the tablet to the patient. The patient should place the tablet between his gum and his cheek. The tablet should not be disturbed as it dissolves. Systemic absorption is rapid across mucous membranes. Doses should be alternated between cheeks to minimize irritation.

Ear Drops (Universal Safeguard: Handwashing)

The ear drops will be labeled otic or auric. They should be warmed to body temperature. Greet the patient orally and check the ID band. Explain the procedure. Place the patient sitting in an upright position, with the head tilted toward his unaffected side, or lying on his side with the affected ear up. Be sure the patient is comfortable. With a dropper, draw the medication up. *Straighten the ear canal by pulling the pinna up and back in the adult, or down and back in a child 3 years or younger.*

Place the tip of the dropper at the opening of the canal and instill the medication into the canal. The

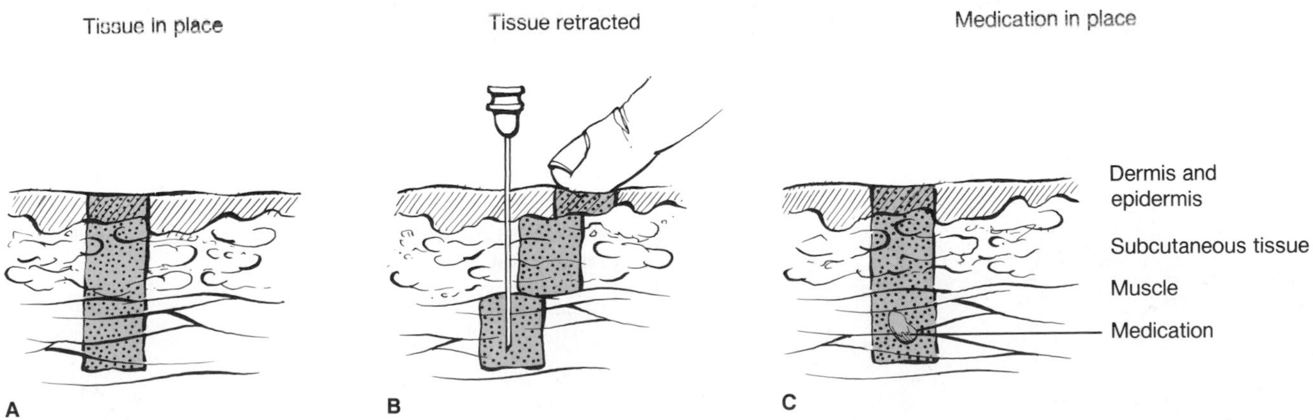

Figure 12-15
Z track technique—dorsogluteal site. The tissue is retracted to one side and held there until the injection is given. When the hand is removed the tissue closes over the injection tract preventing medication from rising to the surface.

patient should rest on his unaffected side 10 to 15 minutes. A cotton ball may be placed in the canal if the patient wishes. Make sure the patient is comfortable. Wash hands. Chart the medication.

Eye Drops or Ointment (Universal Safeguard: Gloves)

Greet the patient and check the ID band. Explain the procedure. Hand the patient a tissue. The patient may be sitting or lying down. If exudate is present, it may be necessary to cleanse the eyelid with cotton or gauze and either normal saline or distilled water for the eye. Any medication placed in the eye must be labeled "ophthalmic" or "for the eye." Eye medications may come in a monodrop container, in a bottle with a dropper, or as an ophthalmic ointment. Gently draw the lower eyelid down to create a sac (Fig. 12-16). Instruct the patient to look up. Instill the liquid medication into the lower conjunctival sac, taking care not to touch the membrane. The ophthalmic ointment should be placed from the inner to the outer canthus of the eye.

Instruct the patient to close his eyelids gently and rotate his eyes. The patient may use the tissue to wipe away excess medication. After instilling eye drops, have the patient apply gentle pressure with his index finger to the inner canthus for a minute. This action inhibits the medication from entering the tear duct.

Each patient should have individual medication containers to prevent cross-contamination. Provide a safe environment if the medication impairs the patient's vision. Make the patient comfortable. Dispose of the gloves according to institutional procedure. Wash your hands and chart the medication.

Nasogastric Route (Universal Safeguard: Gloves)

When possible, obtain the medication in liquid form. Before opening capsules or crushing tablets, check with the pharmacist for alternatives.

Dilute the medication with water. The fluid mixture should be at room temperature. Greet the patient, check the ID band, and explain the procedure. Elevate the head of the bed when possible. Put on gloves. Insert the bulb syringe into the tube. Remove the clamp on the tube. Check the position of the tube in the stomach by (1) aspirating some stomach contents or (2) placing a stethoscope on the stomach and inserting about 15 mL of air. A swishing sound indicates proper placement.

Close off the tube by bending it on itself. Hold the bulb syringe and bent tube in your nondominant hand. Remove the bulb and leave the syringe in place.

Flush the tube with at least 30 mL warm water to ensure patency. Clamp the tube. Pour the medication into the bulb syringe. Release the tubing and allow the medication to flow in by gravity. *Do not force medication to flow by using pressure on the bulb.* If the patient shows discomfort, stop the procedure and wait until he or she appears relaxed.

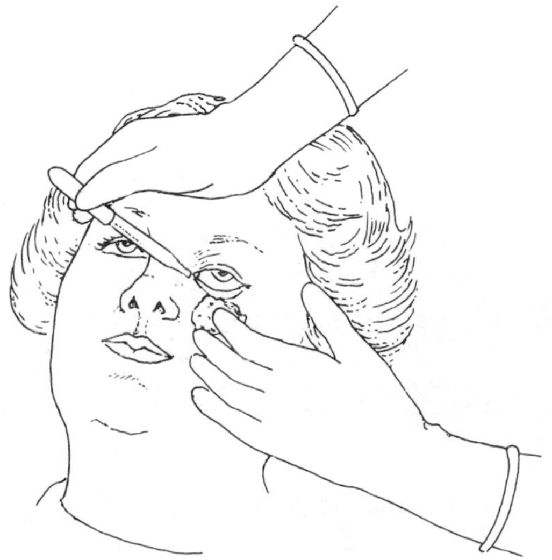

Figure 12-16
Applying eye drops: Gently draw the lower eyelid down to create a pocket. Insert the medication into this pocket.

Before all the medication flows in, flush the tube by adding at least 30 mL of water to the syringe. Shut the tube by bending it on itself before the bulb syringe completely empties. Clamp the tube and remove the bulb syringe. Make the patient comfortable. If possible, leave the head of the bed elevated. Dispose of gloves according to institutional procedures. Wash your hands. Chart the medication.

Nose Drops (Universal Safeguard: Handwashing)

Greet the patient, check the ID band, and explain the procedure. The patient may have to blow his nose gently to clear the nasal passageway. The patient may be sitting or lying down. Have the patient tilt his head back. In bed a pillow may be placed under the shoulders to hyperextend the neck. Insert the dropper about one-third into each nostril. Do not touch the nostril. Instill the nose drops. Instruct the patient to maintain the position 1 to 2 minutes. If the patient feels the medication flowing down his throat, he may sit up and bend his head down to allow the medication to flow into the sinuses.

The patient should have his own medication container to prevent cross-contamination. Make the patient comfortable. Wash your hands. Chart the medication.

If a nasal spray is ordered, push the tip of the nose up and place the nozzle tip just inside the nares, so the spray will be directed backward when the medication is given.

Rectal Suppository (Universal Safeguard: Gloves)

Greet the patient, check the ID band, and explain the procedure. Encourage the patient to defecate (unless the suppository is ordered for this purpose). Position the patient in the left lateral recumbent position (Fig. 12-17). Moisten the suppository with a water-soluble lubricant. Instruct the patient to breathe slowly and deeply through the mouth. Ask the patient to "bear down" as if having a bowel movement to open the anal sphincter. Insert the suppository past the sphincter, using a gloved finger. You will feel the suppository move into the canal. Wipe away excess lubricant. Encourage the patient to retain the suppository. Make the patient comfortable. Dispose of gloves according to institutional procedure. Wash your hands. Chart the medication.

The patient may insert his own suppository if he is able and wishes to do so. Provide a glove, lubricant, and suppository. Check to be sure the suppository was inserted and is not in the bed.

Respiratory Inhaler (Universal Safeguard: Handwashing)

An inhaler is a small, pressurized metal container that holds medication. It is accompanied by a mouthpiece. *The following are general directions to teach the patient:*

1. Shake the inhaler well immediately before use.
2. Remove the cap from the mouthpiece.
3. Breathe out fully; expel as much air as you can; hold your breath.
4. Place the mouthpiece in your mouth and close your lips around it. The metal inhaler should be upright.
5. While breathing in deeply and slowly, fully depress the metal inhaler with your index finger.
6. Remove the inhaler from your mouth and release your finger. Hold your breath for several seconds.
7. Wait 1 minute and shake the inhaler again. Repeat the steps for each inhalation prescribed. (An order might read "Proventil Inhaler 2 puffs qid.")
8. Cleanse the mouthpiece and cap by rinsing in warm running water at least once a day. When dry, replace the mouthpiece and cap.

The inhaler may be left at the bedside stand if the institution's policy permits. Make the patient comfortable. Wash your hands. Chart the medication.

Skin Applications (Universal Safeguard: Gloves)

Greet the patient, check the ID band, and explain the procedure. Avoid personal contact with the medication to prevent absorption of drug. Apply the medication with a tongue blade, glove, gauze pad, or cotton-tipped applicator. Cleanse the area as appropriate before a new application.

Obtain the following information before proceeding, because many kinds of medicines are applied topically.

- The preparation of the skin
- The method of application
- Whether the skin should be covered or uncovered

Drug preparations include the following:

- Powders: sprinkle on your gloved hands and then apply. Use sparingly to avoid caking. Skin should be dry.
- Lotions: Pat on lightly. Use gloved hand or gauze pad.
- Creams: Rub into skin using gloves.
- Ointments: Use gloved hand or applicator. Apply an even coat and place a dressing on skin.

Make the patient comfortable. Dispose of gloves according to institutional policy. Wash your hands. Chart the medication.

Nitroglycerin Ointment (Universal Safeguard: Gloves)

Greet the patient, check the ID band, and explain the procedure. Take a baseline blood pressure and record. Don the gloves to protect yourself from contact with the drug, a potent vasodilator. Remove the previous dose and cleanse the skin.

Measure the prescribed dose in inches on the ruled paper that comes with the ointment. Select a nonhairy site on the trunk—chest, upper arm, abdomen, or upper back. If necessary, shave the area. (Seek advice before doing this.) Spread the measured ointment on the skin, using the ruled paper. Apply the ointment in a thin layer about 6 inches by 6 inches. *Do not rub.* Tape the ruled paper in place over the ointment. Cover the area with plastic wrap and tape the plastic in place. Check the patient's blood pressure within 30 minutes.

If a headache occurs or the blood pressure lowers, have the patient rest until the blood pressure returns to normal. Make the patient comfortable. Dispose of gloves according to institutional procedure. Wash your hands. Chart the medication.

Transdermal Disks, Patches, and Pads (Universal Safeguard: Handwashing)

These products are unit-dose adhesive bandages consisting of a semipermeable membrane that allows medication to be released continuously over time. Some patches are effective for 24 hours, some for 72 hours, and some last as long as 1 week.

The skin should be free of hair and not subject to excessive movement; therefore, avoid distal extremities. The site should be changed with each administration. If the patch loosens with bathing, apply a new pad.

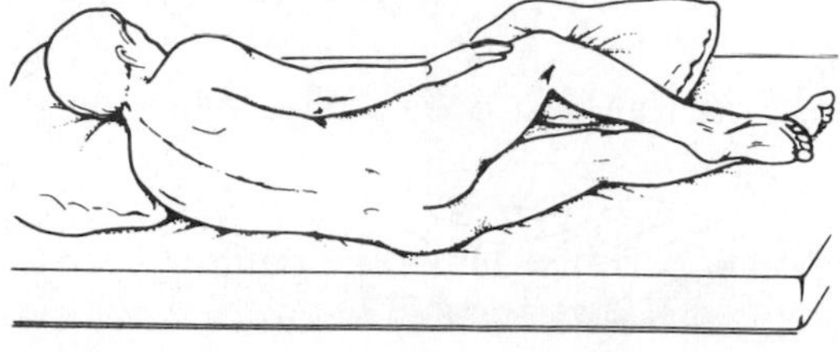

Figure 12-17
Left lateral recumbent position.

Medications that can be administered by this route include hormones, antihypertensive drugs such as clonadine (Catapres), antimotion sickness drugs such as scopolamine, and nitroglycerin.

Greet the patient, check the ID band, and explain the procedure. Select the site. The skin should be clear and dry with no signs of irritation. Open the packet. Remove the cover from the adhesive transdermal drug. *Do not touch the inside of the pad.* Apply the pad to the skin. Press firmly to be certain all edges are adherent. Make the patient comfortable, wash your hands, and chart the medication.

Sublingual Tablets (Universal Safeguard: Handwashing)

The most common sublingual medication is nitroglycerin, which is prescribed to abort an attack of angina pectoris. If relief is not felt in 5 minutes, a second and then a third tablet may be taken. Tolerance to nitroglycerin is common. If the pain is not relieved within 15 minutes, the physician should be notified.

To administer a sublingual tablet, greet the patient, check the ID band, and explain the procedure. Instruct the patient to sit down and place the tablet under the tongue. If the patient is unable to place the tablet under his tongue himself, wear a glove to place the tablet. The tablet should not be swallowed or chewed but allowed to dissolve. The patient should not eat or drink anything because this will interfere with the effectiveness of the medication. Stay with the patient until the pain is relieved. Consult an appropriate text for further information. Wash your hands and chart the medication.

Vaginal Suppository or Tablet (Universal Safeguard: Gloves)

Greet the patient, check the ID band, and explain the procedure. Ask the patient to void in a bed pan. (If the perineal area has much secretion, it may be necessary to perform perineal care after the patient voids.) Insert the suppository or tablet into the applicator. Assist the patient into a lithotomy position (lying on the back with knees flexed and legs apart) and drape her, leaving the perineal area exposed. Don gloves.

Separate the labia majora and identify the vaginal opening. Insert the applicator down and back and eject the suppository or tablet into the vagina. (The patient may do this procedure herself if she wishes.) Place a pad at the opening to collect secretions. Make the patient comfortable before leaving.

Wash the applicator with soap and water, wrap it in a paper towel, and leave it at the bedside. Dispose of gloves and equipment according to institutional procedure. Chart the medication.

Vaginal Cream

Vaginal cream may come in a prefilled disposable syringe, or in a tube with its own applicator. To fill the applicator, remove the cap from the tube and screw the top of the tube into the barrel of the applicator. Squeeze the tube to fill the barrel to the prescribed dose. Unscrew the tube from the applicator and cap it.

Prepare the patient as described above. Insert the applicator down and back and press the plunger to empty the barrel of medication (Fig. 12-18). The patient may do this herself if she wishes. Remove the

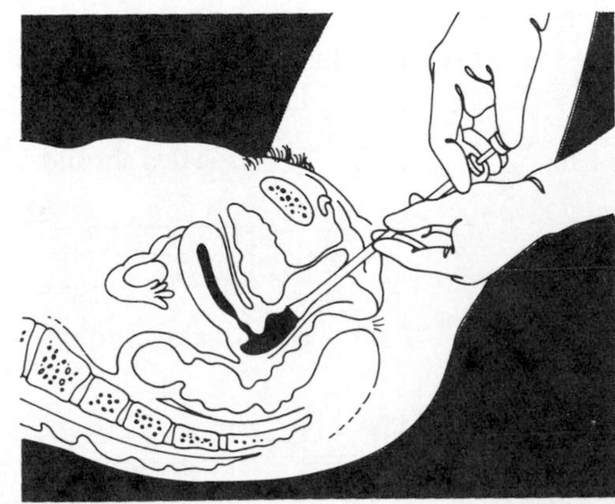

Figure 12-18
Vaginal applicator should be inserted down and back. (Taylor C, Lillis C, LeMone P. *Fundamentals of Nursing*, ed 2. Philadelphia: J. B. Lippincott, 1993, p. 1251)

applicator. Place a pad at the vaginal opening to collect secretions. Make the patient comfortable before leaving. She should remain in bed for a minimum of 20 minutes.

If the applicator is a prefilled unit dose, dispose of it according to institutional policy. If it is reusable, wash it with soap and water, place it in a clean paper towel in the bedside stand. Dispose of gloves. Chart the medication.

Self-Test 1

Give the information requested for universal safeguards in administering medications. Answers may be found at the end of the chapter.

1. Universal safeguards should be applied when administering medications

a. to all patients

b. only to patients with HIV or hepatitis B virus

2. The type of safeguard to be used by the nurse depends upon ______________________

____

3. In administering medications, gloves must be worn when

____ and

____

4. After administering an injection, the syringe should be placed ______________________

____

5. Five safeguards stressed by the Centers for Disease Control are

______________________, ______________________, and

______________________, ______________________

______________________.

6. In administering medications, hands must be washed

a. ____

b. ____

c. ____

d. ____

7. General safeguards in administering medications advise the nurse to use a clamp to ______

____

8. A gown should be worn to protect the nurse's uniform whenever ______________________

____

9. Goggles should be worn whenever ______________________

____

____

10. A mask should be worn when

____ or

____

Self-Test 2

Decide whether the following actions are correct or incorrect according to the safeguards in administering medications; explain your choice. Answers may be found at the end of the chapter.

1. A nurse wears gloves to remove an intravenous heparin lock from a patient's arm. This action is ______

2. A nurse who has just removed a gown and gloves puts them into the proper disposal container in the patient's room and leaves the room. This action is ______

3. In the medication room, a nurse puts on gloves to prepare an IV for administration. This action is ______

4. A nurse puts on a mask to administer an oral medication to a patient on respiratory isolation precautions. This action is ______

5. A nurse applies universal precautions in caring for all patients on the unit. This action is ______

6. A nurse wears gloves to place a transdermal pad behind a patient's ear. This action is ______

7. A nurse puts on gloves and gown to administer 500 mL of a vaginal douche to a lethargic patient. This action is ______

8. A nurse whose finger has been stuck with a contaminated IV needle carefully washes his hands with soap and water and applies a Band-aid to the site. Because the patient's diagnosis is brain tumor, the nurse decides no further action is necessary. This action is ______

9. A nurse giving an injection to a patient makes the judgment *not* to wear gloves. This action is ______

10. A nurse puts on gloves to administer an oral tablet to an alert patient with a positive HIV blood count. This action is ______

11. After administering an injection, the nurse carefully caps the needle. This action is ______

Self-Test 3

Supply the following information. Answers will be found at the end of the chapter.

1. The primary reason patients should have individual eye medication is to ______________________________

2. Two methods of checking the positioning of a nasogastric tube are ______________________________ and ______________________________

3. For administration of a rectal suppository, the patient should lie ______________________________

4. How should each of the following be applied to a patient's skin?
   a. Powders ____________
   b. Lotions ____________
   c. Creams ____________
   d. Ointments ____________

5. How many SL nitroglycerin tablets may a patient take to relieve pain? ____________
   At what time interval? ____________

6. Identify these administration procedures as clean or sterile.

a. SC injection	________	f. Nitroglycerin ointment	________
b. SL tablet	________	g. Urethral suppository	________
c. Vaginal suppository	________	h. Nasogastric route	________
d. Nose drops	________	i. Intradermal	________
e. IM injection	________	j. Rectal suppository	________

7. How should a vaginal applicator be inserted? ____________

8. How should the skin be prepared for an injection? ____________

9. List three reasons for administering medication by injection. ____________

10. What is the difference in administering ear drops to an adult and a 2-year-old child? ____________

Self-Test 4

Choose the correct answer for each of these questions. Answers will be found at the end of the chapter.

1. The purpose of the medication ticket in the ticket system is to identify the drug from the time the order is written until it is

   a. transferred to the Kardex
   b. poured
   c. administered
   d. charted

2. Which of the following is an appropriate action regarding medication tickets in the ticket system?

   a. All tickets are checked against the physician's order sheet.
   b. Tickets are made out only for standing orders.
   c. A new ticket is written each time a drug is given.
   d. The ticket is destroyed after charting a stat order.

3. Checking the Kardex before administering medication by ticket will enable the nurse to determine

   a. the name of the physician who ordered the medication
   b. if some tickets have been misplaced
   c. if a "stat" medication is to be administered
   d. whether the patient can have the next prn dose

4. When pouring an oral liquid medication, the nurse should

   a. place the cup on the tabletop and bend over to get the right level
   b. hold the cup in the hand and pour to the top of the meniscus
   c. hold the cup at eye level and pour to the center of the meniscus
   d. rest the cup on the medication shelf and pour to the mark at the side of the cup

5. Which statement is *false* regarding injections from powders?

   a. Read the label twice before drawing up and once after.
   b. Draw up one medication at a time.
   c. Always use sterile water as a diluent.
   d. Pull back on the plunger before injecting the medication.

6. Withdrawing medication from a vial is facilitated if a specific amount of air is injected into the vial before hand. Which of these statements explains this action?

   a. It creates a partial vacuum in the vial.
   b. It makes the pressure in the vial greater than atmospheric pressure.
   c. It makes the pressure in the vial the same as atmospheric pressure.
   d. It makes the pressure in the vial less than atmospheric pressure.

7. If a patient has difficulty swallowing medications, which oral form of drug may be crushed?

   a. Sugar-coated tablet
   b. Enteric-coated tablet
   c. Buccal tablet
   d. Capsule

8. A major advantage in the unit-dose system of drug administration is that

   a. the drug supply is always available
   b. no error is possible
   c. the drugs are less expensive than stock distribution
   d. the pharmacist provides a second professional check

(continued)

Self-Test 4 (continued)

9. When a drug is to be administered sublingually, the patient should be instructed to

a. drink a full glass of water when swallowing
b. rinse the mouth with water after taking the drug
c. chew the tablet and allow the saliva to collect under the tongue
d. hold the medication under the tongue until it dissolves

10. Ampules differ from vials in that ampules

a. are glass containers
b. contain only one dose
c. contain solids as well as liquids
d. are not used for injections

11. The Z-track technique for injections can be used to

a. administer more than one drug at a single site
b. inhibit hematoma formation by promoting drug absorption
c. prevent skin discoloration by inhibiting drug seepage
d. reduce allergic reactions at the injection site

12. Which action is *correct* in giving a Z-track injection?

a. The skin is retracted and held to one side while the medication is given.
b. The skin is massaged after the injection is given.
c. The plunger is not pulled back when the needle has been inserted.
d. Medication is injected quickly.

13. Which angle of injection is *correctly* matched with the route of administration?

a. Intradermal—45° angle
b. Intramuscular—90° angle
c. Subcutaneous—30° angle
d. Z-track—45° angle

14. A patient asks how he should put drops in his eye. The nurse instructs the patient to place the drops

a. into the lower conjunctival sac
b. under the upper lid
c. directly on the cornea
d. in the inner canthus

15. In administering a vaginal suppository, which statement is *false?*

a. Universal safeguards should be used.
b. The patient may insert the medication.
c. The patient should be lying on her back.
d. The applicator must be kept sterile.

16. In applying the next dose of a transdermal medication, the nurse should

a. shave the new area and prepare with povidone-iodine
b. cleanse the previous area and use a different site
c. rotate the use of arms and legs as sites
d. allow the previous patch to remain on the skin

17. Which is the muscle of choice to be used when an injection is irritating to the tissues?

a. Deltoid—SC
b. Dorsogluteal—Z-track
c. Ventrogluteal—intradermal
d. Vastus lateralis—IM

(continued)

Self-Test 4 (continued)

18. Discomfort of an injection is reduced when the needle is inserted

a. slowly into loose tissue
b. slowly into firm tissue
c. rapidly into loose tissue
d. rapidly into firm tissue

19. After administering an injection, the nurse should

a. immediately recap the needle
b. break the needle off the syringe for safety
c. place the used syringe in a nearby sharps container
d. don gloves to carry the syringe to the utility room

20. Which statement is *incorrect* in the administration of drugs to mucous membranes?

a. Eye medications must be labeled ophthalmic.
b. Patients may insert their own rectal suppositories.
c. Sublingual medications are applied to the space between the teeth and cheek.
d. Eye medications may be left in the client's bedside stand.

ANSWERS

Self-Test 1

1. To *all* patients. There is a risk of potential exposure to hepatitis B virus and human immunodeficiency virus that may not have been detected by standard laboratory methods.
2. The type of contact the nurse has with the patient.
3. When there is any direct "hands on" contact with patient's blood, bodily fluids, or secretions; when handling materials or equipment contaminated with blood or body fluids
4. In a labeled puncture-proof container
5. Handwashing, gloves, gowns, masks, and goggles
6. a. Before preparing medications and after administering medicines to each patient
   b. After removing gloves, gowns, masks, and goggles, and before leaving each patient
   c. Immediately when soiled with the patient's blood or body fluids
   d. After handling equipment soiled with blood or body fluids
7. Hold contaminated IV needles being carried to a puncture-proof container
8. The nurse's clothing may become contaminated with a patient's blood or body fluids
9. A nurse is in extremely close contact with the patient and there is possibility of the patient's blood or blood-tinged fluids being splashed or sprayed into the nurse's eyes or mucous membranes
10. The patient is placed on *strict* or *respiratory* isolation precautions; carrying out a medication procedure may cause blood or body fluids to splash directly on the nurse's face

---

Self-Test 2

1. Correct. As the needle or catheter is removed there is a possibility of bleeding at the site. In addition, the nurse should use a clamp to carry the needle or catheter to a puncture-proof container.
2. Incorrect. The nurse must wash his or her hands before leaving the room.
3. Incorrect. It is not necessary to wear gloves to prepare an IV because there is no contact at this time with the patient's blood or body fluids.
4. Correct. Universal safeguards state that a mask must be worn when the patient is on strict or respiratory isolation precautions.
5. Correct. There is a potential risk of exposure to hepatitis B virus and human immunodeficiency virus. Laboratory testing may not show the presence of the virus or antibodies to the virus.
6. Incorrect. Transdermal pads are applied to intact skin. There is no danger of contact with the patient's blood or body fluids.
7. Correct. In carrying out the vaginal douche there is a possibility of exposure to vaginal secretions.
8. Incorrect. The nurse should squeeze the finger and, after washing his hands with soap and water, scrub the area with povidone–iodine (Betadine) or another accepted antiseptic. In addition, the needlestick should be reported to the proper authority and the protocol for exposure to blood carried out. Universal safeguards apply to all patients regardless of the diagnosis.
9. Correct. It is not necessary to wear gloves in giving an injection. Handwashing is adequate unless there is danger of exposure to blood or body secretions. In injection technique, the alcohol swab acts as a mechanical barrier.
10. Incorrect. Because the patient is alert and can take the medicine cup from the nurse, handwashing is adequate.
11. Incorrect. The CDC guidelines advise the nurse not to recap a needle but to place it immediately in a puncture-proof container.

Self-Test 3

1. Prevent cross-contamination
2. Aspirate stomach contents; *or* place a stethescope on the stomach and insert 15 mL of air. A swishing sound indicates proper placement.
3. On the left side—left lateral recumbent position
4. **a.** Sprinkle on gloved hands and apply; use sparingly to prevent caking
   b. Pat on lightly with gloved hand or gauze pad
   c. Rub into skin while wearing gloves
   d. Use a gloved hand to apply an even coat and cover with a dressing
5. Three tablets; 5 minutes apart
6. **a.** Sterile
   b. Clean
   c. Clean
   d. Clean
   e. Sterile
   f. Clean
   g. Sterile
   h. Clean
   i. Sterile
   j. Clean
7. Back and up
8. Rub the skin with an alcohol pad in a circular motion from the center of the site out
9. The drug would be destroyed orally; a rapid effect is desired; the patient is unable to take the drug orally
10. In the adult, pull the ear back and up. In a 2-year-old child, pull the ear back and down.

Self-Test 4

1. d	**5.** c	**9.** d	**13.** b	**17.** b
2. d	**6.** b	**10.** a	**14.** a	**18.** d
3. b	**7.** a	**11.** c	**15.** d	**19.** c
4. c	**8.** d	**12.** a	**16.** b	**20.** c

Glossary

Adverse effects nontherapeutic effects that may be harmful

Ampule sealed glass container for powdered or liquid drugs

Antagonism interaction between two drugs in which the combined effect is less than the sum of the effects of the drugs acting separately

Apothecary system measurement system using grains and minims, introduced into the U.S. from England in colonial times

Biotransformation conversion of an active drug to an inactive compound

Buccal route of administration in which a drug is placed in the pouch between the teeth and cheek

Capsule a gelatin container that holds a drug in a solid or liquid form

Civil law statutes concerned with the rights and duties of individuals

Contraindication situation in which a drug should be avoided

Cream semisolid drug preparation applied externally to the skin or mucous membrane

Criminal law statutes that protect the public against actions harmful to society

Cumulation the inability of the body to metabolize one dose of a drug before another dose is administered; cumulation leads to increased concentration of the drug in the body and possible toxicity

Diluent a liquid used to dissolve a solid, usually a powder, into a solution

Displacement the increase in the volume of fluid added to a powder, when the powder dissolves and goes into solution

Distribution the movement of a drug through body fluids, chiefly blood, to cells

Dose amount of drug to be administered at one time, or the total amount to be given

Drug a chemical agent used in the treatment, diagnosis, or prevention of disease

Elixir a clear aromatic, sweetened alcoholic preparation

Emulsion suspension of a fat or oil in water with the aid of an agent to reduce surface tension

Enteric coating a layer placed over a tablet or capsule to prevent dissolution in the stomach; used to protect the drug from gastric acid, or to protect the stomach from drug irritation

Excretion the physiologic elimination of substances from the body

Expiration date a drug cannot be administered after the last day of the month stamped on the label

Film coated tablets compressed powdered drugs that are smooth and easy to swallow because of their outer shell covering

Fluidextract potent alcoholic liquid concentration of a drug

Gauge the diameter or width of a needle; the higher the gauge number, the finer the needle

Gel aqueous suspension of small particles of an insoluble drug in a hydrated form

Generic name official name of a drug as listed in the U.S. or other pharmacopeia

Incompatibility mixture of two or more drugs that results in a harmful chemical or physical interaction

Inhaler a device used to spray liquid or powder in a fine mist into the lungs during inspiration

Interaction either desirable or undesirable effects produced by giving two or more drugs together

Intradermal injection given into the upper layers of the skin

Isotonic solutions that have the same osmotic pressure as physiological body fluids

IVPB intravenous piggyback; a medication placed in an infusion set and attached to the main line IV for delivery to the patient

Lotion liquid suspension intended for external use

Lozenge flat, round, or rectangular preparation held in the mouth until it dissolves

Magma bulky suspension of an insoluble preparation in water, which must be shaken before pouring

MDI metered dose inhaler; an aerosol device that consists of two parts: a cannister under pressure and a mouthpiece. Finger pressure on the mouthpiece opens a valve that discharges one dose.

Metabolism the chemical biotransformation of a drug to a form that can be excreted

Military time time based on a 24-hour clock rather than the traditional 12-hour clock

Multidose large stock containers of medication

NDC National Drug Code; a number used by the pharmacist to identify the drug and the method of packaging

Ointment semisolid preparation in a petroleum or lanolin base for external use

Ophthalmic pertaining to the eye

Otic pertaining to the ear

Parenteral a general term that means administration by injection

Paste thick ointment used to protect the skin

Pastille disklike solid that slowly dissolves in the mouth

Pharmacokinetics science of the factors that determine how much drug reaches the site of action in the body and is excreted

Piggyback medication placed in an intravenous infusion set and attached to the mainline IV for delivery to the patient

Placebo an inert substance used in place of a drug for its psychological effect, and the physiological changes caused by the psychological response

Powder a finely ground solid drug or mixture of drugs for internal or external use

Prefilled cartridge a small vial with a needle attached that fits into a metal or plastic holder for injection

Prefilled syringe a liquid, sterile medication that is ready to administer without further preparation

Prolonged release or slow release tablet powdered, compressed drug that disintegrates more slowly and has a longer duration of action

Reconstitution dissolving a powder to a liquid form

Scored tablet compressed powdered drug that has a line down the center such that the tablet can be broken in half

Side effect transient, nontherapeutic reaction to a drug

SI units Systèm International d'Unités; measurement adapted from the metric system used in most developed countries to provide a standard language

Solution a clear liquid that contains a drug dissolved in water

Spansule long-acting capsule that contains drug particles coated to dissolve at different times

Spirits concentrated alcoholic solutions of volatile substances

Subcutaneous the tissue lying between the skin and muscle

Sublingual tablet powdered drug compressed or molded into a solid shape that dissolves quickly under the tongue

Suppository mixture of a drug with a firm base molded into a shape that is inserted into a body cavity

Suspension solid particles of a drug dispersed in a liquid that must be shaken to obtain an accurate dose

Syrup a solution of sugar in water to disguise the unpleasant taste of a medication

Tablet a powdered drug that is compressed or molded into solid shape and may contain additives that bind the powder or aid in its absorption

Timed release small beads of drug in a capsule coated to delay absorption

Tincture alcoholic or hydroalcoholic solution of a drug

Tolerance decreased responsiveness to a drug after repeated exposure

Topical route of administration in which a drug is applied to the skin or mucous membrane

Toxicity nontherapeutic effect that may result in damage to tissues or organs

Trade name a brand or proprietary name identified by the symbol ® that follows the name

Transdermal medication drug molecules contained in a unique polymer patch that is applied to the skin for slow absorption

Troche flat, round or rectangular preparation held in the mouth (or placed in the vagina) until it dissolves

Unit dose individually wrapped and labeled dose of a drug

Universal precautions procedures to protect against infection that are employed in caring for all patients and when handling contaminated equipment

Vial glass container with a rubber stopper containing one or more doses of a drug

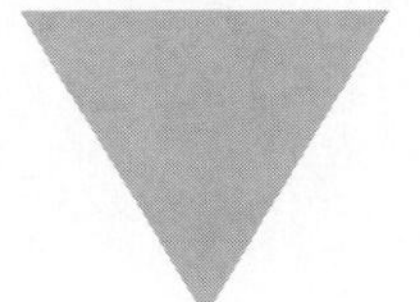

Index

Page numbers followed by *f* indicate figures; those followed by *t* indicate tabular material.

D

E

F

G

H

P

Q

R

S